C000257335

The Distressed Body

The Distressed Body

Rethinking Illness, Imprisonment, and Healing

DREW LEDER

The University of Chicago Press
Chicago and London

Drew Leder is an MD and professor of Western and Eastern philosophy at Loyola University Maryland. He is the author or editor of many books, including *The Body in Medical Thought and Practice* and *The Absent Body*, the latter published by the University of Chicago Press.

The University of Chicago Press, Chicago 60637
The University of Chicago Press, Ltd., London
© 2016 by The University of Chicago
All rights reserved. Published 2016.
Printed in the United States of America

25 24 23 22 21 20 19 18 17 16   1 2 3 4 5

ISBN-13: 978-0-226-39607-1 (cloth)
ISBN-13: 978-0-226-39610-1 (paper)
ISBN-13: 978-0-226-39624-8 (e-book)
DOI: 10.7208/chicago/9780226396248.001.0001

Library of Congress Cataloging-in-Publication Data

Names: Leder, Drew, author.
Title: The distressed body : rethinking illness, imprisonment, and healing /
    Drew Leder.
Description: Chicago ; London : University of Chicago Press, 2016. | Includes
    bibliographical references and index.
Identifiers: LCCN 2015051193 | ISBN 9780226396071 (cloth : alkaline paper) |
    ISBN 9780226396101 (paperback : alkaline paper) | ISBN 9780226396248 (e-book)
Subjects: LCSH: Human body (Philosophy) | Medicine—Philosophy. | Imprisonment—
    Philosophy. | Factory farms—Philosophy.
Classification: LCC B105.B64 L433 2016 | DDC 128/.6—dc23 LC record
    available at http://lccn.loc.gov/2015051193

♾ This paper meets the requirements of ANSI/NISO Z39.48-1992 (Permanence of Paper).

For Janice McLane,
my wife, fellow-philosopher, and best friend

What do I mean when I say "Respect great distress as you do your own person"?
The reason why I have great distress
Is that I have a body.
If I had no body, what distress would I have?
TAO TE CHING, Verse 13 (trans. Robert G. Hendricks)

Contents

We all know what it means to have a "distressed body." Or to *be* a distressed body. The former phrase—to *have*—posits the body as something separate from the essential self. This is how it can feel, for example, when in pain. The body seems *other, alien*—like a possession now uncomfortably possessing us.

Yet the depths of this mutual possession also suggest that who I am is inescapably embodied. I wouldn't quite know how to live a bodiless life, nor would I usually choose to. It is with, and through, and as a body that I play, desire, love, travel, enjoy delicious food, listen to thrilling music—even read and ponder, as you are doing now.

For our bodies are naturally *ecstatic*, from the Greek roots *ek* and *stasis*, meaning to "stand outside." As a Greek term, *ekstasis* also can refer to "astonishment" or "amazement." The body does have an astonishing capacity to stand outside itself, to fling itself across the universe through the projective powers of desire, perception, movement, contemplation—whether we gaze at stars billions of light-years away or stroke the cheek of a lover. The body is not just a piece of *meat*, but the way we rush out to *meet* the world. We ever leap beyond our fleshly limits through the agency of the flesh.

Yet to have/be a *distressed* body changes things. To be sick, hungry, in pain, fatigued, afraid for one's safety, scorned by others, immobilized, incarcerated—these are variants on a theme. Again, etymology provides clues to experience. The word "distress" comes from the Latin *dis*, meaning "apart," and *stringere*, to "press together," "stretch," or "bind."

When distressed, we are *stretched apart* from our customary lives, and from one another. For example, in the case of imprisonment we are seized from our home, family, habitual scenes and routines, and confined behind bars and barbed wire. We are *dis-placed*, pulled away from our usual place in the world. Yet chronic illness or pain does something similar. No one else can share our inner experience, let alone fix it. To even put into words what we're feeling is a struggle. We begin to drop away from our customary rounds— stay home from work, give that movie a miss—increasingly drifting apart from the world and our fellows. We sit alone at night with our painful body, but are even "stretched apart" from that. The body is no longer the taken-for-granted seat of our powers but a distrusted *other*. Who knows when it will flare up, that torturer?

This is all suggested by the etymology of "distress." On the face of it, "distress" should mean the opposite of "stress"—since *di* or *dis*, meaning "apart, away from," suggests the privative of what is being modified, as in words like "dis-ease" (the opposite of ease) or "dis-pleasure" (the opposite of pleasure). But paradoxically, in English "distress" is *not* the opposite of "stress." In fact, their sense is quite similar, each word suggesting worry, pressure, struggle, and tension.

Imprisonment provides a clear example. It creates stress—again, from the Latin *stringere*, to "press together" or "bind." Prisoners are pressed together in overcrowded spaces. Two persons might be forced to share for decades a nine-by-twelve-foot cell. Even worse can be the pressure caused by prolonged solitary confinement, a form of disciplinary torture vastly overused in American prisons. Chronic pain or illness can do something analogous. The sick person is pressed together—with her body, source of suffering; with a disease that cannot be eased; with the narrow confines of her bed and restricted view; with the very fact of bodily vulnerability, aging, and death. Her world presses inward, becoming constricted by limitations of energy, movement, even of interest in outward things. It is not surprising that prisoners, and the chronically ill, can become *depressed* (etymologically, "pressed downward").

In this book I will look at illness and pain, and the medical response thereto; the experience of being imprisoned in our "age of mass incarceration"; and also the mistreatment of animal bodies, as in modern factory farms. These are bodies that are *stressed*—pressed inward—but thereby also *distressed*—pulled apart. They dwell in that paradoxical tension of forces.

Yet to focus only on distressed bodies would be too distressing. This book is not just about suffering, but its relief. To engage in a phenomenology of experiences of distress, and a hermeneutics of its contexts—how it is culturally interpreted and the institutional practices that surround it—can help locate pathways to healing. (Not to "solutions" exactly—the vulnerabilities of embodied existence are not exactly "solvable," though modes of re-solving and dis-solving distress remain possible.)

"Healing" shares an etymological root with "wholeness" and "holiness." Is it possible that even when stuck in prison for an unimaginably long sentence, or mired in chronic pain or illness, that one can yet heal? Or that imprisonment and illness can at times be agents of healing, prods toward growth and wholeness? Can we also think about healing dysfunctional institutions—like the prison system or the modern medical system, which share some distressing similarities? To heal is to reintegrate what has disintegrated, to enlarge what has shrunk. One can reclaim wholeness even in the face of massive disruption. This book will not simply survey distress but search for individual and communal healing.

The methods of analysis I use will be varied. Primary is a reliance on phenomenological analysis as developed by Continental philosophers such as Edmund Husserl, Martin Heidegger and, most important for my purposes, Maurice Merleau-Ponty. They attempt to uncover essential structures of lived experience, especially experience-*as-embodied* in Merleau-Ponty's case. Michel Foucault's work on the history of "biopower" also proves useful, as well as that of others who thematize changes in the life-world wrought by contemporary technology. At times I also turn to literary, psychosocial, and medical studies, and even my personal struggles, to unpack the texture of lived experience. I also utilize "hermeneutical" methods as developed by Heidegger, Hans-Georg Gadamer, and others. I discuss not only the *texts* constituted by the ill body and aspects of the medical workup, but the larger social, historical, and philosophical *contexts* that shape our modes of experiencing, understanding, and treating distressed bodies. Particularly important contexts include the Cartesian mechanization of the natural world (human body included) and the capitalist tendency to view the body as commodity, consumer, and producer rolled into one.

Throughout I avoid spending too much time presenting and critiquing theory as such. Husserl wrote of the need for phenomenologists to go back "to the things themselves," the structures of actual experience. So I have focused on certain "things themselves"—the experience of illness and of imprisonment, the use of pills in medicine, the nature of touch and its healing powers, and so forth. Various authors and theories have been invoked to the extent necessary but I have tried to stay away from technical "in-house" debates, for example, about subtleties in Merleau-Ponty's scholarly trajectory. I wish my writing to be accessible to the interested generalist and to resonate with the reader's own life-experience.

The book also refrains from the linear argumentation characteristic of some scholarly monographs. It does not set forth a series of systematic categories, definitions, and explanations that neatly interlock. Rather, chapters are based on pieces that were published in a variety of venues, originally designed to address different issues and audiences. Here they have been revised and unified in such a way that they now present a continuous exploration of the sources of bodily distress—in our biology, lived experience, culture, institutions—and their potential remedy through more humane and transhuman practices. Yet while the journey has been unified, the reader may still sometimes feel that he or she is leaping from stone to stone, occasionally in unexpected directions. Hopefully, this will be perceived not simply as a defect of the book but a virtue. Each chapter can, to a degree, be approached as a "stand alone." That is, it takes up a single topic—be it the experience of pain, the use of pills, organ transplantation, factory farming, shape-shifting—employing interpretive tools appropriate to that issue. The reader is thus free to choose a traditional linear path—each chapter does lead to the next, and there are cross-references between them—or to skip around at will. (Notice how many of our linguistic metaphors derive from the lived body—chapters *stand alone*; readers *under-stand* them; one might *grab* your interest as you *move around* the book, *skipping* other chapters—though hopefully not too many.)

Each chapter is titled, as the book is subtitled, a "rethinking" of a particular topic. It may seem anomalous to use the language of "thought" in a book so focused on embodiment. This is so only if one accepts a mind-body dichotomy. Not only can thought be about, but also arise from, the lived body as it grapples with its world and reflects back on itself. I also use the notion of "thinking" in a somewhat Heideggerian sense. He means by this a kind of philosophical-meditative inquiry, distinct from the calculative rationality characteristic of our technological age. This thinking, which is necessarily a rethinking, seeks to be attentive to what is and what is needed; to reveal that which has been concealed by our settled views and practices; and which is necessarily meandering and responsive to the phenomena in their interwoven complexity, not linear and prescribed. This book thus follows the path of (re)thinking where it may lead, including to a multiplicity of methods and topics.

For such reasons, this book also embraces multiple voices. It is meant to be *dialogical*, from the Greek *logos* ("speech, reason") and *dia* ("between, through, across"). I have said the book "speaks across" a number of issues and disciplines. But to achieve this I needed dialogue partners who could provide challenge, clarification, and expertise. In three chapters on medical practice, alternative and conventional, I worked with Dr. Mitchell Krucoff, an eminent Duke University cardiologist. I have an MD myself but do not practice. Dr. Krucoff was able to draw on real-world clinical examples, as well as

his enlightened vision of what could be. Something similar migh
the incarcerated men whose voices permeate chapters toward t'
book, two originally coauthored, one with thirty members of m. ,
and one with Vincent Greco, recently released after thirty-three years. .
experience in maximum-security prisons makes them stone-cold realists. Yet
they are also visionaries concerning how prisons might be transformed and
what persons might achieve even while incarcerated. It is important their
voices be heard in a society that systematically silences them.

Though I serve as the primary author of all chapters—when they first appeared and in their revision for this book—I also try to speak not only for but
with others. I would say the same to you, now the book's primary reader.
That is, I hope the words will speak to you of distressed bodies you have
known, your own or others, including institutional bodies. I hope you will
also feel free to contradict or supplement the arguments and voices found in
this volume. Only in this *dialogue*, the "speech-between" the text and reader,
does a book leap to life. But let me start off the conversation by supplying a
brief guide to the book's contents.

The first part is entitled "Illness and Treatment: Phenomenological In-
vestigations." It primarily (though not exclusively) uses phenomenological
methods to examine what it is to be ill or in pain, and how modern medicine
does—and could—respond.

Chapter 1 begins with a classical literary example. On the way to fight in
the Trojan War, Philoctetes develops a foul-smelling, agonizing foot wound
that provokes revulsion in others. He is abandoned for ten long years on the
desolate island of Lemnos until a prophecy suggests that he must be brought
back. I read Sophocles' play as a reflection, literal and metaphorical, on how
illness places us in exile—from our own body, our comrades, the cosmos.
Again, it is in the nature of *distress* that one is pulled apart, displaced—and also
pressed inward (*stressed*). Philoctetes, moored on his isolated island, serves as
a launching point for our explorations.

In chapter 2 I turn specifically to the issue of chronic pain. In this case I
draw on my personal (rather unpleasant and ongoing) experience, as well as
multiple studies and authors that have surveyed the theme. Pain proves to
be far more than an aversive sensation. Chronic pain, in particular, involves
the sufferer in a complex experience filled with ambiguity and paradox. The
tensions thereby established, the unknowns, pressures, and oscillations, form
a significant part of pain's *painfulness*. I examine nine paradoxes that surface
in lived experience. For example, pain can seem an immediate sensation but
elicits complex interpretation; it pulls one to the present but also projects one
outward to a feared or desired future. Chronic pain can seem located in the

body and/or mind; interior to the self or an alien other; confined to a particular point and/or radiating everywhere. Such paradoxes, epistemological and existential, are an ever-present challenge for those in long-term pain.

The next three chapters, originally cowritten with Dr. Krucoff, examine the therapeutic responses to distressed bodies. This analysis remains for the most part within a modern, Western context. Work in the history of medicine, and medical sociology and anthropology, have shown that sickness and healing can be understood and treated in widely variant ways in different time periods and cultures. However, for we in the contemporary West, propagating a medical model that is now circulating the globe, it is a pressing task to understand where we have arrived, how we got there, and where we might travel in the future.

Chapter 3 explores the healing role of *touch* in the clinical encounter. All too often modern medicine is characterized by the "objectifying touch" of the physical exam or an "absent touch" insofar as technology has altogether replaced embodied contact. Yet for an ill person, feeling exiled from others, even from one's own painful body, touch can play a crucial reintegrative role. Unlike other sensory modes, touch unfolds through an impactful reciprocity between the toucher and the touched. For the ill person this can serve to reestablish human connection and assist therapeutic change at the prelinguistic level. Chapter 3 is a rallying cry for the recovery of touch as a diagnostic and healing modality.

Chapter 4 examines a polar opposite approach—the ubiquitous use of *pills* in modern medicine. I discuss four properties that characterize the material nature of pills: they are ingestible, potent, reproducible, and miniaturized. This allows them to serve as ideal consumer items for distribution and sale, and also as model technological "devices" capable of downloading into the body needed chemicals. As such, they seem to promise a solution to many of life's ills. In our cultural fantasy, pills can be used not only to treat and prevent disease but to raise energy, lose weight, lessen pain, lift mood, cope with stress, and enhance sexual and athletic performance. This chapter explores the many adverse side effects of pills themselves as well as of the exaggerated cultural fantasy that accompanies them. I suggest an alternative way we can view and take our pills—or, in some cases, not take them.

Chapter 5 steps back to take an overview of the modern medical paradigm—and how our phenomenology of illness has suggested it could and should transform. A conventional critique of medicine is that it is "too materialistic" and therefore insufficiently holistic and effective. Yet this critique may be ambiguous and misleading. "Materialism" can denote the way financial concerns drive medical practice (as in capitalism). It can also refer to the mechanistic model that treats the patient as a body-machine (Cartesianism). I suggest that neither is a true "materialism," but actually signify the dominance of high-level *abstractions* in medicine (such as financial and diagnostic-coding numbers) rather than a focus on the needs of the embodied, sick person. In a sense, medical practice is *not materialist enough*. Using examples—prayer/ comfort shawls, an unusual Indian hospital, a popular alternative to nursing homes—we see how an authentic materialism might humanize, even spiritual- ize, medical devices and environments.

This leads us into part 2 of the book, on "Medicine and Bioethics: Her- meneutical Reflections." In this part I draw on thinkers like Heidegger and Gadamer, who teach us of the import in human existence of interpretive acts. Chapter 6 suggests that clinical medicine can best be understood not as a pu- rified science but as a hermeneutical enterprise. A diagnosis and treatment plan are pieced together from ambiguous signs and symptoms. The interpre- tive process is rendered complex by a wide variety of textual forms. I discuss four in turn: the "experiential text" of illness as lived out by the patient; the "narrative text" constituted during history taking; the "physical text" of the patient's body as objectively examined; the "instrumental text" constructed by diagnostic technologies. I argue that certain flaws in modern medicine arise from its refusal of a hermeneutic self-understanding. Seeking to escape all in- terpretive subjectivity in favor of a purified vision or mathematics, medicine has threatened to expunge its primary subject—the living, suffering patient.

How would a hermeneutical self-understanding shift not only clinical prac- tice but the field of bioethics? This is the subject of chapter 7. Frequently, the bioethicist seeks to resolve a quandary by applying an overarching theory—for example, Kantian "respect for persons"—to the particulars of a case. I suggest something of a reverse approach. Paying careful attention to the interpreta- tions of, and the dilemmas faced by, real-life participants—clinical, emotional, social, financial—can deepen and change our case reading. I use the examples of "truth telling" and "autonomy." Seen from the heights of Kantian theory, it may be clear the doctor should "tell the truth" to enhance the patient's "au- tonomy." But what if "auto-nomy" ("self-rule") is already disrupted by disease and therefore in dire need of repair? What if medical language and institutions are disempowering? In "telling the truth" medically, the doctor may yet desta- bilize the patient's own narrative quest for meaning. A hermeneutical bioeth- ics seeks to disclose such contexts and deepen reflection, rather than simply to provide "the answers." Along the way it may also generate new questions that a traditional "top-down" bioethics has overlooked.

Chapter 8 applies this approach to issues in organ transplantation. Should a person be allowed to sell a kidney to an eager buyer? Should a government "presume consent" to harvest cadaver organs unless a person deliberately opt outs, or is this state intrusion? Rather than engage in standard ethical theorizing, I look at the contexts that shape practice. These include the capitalist model of the body as a producer, consumer, and commodity for purchase, and the Cartesian notion of the body as a machine with replaceable parts. (I here return to themes from part 1.) I propose instead a phenomenological model of the body as in deep connection, even interpenetration, with other bodies from before the time of birth until after death. I suggest ways this would reframe our very understanding and practice of organ transplants. Chapter 8 completes our discussion of matters medical and involves the most sustained *philosophical* treatment of the paradigms underlying the modernist view of the body, as well as a possible alternative.

In part 3, "Discarded and Recovered Bodies: Animals and Prisoners," the book takes its analysis in new directions. Parts 1 and 2 focus on the ill body and its treatment by the medical system. But this is far from the only sort of "distressed body." We can imagine any number of others, each worthy of an extended phenomenological/hermeneutical workup. Such include the bodies of domestic abuse victims, displaced refugees, those who feel shame around physical appearance, people coping with challenging disabilities, the aged struggling with late-life breakdowns, people of the "wrong" gender or skin color living in sexist and racist societies, and on and on. Such crucial topics are taken up by many other authors and disciplines. My personal interests and engagements, along with developments I witness in the larger culture, lead me here to write on issues concerning prisoners and animals.

I call theirs "discarded" bodies. In the United States, more than two million men and women are incarcerated. Many billions of animals live out brief, and often painful, existences in our factory farms. These lived bodies are displaced from our society and our consciousness; they reside in conditions we are largely unaware of and, in fact, are often prohibited from knowing. It is important to remember the forgotten, to penetrate beyond the walls, bars, and razor wire that conceal them. In this way we reclaim our fellow beings in the circuit of compassionate connection. Examining the situation of prisoners and animals together also creates a reverberating circuit for reflection. How is it that we treat so many people as if they were "nothing but animals," removing human rights and placing them in cages? Conversely, how is it that we can cage and abuse these animals, disconnecting from them and from our own humanity?

Chapter 9 starts with the peculiar institution of the factory farm. Somewhere along the line the traditional farm was reconfigured according to the model of an industrial factory. As in the previous chapter on organ transplantation, I address how capitalist modes of production, and Cartesian mechanism, have operated synergistically. The animals, as worker-machines, suffer from all four forms of "alienated labor" that Karl Marx describes. I also examine another factor—the anthropocentrism dominant in Western culture (and many others). This prohibits our viewing animals as moral subjects, allowing cruelties more unrestrained than those directed at people. But reforming factory farms involves more than seeking to "humanize" conditions. It involves questioning our very categories of "human," "animal," and "machine" so that we might attend to and respect other living creatures as they are.

Chapter 10 turns to incarcerated persons. A phenomenological analysis reveals how imprisonment constricts, disrupts, and fragments lived time and space, and one's experience of embodiment. Yet the prisoner is not passive in all this. He or she constructs strategies of response. Working with dialogues from my prison class, I give examples of two such strategies that I respectively call *escape* and *reclamation*—that is, imaginatively flying beyond the constraints of prison or working with them in a positive fashion. There is also an *integrative* approach that combines elements of both. Even in situations of severe restriction, the human being retains some freedom and responsibility— that is the *ability to respond.*

Chapter 11 switches focus from the way an individual can reform his or her personal experience to the reform of penal institutions themselves. Discussion with a class of thirty men (who served collectively as coauthors of an original version of this piece) shapes these reflections. Prison was not something they had studied but *lived.* They draw on personal experience of what damaged—or occasionally assisted—their quest for positive change. They are critical of the typical "endarkened" prison: Marked by despair and stasis, it classifies and isolates inmates, judging and punishing them for demerits. The "enlightened" prison would embody opposite values: support for hope, growth, individuality, and community, with merit recognized and rewarded. Perhaps this is a utopian ideal. Yet the values of the "enlightened" prison begin to manifest, in some small way, in our classroom and other such supportive communities.

Chapter 12, originally written with Vince Greco, a prisoner who was recently released, synthesizes the topics of previous chapters—that is, prisoners and animals. Its first part explores the correlation between the two in the public imagination. Prisoners are often portrayed as savage and animalistic.

This justifies the caging, and sometimes brutal treatment, to which inmates fall prey. More positively, the second part of the chapter looks at the surprising relationships that inmates are able to form with actual animals, sanctioned or illicit. I explore how cross-species communication nurtures an ethos of mutual protection, care, and growth. The "endarkened" prison comes back to life. If prisoners and many animals are *discarded bodies*, they can yet reclaim and rescue one another.

Perhaps it is not just prisoners and animals, but all of us, that need rescue—from our flattened world with its anthropocentric focus on screens, devices, material gratifications, and monetized relationships. The final chapter of this book explores a way in which we heal and expand by *shape-shifting* with animals and other natural beings. "Shape-shifting" refers to the human ability, through imagination and praxis, to merge our bodies with those of the more-than-human world. I explore how this is accomplished in areas as diverse as children's play, mythical and religious iconography, spiritual practice, sports, fashion, the performing arts, even blockbuster movies. This potential for shape-shifting with other creatures is grounded in our evolutionary history and biological kinships. It is also revealed through a phenomenology of the lived body, so central to the entirety of this book. The body ever leaps beyond itself to communicate with and incorporate its surroundings. Too often this is simply a human-constructed world of buildings, cars, computers, and TVs. Cyborg-like, we merge with our own machines. But when we shape-shift with other creatures (and rivers, trees, and mountains), we recover our animality and, paradoxically, our humanity. We also regain an eco-spirit of valuing the earth.

Distressed bodies can be de-stressed. Discarded bodies can be reclaimed. At times, this is a solitary quest: a person rendered lonely by pain, illness, or imprisonment must often summon up resources within the self. But this pursuit need not and cannot be only an individual one. A communal effort is needed to assist one another and to remake environments—the modern medical hospital, or worse, the prison or factory farm—that can severely stress already distressed bodies. This we do by "putting our minds together," but also by "walking shoulder to shoulder," "working hand in hand" (or even "hand in paw"). We are not just minds, but embodied creatures. This can be our curse, yet also a great blessing.

PART 1

Illness and Treatment:
Phenomenological Investigations

Rethinking Illness:
Philoctetes' Exile

Sophocles' play *Philoctetes* is set on the desolate island of Lemnos. The protagonist has lived there alone for ten years, devoid of companionship and the comforts of home. It is illness that has brought him to such a state. Bitten by the snake that guarded the sanctuary of Chryse, Philoctetes has sustained a foul-smelling, suppurating, agonizing foot wound. His companions, on the way to battle and unable to bear his groans, abandon him on Lemnos. The play begins with the arrival there of Odysseus and Neoptolemus, Achilles' young son. But they come only under compulsion; the Greeks have learned by prophecy that they need Philoctetes and his bow before they can conquer Troy.

Through a causal chain of events, illness has given rise to an exile. But the play, for this reader, suggests something more: that *illness is an exile*, a banishment from the customary world. Such a metaphoric equation may have been far from Sophocles' intent. Yet his text provides us with a rich set of images to commence a phenomenology of illness and therefore to start off this book. The wild and isolated Lemnos evokes the distant country of the sick that we all may one day come to inhabit.

> Boy, let me tell you of this island.
> No sailor by his choice comes near it.
> There is no anchorage, nor anywhere
> that one can land, sell goods, be entertained.
> Sensible men make no voyages here.
> Yet now and then someone puts in. (lines 300–305)[1]

To speak of *illness* is not the same as to speak of *disease*.[2] The latter term refers to an entity defined by means of medical categories. Were a contemporary physician present, Philoctetes' problem might be diagnosed as a chronic localized infection, perhaps actinomycosis, extending into the bone. (I thank Dr. Richard Selzer, the surgeon-writer, for this hypothesis—I'll speak more of him in chapter 3.) As *disease*, the condition is objectified, identified with an anatomical lesion or disordered physiology. Implicit reference is made to etiological agents, epidemiological distributions, predictions of outcome, diagnostic and therapeutic techniques.[3]

The term *illness* here refers instead to suffering and disability as experienced by the sick. To fall ill is not simply to undergo a physiological transformation but a transformation of one's experiential world.[4] (I here refer in endnotes to a few of the many works on the phenomenology of illness. In the main body of this chapter, I confine myself largely to Sophocles' own *footnotes*, so to speak, concerning Philoctetes' foot wound.) When seriously ill, space is constricted, time slows to a stop, the future grows uncertain, habitual roles are abandoned. Concerns that once were paramount now seem trivial, and vice versa. It is incumbent on physicians to be aware of the experienced illness that lurks behind the disease; it is the illness, after all, for which the patient seeks relief. Yet, on the nature of illness, medical journals have little to say and Sophocles much.

As we'll see in chapter 2, medical knowledge is so ubiquitous in our modern world, as solicited on Internet, in chats with our friends, and through visits to practitioners, that our experience of illness is often vectored by clinical interpretations. The distinction between "illness-as-experienced" and "disease-as-diagnosed" can thus become complex and provisional. But Lemnos has no physicians and hence no "diseases." The play allows us to examine illness in the raw. We find that the *distress* (to be "stretched apart") associated with serious illness involves a threefold exile: from the cosmos, the body, and the social world. Let's examine each in turn.

Philoctetes' illness first involves a falling out with the cosmos, the universe at large. He has violated the divine order by coming too near Chryse's shrine. Inflicted by a guardian-snake, the "sickness is of God's sending" (line 1326). Throughout history, sickness has been associated with divine punishment, from the Black Plague of the fourteenth century to the AIDS epidemic.[5] The very word pain arises from *poinē*, the Greek word for "punishment." This association, pernicious as it may be, has roots deep within the illness experience. The person who develops a serious disease often feels he or she must have done something to deserve it. Pain is the very immediate bodily sense of something bad or wrong. It is natural, then, to look for its origins in something bad or wrong about the sufferer. This is not restricted to the religious enthusiast concerned with being a sinner. The cancer patient, surveying her smoking history or "cancer-prone" personality, may feel the same sense of sickness-as-retribution. To be ill is to feel oneself out of joint with the cosmos, an exile from the harmonious totality of the world.

But illness can also raise a different specter: that the world itself is not, after all, a harmony. To the chorus of Sophocles' play, Philoctetes is no sinner, his illness, no proper recompense.

> But I know of no other,
> by hearsay, much less by sight, of all mankind
> whose destiny was more his enemy when he met it
> than Philoctetes, who wronged no one, nor killed
> but lived, just among the just,
> and fell in trouble past his deserts. (lines 680–85)

He intruded on Chryse's province unwittingly, without malicious intent. As such, Philoctetes' wound has a senseless quality that may remind us of the biblical Job's unmerited tribulations. Here Philoctetes is the victim of a chance occurrence, and then the unfolding of inexorable necessity.

So it is for the sick, to whom the universe can appear lacking in elementary kindness or justice. In the midst of a happy and successful life, on the afternoon of a glorious day, we may suddenly feel a pain, and that pain may lead to tests, and those tests reveal the onset of a disabling, progressive, even fatal, malady. Where then is the justice, where the meaning? Sickness can shatter all faith in an ordered universe. This sense of the arbitrariness of illness can bring its own form of suffering as or more powerful than that introduced by the punishment model. If illness is a form of retribution, at least justice remains operative and atonement can restore health. But what if one is not simply out of joint with the world, but the world itself is out of joint? This sense plagues Philoctetes, compounding his physical agony with rage and despair:

> [The Gods] find their pleasure in turning back from Death
> the rogues and tricksters, but the just and good
> they are always sending out of the world.
> How can I reckon the score, how can I praise,
> when praising Heaven I find the Gods are bad? (lines 447–52)

While this is not Sophoclean theology, it is psychologically acute. When we are seriously ill the gods can seem bad or nonexistent. We no longer feel at home in such a universe. It appears, like Lemnos, "a shore without houses or anchorage" (line 221).

If illness can effect an exile from the cosmos, so too from our small piece of it, the body. In health, we simply *are* our body. We gaze, speak, move our way through the world, taking for granted our physical capacities and all they render available. The body is largely transparent, simply who we are in action. But in illness the body surfaces as strangely *other*.[6] It asserts an autonomous life, refusing to obey our commands. For Philoctetes, "neither of foot nor of hand nor of anything is he master" (line 860). Those organs that once were compliant, the very agents of one's identity and capacities, for the sick person are now felt an external threat. A chasm opens up between Philoctetes and his "habitual body" with its range of predilections and abilities.[7] Now he is *dis-abled*. Philoctetes' foot becomes a thing he must laboriously drag behind, and the cause to him of unspeakable pain. He longs for nothing more than escape, whether through sleep, death, or amputation.

> By God, if you have a sword, ready to hand, use it!
> Strike the end of my foot. Strike it off, I tell you, now. (lines 748–49)

But the body cannot simply be cast off as we would an offending object. The ill person knows better than the complacently healthy of the inescapable force of embodiment. Here then is the paradox of illness: we are brought home to a heightened awareness of the body, but it is a body in which we no longer feel at home. As we will see in succeeding chapters, medical treatment can often exacerbate rather than heal this sense of division: the body is objectified, examined, probed and needled, scanned and measured, while the patient must be patient.

Illness and disability are an exile not simply from the cosmos and the microcosmos of the body, but from the social world that mediates between them.[8] When we fall sick, we are banished from the daily round of roles and duties on which so much of our conventional identity is based. From our bedroom window we hear the bustle of the street, the sound of people on their way to work, but now as if from a great distance.[9] The world is there just as it was the day before, with one exception—we are no longer a part of it. We dwell in our bed, the sole inhabitants, like Philoctetes, of a far-off island. This banishment is not simply the result of physical immobilization but of a shift within our framework of meaning. We are no longer a party to the concerns that absorb the outer world. The tenuous condition of our physiology has taken precedence. Sophocles' play well represents the solipsism of the ill. Its protagonist knows nothing of the momentous events taking place in Troy. While gods and heroes battle, the destiny of great city-states hanging in the balance, Philoctetes remains oblivious for ten long years. His life is bounded by an injured foot and private rage.

The ill person sometimes compounds this isolation through a self-imposed exile. When sick, we may purposefully shun the company of the healthy. Their vibrant energy seems almost repugnant, a taunting reminder of all we have lost. Then too we may wish to conceal our own reduced state. The sallow look, unpleasant odors, and physical dysfunctions of illness can lead the sufferer to a shamed seclusion.

Even when standing in the midst of others, the ill person, to some extent, stands alone. The healthy may be solicitous, yet cannot fully understand, alleviate, or share in the suffering. The sick one is singled out, by the long-term threats posed by serious illness and by the immediacy of present pain, a private sensation. While sight and hearing reach out to a common world, pain is largely enacted within an interior theater. Moreover, lacking any referential object in the world, pain is difficult to translate into speech,[10] a theme I will explore more in the next chapter. It can, in fact, actively destroy speech; Philoctetes is reduced by a severe attack to cries and shrieks.

Because illness renders communication so problematic, the latter can take on heightened value for the ill. Far from shunning others' company, the sick person may seek it out with desperation. In Philoctetes' words:

> I have been alone and very wretched,
> without friend or comrade, suffering a great deal.
> Take pity on me; speak to me; speak,
> speak if you come as friends.
>   No—answer me.
> If this is all
> that we can have from one another, speech,
> this, at least, we should have. (lines 227–31)

Yet the plea of a Philoctetes does not always meet due response. After all, he has a repulsive effect on others. Odysseus explains why Philoctetes' own comrades-at-arms abandoned him on Lemnos:

> We had no peace with him: at the holy festivals,
> we dared not touch the wine and meat; he screamed
> and groaned so, and those terrible cries of his
> brought ill luck on our celebrations; all
> the camp was haunted by him. (lines 6–10)

Stray sailors who have wandered onto the island have offered Philoctetes scraps of food and cast-off clothes, but none of them will give him passage home (lines 308–11). His wound gives off a great stench and leaks a black flux of blood and matter. His personality has been twisted by long frustration. The screams and moans of his agony are hard to bear. Who would want him as a companion?

Most of us share to some degree a secret, perhaps subconscious, wish to avoid or banish the ill. Rather than condemn such feelings we need to recognize them as natural. For illness can be contagious, not only physically but experientially: the very presence of the sick person threatens to infect the world, reminding the healthy of all they would most like to forget. Here is a specter of the extremes of pain, ugliness, and helplessness to which the human being can fall prey. We are recalled to the acute vulnerability of embodied life and the inevitability of our own death. It is natural to wish to escape from such thoughts, perceptions, and feelings. We thus find ways to quarantine the distressed. Hospitals, nursing homes, mental institutions can all serve such a function. Nor must quarantine take a physical form. It is there in the cheery smile we put on with a dying friend, the impersonal professionalism of her attending physician, coupled with a subtle refusal to touch the sick person (touch is the focus of chapter 3).

Yet if, as I have suggested, *illness is exile*, to compound the exile is to compound distress. The world disruptions effected by illness are hardened into place through the reactivity of others. This is true for Philoctetes. The primary cause of his isolation and rage is not physical pain per se, but the way his companions have cast him off:

> Think, boy, of that awakening when I awoke
> and found them gone; think of the useless tears
> and curses on myself when I saw the ships—
> my ships, which I had once commanded—gone,
> all gone, and not a man left on the island,
> not one to help me or to lend a hand
> when I was seized with my sickness, not a man!
> In all I saw before me nothing but pain;
> but of that a great abundance, boy. (lines 276–84)

Even the strong-willed Philoctetes is reduced by illness to childlike need: he begs Neoptolemus not to leave him alone (lines 808–9). If abandoned at a time of acute vulnerability, we feel pulled apart (*di-stress*) from others, and pressed inward (*stress*) on our solitary pain.

For a more contemporary example, we might reflect on the treatment of those with AIDS. Especially when the disease was first manifesting, clinical suffering was often intensified by social exile. This reaction toward AIDS patients took an exaggerated form for several reasons.[11] First, groups in the United States initially associated with the disease—homosexuals, IV drug users, Haitians—were already viewed as marginal members of society. It is then easier to turn away from, or vilify, their suffering. The primary perceived modes of transmission, needles and gay sex, were often regarded as illicit. Hence, some portrayed AIDS as a form of divine retribution, illness-as-punishment. Social exile is justified by reference to an exile from the cosmic order. Moreover, full-blown AIDS began as an almost uniformly fatal disease, spreading at an epidemic rate with no cure in sight. Widespread fear was thus also a factor intensifying the urge to banish the ill.

To take one Philoctetes-like example from the 1980s, Robert D., living in Baltimore, was turned down by nursing homes and hospices after he developed AIDS-related pneumonia.[12] His family rejected him, and his lover demanded he move out of the apartment. With only months left to live, he rented a room in a rundown hotel. The staff refused to enter his room, leaving food for him in the hallway. After reading a newspaper account, a stranger took him into her home, but asked him to leave a few days later. Next, he went to live with an elderly couple, but threatening phone calls and vandalism again forced him to go. He finally found a home with three adults, one also an AIDS patient, before returning soon thereafter to the hospital to die. So with Philoctetes:

> He was lame, and no one came near him.
> He suffered, and there were no neighbors for his sorrow
> with whom his cries would find answer,
> with whom he could lament the bloody plague that ate him up.
> No one who would gather
> fallen leaves from the ground
> to quiet the raging, bleeding sore,
> running, in his maggot-rotten foot.
> Here and there he crawled
> writhing always—
> suffering like a child
> without the nurse he loves—
> to what source of ease he could find
> when the heart-devouring suffering gave over. (lines 691–707)

When philosopher Havi Carel fell victim to a very rare, severely disabling, and predictably fatal disease (a form of lymphangioleiomyomatosis), she reflected on this sort of abandonment:

> Empathy. If I had to pick the human emotion in greatest shortage, it would be empathy. And this is nowhere more evident than in illness. The pain, disability and fear are exacerbated by the apathy and disgust with which you are sometimes confronted when you are ill. There are many terrible things about illness; the lack of empathy hurts the most.[13]

Philoctetes would no doubt agree. The Greeks callously abandon him to pursue, unhindered, the siege of Troy. But they discover by prophecy that they cannot win victory until the man and his bow are restored. There may be a lesson here well worth learning in our troubled times: a society can be judged, can even stand or fall, on how it chooses to treat or neglect its sick.

I have traced out the theme of exile in *Philoctetes*, the exile from cosmos, body, and society that serious sickness can cause. Illness brings about a profound experience of "unhomelike" being-in the-world.[14] But other modes of trauma can as well. The *Theatre of War Project*, with a $3.7 million dollar grant from the Defense Department, has conducted dramatic readings of Sophocles' *Philoctetes* and *Ajax* in dozens of US military bases, the Pentagon, a shelter for homeless veterans, among many other places, reaching some forty thousand military service members, veterans, and their families.[15] Sophocles was himself a general, his audience members often citizen-soldiers. In this context *Philoctetes* can also be seen as highlighting the effects of war and its aftermath, which can inflict profound physical and psychological trauma. Speaking of a recent veterans-care scandal at Walter Reed Army Medical Center, Byran Dorries, the mastermind behind the *Theatre of War Project*, says:

> On every front page there were pictures of modern Philocteteses, waiting for treatment, abandoned on islands, just like the character in the play. And all of a sudden it became a revelation that this play was about a wounded vet who was waiting for treatment and had to accept it from a medical establishment he no longer trusted.[16]

This theme of abandonment is also relevant to the men in a maximum security prison whom I turn to later in this book. Like the traumatized warrior and the chronically ill, prisoners can undergo a threefold exile from cosmos, body, and society. We will also discover ways in which the imprisoned men seek healing, with help from one another. So, too, the attendees of *Theatre of War* performances, who discuss the material afterwards in open forums. This allows hidden distress, as well as mutual compassion, to be *expressed* (pressed outward). *Philoctetes*, too, is a play not only about exile but about repatriation—the act, helped by others, of *coming home*.

To assist this process, empathy for those suffering is key. But as Carel says above, it can be in short supply. So many things get in the way: fear of our own vulnerability and death, and of being overwhelmed by the other's neediness; visceral feelings of repulsion; an inability to understand and enter into the other's experience; a social training toward polite distance; our natural self-absorption; and on and on. Yet the miracle is that a light does sometimes shine through all these blocks. There is something in the human spirit responsive to the call of anguish. The Greek word is *oiktos*, translated as "pity" or "compassion." Just as it is natural to want to escape from suffering, so too is it natural to feel compassion for those in distress.

The sailors who put into Lemnos over the years express pity for Philoctetes (line 308), as does the chorus (lines 169, 507). Neoptolemus cannot go through with a plan to deceive Philoctetes and capture his bow:

> A kind of compassion,
> a terrible compassion, has come upon me
> for him. I have felt for him all the time. (lines 965–66)

Even the very bow that the Greeks need first came to Philoctetes through an act of compassion. He had built the lethal fire that released Heracles from his torment and was given the hero's weapon in gratitude.

It is thus not merely exile but compassion that turns the plot of Sophocles' play. In English, the word "compassion" derives from *pati*, "to suffer," and *com*, "together with." To feel compassion is to suffer together with another, the one who is the "pati-ent," the sufferer. We are capable of this; at times it is almost unavoidable, unless we are trained out of it (alas, like many medical students). Just as laughter is infectious, passing from person to person, so we experience within ourselves the sorrow, pain, or fear of another. We simply respond on a pre-intellectual basis. Our "heart goes out" to the bedridden, the lonely, the dying. We want to ease this suffering, no longer sure, perhaps, to whom it belongs. As Neoptolemus says to Philoctetes:

> I have been in pain for you; I have been
> in sorrow for your pain. (lines 805–6)

We thus echo one another. The space between two faces is not empty but a rich membrane across which speech, emotions, and experiences ceaselessly flow. Pain need not remain a fully private thing: it can be transformed into a bond of communion. Through this mutual echoing, the repatriation of the ill begins.

However, compassion is indeed but a start. The sailors who strayed onto Lemnos for the past ten years had expressed empathy for Philoctetes, but little came of it. To be fully efficacious, compassion must issue in proper action. In a modern context such action can take many forms: visiting the hospital, conversing with a sick friend, taking an aging relative into our home. On a social level, we need to work to establish more humane healers and institutions, as well as forms of health insurance and care that leave no one an exile—financially, medically—during their time of distress.

Within Sophocles' play, only Neoptolemus is willing to act on his compassion. He finally agrees to return Philoctetes to his native land. Such is not to be, for at this point the demigod Heracles appears and intervenes, command-ing Philoctetes to Troy where he will be cured by Asclepius, the Greek god of medicine, and will assist the Greeks to win their war. This is a classical *deus ex machina* ("god from the machine," referring to the device used on the an-cient stage). As Philoctetes' illness was first brought on by a god, so only a di-vine visitation can fully restore him to body, society, and cosmos. Sickness and healing do have something sacred about them, something that transcends human command. (We will explore this in later chapters on pills and organ transplantation—at the heart of these Promethean technologies we find reso-nances of the sacred gift.) Nevertheless, it is a humane act that begins the healing. When Neoptolemus offers to take Philoctetes home, the stalemate is broken, the way prepared for the god to appear.

Sophocles also shows that compassion is embodied in *right speech* as well as right action. In the first half of the play, Neoptolemus participates in Odys-seus' plot to deceive the protagonist. The goal is to capture Philoctetes and his bow and bring them to Troy. According to prophecy, this will allow the Greeks to take Troy and will occasion the healing of Philoctetes' foot. But the Greeks know that his bitterness at his exile will lead Philoctetes to reject this resolution. Hence, a "healing lie" is constructed—one that seems best for this "patient" as well as all others concerned.

The plot turns when his "terrible compassion" leads Neoptolemus to un-equivocally reject this deception. Instead he tells Philoctetes the truth. A res-toration based on deceit, the play suggests, is no restoration at all. We are reminded of the link between compassion and honest speech, and the im-portance of the latter in the project of healing. Within bioethics, discussions of truth in the doctor-patient relation have often revolved around questions of abstract rights and duties. But such is not Neoptolemus's primary concern. He is called to truth by a confrontation with raw suffering. He cannot bear to deceive a man so vulnerable, so in need of a trustworthy companion. Truth takes on a heightened import in the context of extreme distress.

For truthful speech works to restore precisely those things that illness-as-exile has undermined. It fosters knowledge on the part of the listener, trust to-ward the speaker, a communicative bond between the two. *Knowledge, trust, communication*: these have all been rendered problematic by illness. The sick person often does not fully know the causes or future consequences of the dis-ease. Trust in one's own body and the cosmos are damaged. Communication with others is undermined by the private nature of pain. There is a sense of re-verberating epistemological and existential crisis. Here we see the healing force of truthful speech and how it helps repatriate the ill person. Such is relevant as well to the plight of the prisoner, and also the soldier. The *Theatre of War* performance of *Philoctetes* is meant to provoke truthful speech to and with the audience about the traumas of war and its aftermath.

Neoptolemus cannot fully enact "com-passion" ("to suffer together with") when he strategically lies to Philoctetes, even in a good cause. One man knows what is taking place while the other does not. One man is controlling the course of events while the other has only the illusion of decision. They seem to be suffering together, but in fact the sick person remains an exile, excluded from the other's knowledge and the true situation. Extrapolating to the present, one might say that honesty in medicine is not a mere preliminary to proper treatment, but integral to the healing process. But what does it means to "speak the truth"? How much, and how best to do so? What kinds of "truth telling" assists the patient to reclaim genuine "autonomy"? In chapter 8 I will return to these clinical/bioethical issues.

✳

In the wild landscape of Lemnos we have seen the face of suffering writ large. *Philoctetes* teaches us of the many-dimensioned exile of the ill: the sense of sickness as punishment, the loss of trust in the gods, estrangement from one's own body, the obliteration of social roles, the struggle even to speak. We witness the power of others to compound or alleviate distress. The instinct to banish the sufferer is exemplified in the unscrupulous figure of Odysseus. In Neoptolemus, we see the converse personified: he feels compassion and finally accords due respect and honest language.

But this is not simply a matter of heroes and villains. Clashing urges coexist within the human heart. In the presence of the ill we feel both revulsion and sympathy. We have a reflex to withdraw and to reach out in aid. Most of us arrive at an uneasy compromise. Yet recognizing this battle, maybe even winning it from time to time, is core to any project of healing. Over the course of a lifetime, we will have many occasions to be Neoptolemus—and also, alas, Philoctetes.

Rethinking Pain:
The Paradoxical Problem

Chapter 1 introduced the experience of illness with a literary example. Poets and dramatists often probe more deeply into the human predicament than do academicians. At the same time, there is merit to a more formal, structural exploration of experience. In this case I will not try to take on "illness" in its totality. The first chapter made some provisional generalities. Yet there are so many different kinds of diseases and injuries, each invoking its own special modes of distress and disability, as well as different individuals experiencing them in unique ways, that it would be an indefinitely large project to explore illness in all its forms. One can imagine a series of textbooks, not simply of *diseases*—diabetes, rheumatoid arthritis, chronic ulcerative colitis—but of *illnesses*, that is, of the experiential correlates that often accompany each of these syndromes.

In this chapter I will narrow my theme to that of physical pain. It is both particular in nature, yet wide-ranging in its manifestation across a range of injuries and diseases (and life in general). I specify *physical* pain to distinguish it from other modes of psychological, existential, and social suffering—grief, depression, and the like. Yet I will also call into question the very distinction just invoked. "Physical" pain is an experience, and one in which grief, depression, isolation can provide its very texture and intensity.

I will also focus primarily on *chronic* physical pain, rather than brief, acute, and perhaps medically resolvable pain. However, again, this distinction is ambiguous. "Chronic pain," which can feel quite acute, is defined by different sources as pain lasting more than twelve weeks, six months, or a year. It can also be understood as pain that no longer has a clear etiology or telos, but "persists after all possible healing has occurred, or, at least long after pain can serve any useful function."[1] But while both medically and experientially imprecise, the notion of "chronic pain" does capture something—a pain that persists, and persistently raises questions such as "what is going on here?," "will this ever end?," and "why me?".

Instead of employing a literary account, like that supplied by Sophocles, I will use a personal example concerning a recent and ongoing pain experience. This taken by itself would be methodologically questionable given the idiosyncrasies of any individual case. The numbers of people suffering from some form of chronic pain is huge—according to the Institute of Medicine in the United States, about 100 million adults.[2] There is also an extensive literature on pain—philosophical, clinical, and sociological—utilizing and supplemented by many individual "pathographies" written by those grappling with serious illness. I will draw on that substantial literature. Yet using the method of phenomenology—the careful examination of the structures of experience, having "bracketed" (set aside) any precommitments to metaphysical or scientific-causal structures of explanation[3]—there is something to be gained through reflecting on one's own experience. We have seen that pain, immediately present to the sufferer, is difficult to objectify and communicate. I will supplement my reading of others' descriptions with what persistent pain has felt like from within, speaking about it as best I can.

The methodological ambiguities mentioned above—pain as physical/psychological, chronic yet acute, accessible in different third-person/first-person ways—I take to be ingredient in the topic itself. In fact, such ambiguities *are* the topic. Pain, I will suggest, and especially persistent pain, involves negotiating a series of dialectical tensions and experiential paradoxes. These can be the source of doubt, struggle, frustration, and confusion that greatly add to the painfulness of pain. In this chapter I will examine no less than *nine paradoxes* associated with fundamental questions that arise for the person in distress. In such a way I will take off from, but deepen the analysis originally triggered by Philoctetes' painful wound.

1. Sensation and Interpretation

First, what is this pain? In a certain way, the answer to this question is clear— *this* is the pain, this immediate, unpleasant, somewhat inexpressible, sensation. Elaine Scarry, in her influential *The Body in Pain*, characterizes it as a unique bodily experience. Senses such as hearing and sight apprehend objects. Even intentional states such as hunger or fear remain "hunger for" or "fear of" something. But she writes "pain is not 'of' or 'for' anything—it is itself alone. This objectlessness, the complete absence of referential content, almost prevents it from being rendered in language."[4] Hence, we can be reduced to grunts and cries like Philoctetes. Only subsequently, and often analogically, does pain come to be connected with objects in the world.

There is a phenomenological truth here—pain can suddenly seize us from within, collapsing our complex world of involvements. Still, I would challenge Scarry's characterization of pain as nonreferential.

My own pain was consistently a "pain of." As the content of what it was "of" shifted, so too the experience. Consulting orthopedists about a lower leg pain, and then vascular surgeons, neurologists, a pain specialist, an acupuncturist, and a plastic surgeon—along with my own, sometimes obsessive, skimming of webpages—led me to many different answers concerning what this was a "pain of." With each new interpretive perspective, the sensed pain itself changed in quality, intensity, meaning, and affective content. The pain of a possible stress fracture felt sharp, as if something inside was indeed broken. When viewed as ankle "inflammation," it exuded warmth. When varicose veins seemed the cause, I felt a heaviness in my leg. The ultimate diagnosis of a "peripheral neuropathy" highlighted the pain's stinging and burning qualities. Also, based on the shifting prognoses, these pains felt at times more serious or less so, on the way to recovery or depressingly untreatable. Each different pain also cried out for a different response. You do not, for example, walk on a stress fracture. My leg pain then seemed to be telling me in no uncertain terms to *rest*. But when the diagnosis shifted to a focus on varicose veins (where exercise is important to keep blood from pooling), my pain now felt like a call to *get up and move*.

Pain thus partakes both in the immediacy of sensation and the mediacy of complex referentiality and interpretation.[5] We realize this as well through biological reasoning. Pain serves as a protective mechanism whereby a living creature is made aware of actual or potential tissue damage and is motivated by the aversive quality of the sensation to take corrective action.[6] As such, pain calls for creatures to feel, investigate, respond. Wall, a neuroscientist and pain expert, writes, "I have never felt a pure pain. Pain for me arrives as a complete package. A particular pain is at the same time painful, miserable, disturbing, and so on. I have never heard a patient speak of pain isolated from its companion affect."[7]

The neuroscientific "gate control" theory Wall helped introduce also suggests that pain experience is not simply the result of a peripheral stimulus but is filtered and modulated by spinal and cerebral centers of the central nervous system. This theory, "with its emphasis on parallel processing systems, provided the conceptual framework for integration of the sensory, affective and cognitive dimensions of pain."[8] I will not dwell further on such scientific theories. They are suggestive but also likely to change as research continues, and in any case, should be "bracketed" from a phenomenological perspective, such that second-order explanatory accounts not displace our investigation of "the things themselves."

In the first chapter I contrasted "illness" (experiential) with "disease" (medical category). *Yet I have said that this division is provisional.* Scientific interpretations sink into and vector our life-world. Pain experience can oscillate between the pole Scarry emphasizes—that of nonreferential sensation—the pure "ouch!"—to that of complex interpretation, as when the doctor tells you this "ouch" may be a sign of diabetic neuropathy. The "ouch" can even be created out of the diagnosis. Groopman, himself an expert oncologist, describes an occasion where a bone scan he underwent for a hand problem revealed what seemed to be metastatic cancer in his ribs. "I generally think of myself as reasonably well put together psychologically, but within moments my chest began to ache. When I touched my ribs, they hurt." Further tests revealed no such cancer, but it took several hours for the ache and tenderness to subside.[9]

Diagnosis changes our sensations. New sensations can also change our diagnostic picture. Chronic sufferers who repeatedly survey and evaluate their pain, in dialogue with the medical community, may find themselves in a hermeneutical circle that has no clear terminus.[10] Chapters 6 and 7 will examine in more depth the complex hermeneutics of diagnosis and the way it arises from and impacts the treater-patient relation.

2. Certainty and Uncertainty

This all leads us to a second paradox of pain: that between certainty and uncertainty. Again, Scarry provides a way into the topic, though one I will again challenge. She writes:

> Pain enters into our midst as at once something that cannot be denied and something that cannot be confirmed (thus it comes to be cited in philosophic discourse as an example of conviction, or alternatively as an example of skepticism). To have pain is to have *certainty*; to hear about pain is to have *doubt*.[11]

Scarry is surely right about this existential/epistemological split dividing the sufferer from others. Though my family never actively doubted my complaints—in this I was fortunate because there are skeptical families, employers, doctors, and government officials—they couldn't know it from within as I did. I either kept quiet (which increased my sense of isolation) or tried to convey my pain through groans and words (which made me feel like a complainer). In either case, though they behaved with compassion, I remained experientially on my own. That is, I dwelled on Philoctetes' island. This was true as well in my relationship with doctors, including the many who were kindly. My suffering, so searingly present for me, was to them an interesting puzzle—until it proved insolvable by or irrelevant to their particular discipline, in which case their interest might wane.

But is Scarry right to assert that "to have pain is to have *certainty*"? True, one has privileged and indubitable access to one's own mental states. This was at the core of René Descartes's *cogito ergo sum* realization. Clinically, one can and should respect the patient's self-report. Yet I would contend that there are features of radical *uncertainty* for the experiencer of pain, not only for the one hearing about it. I found my own pain states often opaque and ambiguous in any number of ways.

"On a 1–10 scale how would you rate the intensity of your pain?" This common doctor's office question can lead to bafflement. My pain would shift moment to moment or at different times of day. And at any time how intense is it really? Am I being a big baby, exaggerating a minor ache, or am I someone with high pain tolerance (something I was once told), soldiering on in the face of a major assault? Is it *really* a 3 . . . or a 6?

And where is this pain exactly? There were surface stings and stabbings, along with burns and deep aches difficult to locate in the nether-space of the bodily interior. This was like the coenesthetic equivalent of seeing a shadow move, uncertain whether it was a menacing stranger or simply curtains waving in the wind. The pain can take on an uncertain and therefore uncanny nature—what did I just feel? Neither friend, doctor, nor technological device can step in to answer that question.

Hence, the radical doubt that Scarry refers to is not simply the property of the "other" but can also permeate the world of the sufferer. Even the absence of pain is open to question once chronic pain has become the norm. "I don't remember being in pain this afternoon," I would think to myself. "Maybe my ankle is finally healing. But I was busy teaching class. Was I really not in pain or just too distracted to notice it? But if I didn't notice it, was it still pain?" This is a version of the old question, "if a tree falls in the forest but no one hears it, did it make a sound?" but now referring to one's own unclear, interior forest.

3. Present and Projective

An associated question arises: "*When* is this pain?" Here I do not refer to calendar time—one can often know with great precision, as I did, what day pain first appeared or when in the evening it worsens. But this sidesteps the issue of what pain does to time-consciousness itself—the "when" of it in this sense.

This is a complex and multidimensional issue, which I have not the time—
paradox intended—to treat fully in this chapter. But, returning to the literary
world, here a poet such as Emily Dickinson, famous for her own brevity, may
get us started:

> Pain—has an Element of Blank—
> It cannot recollect
> When it began—or if there were
> A time when it was not—
>
> It has no Future—but itself—
> Its Infinite contain
> Its Past—enlightened to perceive
> New Periods—of Pain.[12]

Dickinson articulates an alteration of normal time-consciousness. Though she
refers to past and future—the projective "*ecstases*" of time, to use Heidegger's
term[13]—the "now" of pain is never explicitly mentioned. Yet this is because
present pain is *everything*, has swallowed up the world, until it "cannot recol-
lect . . . A time when it was not" and "has no Future—but itself."

When pain is severe or persistent, it can feel like this. It is very difficult,
though perhaps not impossible, to project beyond it—that is, to use one's powers of recollection, imagination, positive anticipation to escape its grasp.
Physical pain—in my case, specific nerve shocks and spasms—kept seizing
me back to the here and now. This lived present may also slow and expand.
In Brough's words, "Thus the now of the pain I live through may appear to
me to be endless, while the procedure inflicting it may by the clock take only
45 seconds."[14] Concurrently, for the person in pain, "Hopes, dreams, and aspirations for the future might seem to disappear, stranding the person in the
unsatisfactory present."[15] In my case, this led me to the edge of desperation,
from the Latin *desperatus*, meaning "without hope." Even making one's way
through a single painful evening—until the clock renders permission to call
it bedtime—can be like slowly swimming through a thick tide, time itself a
resistant medium.

This immersive present need not always be so negative. Forced by my
painful ankle to slow down, sit down, and eventually to calm down, I have
done deeper reading and contemplation than I would otherwise. Ironically,
I've been working my way through Marcel Proust's multivolume *In Search of
Lost Time*, a work I set aside some twenty years ago. I just didn't have the time
then—but do now, thanks to the way my injury slowed and emptied time.

It can also be healing, particularly when facing an illness with an uncertain, or even fatal, prognosis, to choose to remain firmly rooted in the now.

Carel writes, "Focusing on present abilities, joys and experiences instead of worrying about a no-longer-existing past and a not-yet-existing future, is a way of avoiding some of the suffering caused by illness."[16]

True, but chronic pain can also poison the "now" with suffering. Rather than returning to the present as a joyful home, it may appear quite "unhomelike."[17] With no clear end in sight, time's briefest slice can expand into Dickinson's harsh "infinite," a prison sentence of indefinite length. Pain thus motivates a variety of attempts at jail break. That is, its felt aversiveness not only fixes us to the present but compels us to run away. We project outward to other time realms in search of relief. Some might turn to comforting memories. A life review can recall happier times and place the pain episode in broad perspective.

In my case, I turned my attention more to the future. *When* will I find a proper diagnosis and treatment? *When* is the appointment with the next specialist? *When* will this pain go away and real life recommence? On such questions I focused with the intensity of a dog staring fixedly at his master's hand, hoping it holds a treat, yet afraid of a beating. This search for a pain-free future can be freeing (there is hope) but also limiting and solipsistic. "The focus becomes entirely directed on the self. All purpose becomes directed at the relief of pain, sickness and suffering."[18]

The temporality of pain thus unfolds in paradoxical tensions—the "now" both summons and repulses; the past can comfort but ever recedes from our reclamation; the future opens up horizons of possibility, but it can neither satisfy our higher aspirations nor provide certainty of relief, and may in fact threaten a worsening of symptoms.

4. Never-Changing and the Ever-Changing

Chronic pain introduces another temporal paradox: it can seem simultaneously both never- and ever-changing. The term "chronic" from the Greek word for time, *khronos*, suggests that certain modes of suffering are set off, made different, by the long passage of time. Again, this is not just the calendar times—three months, six months—referred to by clinical definitions. To the sufferer, chronic pain can seem to go on and on repetitively, like a nightmarish version of Friedrich Nietzsche's eternal recurrence.[19] To reawaken each morning to the same constricting pain, no matter how freely one moved in one's dreams; to know that it gathers intensity each evening starting around 7 p.m.; to find that after a certain amount one can walk no more because the pain has arrived to enforce its restrictions; to survey hours, days, weeks, months, and be unable to discern demonstrable improvement: this is to feel oneself trapped in a never-changing time. In Dickinson's words, "It has no Future—but itself— / Its Infinite contain . . . / New Periods—of Pain."

Yet, and paradoxically, this "never-changing" pain is constantly fluctuating. As the above examples suggest, pain can alter according to time of day, exercise, body position, a texture that brushes up against the skin, even a passing thought or mood. In longer terms, one's condition may be improving or degenerating according to the specific nature of the illness and treatment, which impose their own temporal progressions.

At times, pain may entirely disappear. The experience then of *not-being-in-pain* differs from the pain-free state that is taken for granted when one is healthy and therefore rarely thematized. This *not-being-in-pain* is noticeable, perhaps startling, inducing both hope and fear given its precarious nature.

I found, though, that what Dickinson says about the temporality of pain works equally well when inverted:

> *Not-Being-in-Pain*—has an Element of Blank—
> It cannot recollect
> When it began—or if there were
> A time when it was not—

That is, when my leg pain went away, in my blessed relief I had difficulty reconnecting with past experiences of pain (even if I retained an intellectual memory thereof). Pain is such an intense *presence* that when it disappears for a time it can simply feel *gone*. This actually proved problematic for me because those better times would lead me to incautiously overdo my walking and climbing, no doubt hastening the return of serious pain. Amnesia concerning past agonies was associated with deficient anticipations concerning the future—I lacked clarity that pain could and would return, especially if I wasn't careful.

Thus chronic pain can oscillate in ever-changing patterns. It is boring and unremitting, yet also endlessly novel in its play of forms. The author Alphonse Daudet (a close friend of Proust), when dying of tertiary syphilis, wrote, "Pain is always new to the sufferer, but loses its originality for those around him. Everyone will get used to it except me."[20] This ever-newness can trigger "the start of an obsessive process of self-observation in our painful bodies"[21] that further isolates us from others and from life's richness.

More positively, moment-to-moment awareness of shifting sensations can also yield beneficial results. What Carl Jung said of life and the process of aging is also true of even a day spent in pain: "But we cannot live the afternoon of life according to the programme of life's morning; for what was great in the morning will be little at evening, and what in the morning was true will at evening have become a lie."[22] I found literally that what in the morning might lessen my pain (for example, exercise) might in the evening increase it. Akin to Buddhist mindfulness practice, I learned to listen carefully for the body's changing messages and the shifting strategies that might best serve each moment.

Yet this dialectic of the "ever-changing" and the "never-changing" dimensions of chronic pain can lead to (very un-Buddhist-like) cycles of hope and bitter discouragement, and sometimes the sense of doing much but accomplishing nothing. Then "chronic pain" is truly the pain of time itself (*khronos*), unless and until the sufferer can make peace with this three-faced god of past, present, and future.

5. Mind and Body

I have been discussing the "when" of pain—its temporal profile. But *where* does the pain unfold? At least within our culture, steeped in a dualistic religious and philosophical heritage, two options immediately present themselves: it is in my body or mind. Paradoxically, both seem experientially confirmable.

It is clear, in one sense, where my ankle pain is located—*in my ankle*. I can reach down and touch the site of pain. This injured body seems largely recalcitrant to my mental intentions and desires. Yet when I probe experience more deeply, as Descartes did in his famous meditations, I can also arrive at a seemingly opposite conclusion: pains are actually in the mind, events (or "qualia," to use contemporary philosophical language) that present themselves within my stream of consciousness. Such may be triggered by physical forces—for example, tissue or movement compressing my saphenous nerve—but the pain itself, the aching and burning, is an object of conscious experience.

These two perspectives on the "where" of pain tend to re-present themselves in the causal analyses and treatment options available to the pain patient. As Kleinman et al. write:

> The medical literature privileges objective somatic processes, and it enshrines them as the agent that produces pain. The psychological literature takes the opposite position: it imputes agency to the subjective mind (as affected by specific behavioral contingencies and family dynamics); these mindful processes then produce physical pain. The Cartesian dichotomy remains unquestioned.[23]

More holistic understandings try to bridge this Cartesian dichotomy by variously blending, or attending to, both sides. The International Association for the Study of Pain, for example, defines pain as "an unpleasant sensory and emotional experience associated with actual or potential tissue damage, or described in terms of such damage."[24] With both mental and physical components playing a part, pain management guides often recommend multidimensional interventions: medication and meditation both have their uses and often work well in synergy.

However, for the patient in pain, the "mind-body question" may remain a lived, perhaps irresolvable, paradox. Good records an interview with a young man, Brian, who has long suffered from intense pains in his head, throat, and ears. Temporomandibular Joint Disorder (TMJ) has been offered as a possible physical diagnosis, but Brian remains unsure: "Is it my body? Is it my thinking process that activates physical stresses? Or am I, or is it the other way around? It's all that uncertainty."[25]

Many in chronic pain can relate to "that uncertainty." At times, my ankle pain seems something mechanically produced by the forces involving in weight-bearing joints, nerve transmission, and the like. There then seems little I can do except stay off my feet. At other times I understand pain more as an object and product of my consciousness, and therefore one that can be modulated by positive reframing, healing imagery, even self-hypnosis.[26] This mentalizing of pain can feel empowering (I can alter my experience) or guilt-producing (the pain is worse today; I must have been thinking wrong thoughts). Physicians have learned, quite rightly, not to label chronic pain syndromes "psychogenic," which tends to be stigmatizing, implying "it's all in your mind."[27] But with the causative factors of chronic pain complex and unclear, what exactly is initiated by mind and what by body may be puzzling for patient and physician alike.

6. Self and Other

Part of the problem may lie in the flawed metaphysics of mind-body dualism. Phenomenologists, such as Merleau-Ponty, have proposed that it is more experientially illuminating to understand the person as a unitary "lived body." We do not just *have* a body, as if it were some object in the world to which our intellect is mysteriously attached. We also *are* our bodies. Our subjectivity, that is, our powers of perception, movement, desire, communication, are all profoundly embodied modes through which we inhabit our surroundings. In short, "The body is our general medium for having a world."[28]

Yet viewing ourselves in this more unitary fashion does not fully resolve the experiential paradox of where pain is. We may no longer frame this in relation to the mind-body question, but there remains an issue of whether pain is experienced as fundamentally *within the self* or as *other*. For the sufferer, the answer may be *both*.

The healthy body serves as a largely transparent medium through which we explore and act upon the world.[29] When striding along the trail, I am free to enjoy the blustery spring day, birdsong, and early leafing trees. Yet my leg injury shifts focus. My attention now folds back upon my own body as a problematic object—*how is my leg doing?* I wonder, step by uncertain step, noticing with foreboding its twinges.

As such times, the body reveals itself as both an inescapable part of me and an uncanny "alien presence."[30] In Scarry's words, "Even though (pain) occurs within oneself, it is at once identified as 'not oneself,' 'not me,' as something so alien that it must right now be gotten rid of."[31] There are biological benefits associated with such an attitude: objectifying the bodily process enables one to offer it up for study, repair, or even amputation.[32] Yet this is not always easy since the "other" in question is very much a part of me and mine.[33] This, in Slatman's words, is the deep existential "strangeness" of the body: it is both the source of one's identity and powers, and yet also meat, machinelike, weighty, resistant.[34]

The person in chronic pain must negotiate this ambivalent relationship with his or her body, even specific parts. In my case, over time, instead of viewing my damaged nerve as an enemy, I sought to befriend it, ask it what it wanted, thank it for its good service even in challenging periods. I wondered, if it came time, as a last-ditch method of ending the pain, to chemically or surgically lesion the nerve, could I bear to kill my friend? Yet even viewing the painful body-part as friend does not eradicate the sense of duality—of "me" and "it." This merely modulates our complex affiliation.

Friend? We can try to take this attitude. Yet in chronic pain one may wonder whether this body will not only torture but kill me. This is a clear issue for those with degenerative or fatal illnesses. Even in a less dire case, such as my own, a foreshadowing of mortality occurs. "Pain is a harbinger of death," writes Bakan.[35] Its sensory seizure tells us of the vulnerability of the flesh and seems a seed of our demise ever growing from within.[36] My nerve problem affected my foot area, and I remember one day being struck by the metaphor, "I have one foot in the grave." The whole rest of my body longed for activity, adventure, *life*, but that one foot was dragging me down into Hades.

Pain thus initiates a profound and paradoxical *double alienation*. As interior to the self, unshareable, inexpressible, pain brings about "this absolute split between one's sense of one's own reality and the reality of other persons."[37] Alienated from others, one is also alienated from an embodiment that now surfaces as *another other*. Our own body opposes our will, can even pull us prematurely toward death. This double alienation is not necessarily the endpoint of chronic pain.[38] For example, I have mentioned my ability to befriend my injured ankle, and have also found others—compassionate family members and professional healers—to help me with that process. Philoctetes found a caring friend in Neoptolemus, and a divine healing. Yet as we saw in chapter 1, pain has the power to dis-integrate one's relation to others, to one's own body—and as we will now explore, to the world as a whole.

7. Here and Everywhere

For another paradox arises in response to the question of "where is the pain?" In most cases, pain has a location, a "here" that one can point at. In my case, there was a small oval area two inches above the left medial malleolus (ankle bone) that formed the epicenter of my suffering. I would even outline this region with a marker before visiting a doctor. Yet insistent pain can also globalize itself throughout our attentional field. As Proust writes, "Is there not such a thing as diffused bodily pain, radiating out into parts outside the affected area, but leaving them and disappearing completely the moment the practitioner lays his finger on the precise spot from which it springs?"[39] Proust has himself laid his finger on an interesting point—that pain can have definite location and/or be diffused, a generalized place in which we dwell as when we simply say "I am *in pain*." Both can be true simultaneously, or we can oscillate between these poles of precision and diffusion as in Proust's example.

Since one's world is always experienced with and through the lived body, we find that pain can even overrun fleshly limits and saturate one's environs.[40] To use Heidegger's term, pain can be a kind of "mood" or "attunement" (*Stimmung*) through which our being-in-the-world is disclosed.[41] In my case, when on the edge of pain, a path I used to stride with ease was now revealed as filled with crevices, rocks, and other potential hazards. The shrieks of nearby children could take on a harsh quality. The world as a whole might feel vaguely menacing; or drained of all color and warmth; or something muffled and far away, as if one dwells on that isolated island of Lemnos. In such ways, the pain in my left ankle could totalize itself. It diffused like a malignant mist throughout the experienced world. Conversely, when my ankle felt better, not only did I feel like a new person—my self-esteem rising, my voice becoming stronger—but the world opened its doors and windows, beckoning me to cheerful adventure.

Thus a full-scale phenomenology of pain (this is but a partial version, honing in on certain paradoxes) leads us far beyond the perimeter of specific sensation. We see how pain reconfigures our sociality, creating zones of isolation, others of empathic call and response; it severs space into regions of the near and far, those objects and activities that remain accessible, and others withdrawn from reach, given the limitations of function; it causes contractions of spatiality around the sickbed analogous to the way, in relativistic physics, that mass curves space around itself, exerting a gravitational pull difficult to escape. "Chronic" pain (the pain of *khronos*, time) is also the pain of *topos* (place), changing our place in the world. Analogous to Einsteinian physics, the fabric of experiential space-time is multidimensionally warped.

8. In-Control and Out-of-Control

I conclude here with issues concerning the "how" and the "why" of chronic pain. First, a question paramount for the sufferer: *How* do I gain mastery over the pain? Or must it always have mastery over me?

In one sense, as per the discussion above, pain seems quite out of our control. It may continue despite all our attempts at diagnosis and treatment; tests and medications; the alterations of rest, diet, and exercise; even alternative therapies and petitionary prayer. The pain manifests as a foreign agency, one more persistent and powerful than our paltry efforts. Brian, the patient discussed earlier with possible TMJ, says that when his pain comes on, "It seems like there's something very, very terrible happening. I have no control over it, it's ah . . . I really don't have any control over it, although I like to believe I do."[42] Pain, if anything, has control over us, determining what we can do and must feel. The Latin word *pati*, meaning "to suffer," is the root of the English words "patient" and "passive," suggesting this lack of agency.

However—and here is the paradox—chronic pain can also create a sense of *hyper-agency* in the sufferer. In my case, far from being absolved of responsibility by my injured leg, I had to exert a level of vigilance and decision making on both micro- and macro-scales that I was unaccustomed to during the comparative ease of health. Before, I could heedlessly head out on a two-hour hike—no big deal. Now I had to be careful with each step, making sure I was leaning to the outside of the foot in a way that would minimize pain on impact. I would decide to ice after a short walk and perhaps try a nerve-cream. I had to stop computer work periodically to rest and elevate my leg, decide whether it felt wise to go to a movie at night or to schedule travel to a conference a few months hence. On many occasions, these decisions were seemingly revealed as "good" or "bad" based on the level of pain control I maintained.

There are hazards to overemphasizing this exercise of control. Arthur Frank, a medical sociologist, reflects on his own experience living through a heart attack and then cancer: "In society's view of disease, when the body goes out of control, the patient is treated as if he has lost control. Being sick thus carries more than a hint of moral failure; I felt that in being ill I was being vaguely irresponsible."[43] Doctor and patient can collude to "blame the victim."

Such can serve as a defense mechanism on the part of the clinician. Patients often arrive with an unrealistic fantasy that modern medicine, with all its high-tech diagnostic and therapeutic powers, must be able to fix any problem or at least remove its associated pain. Sadly, that is not always the case. It is painful for doctors, not simply their patients, to be unable to fulfill this fantasy of absolute control.[44] Frank's illnesses finally taught him that "giving up the idea of control, by either myself or my doctors, made me more content."[45] It probably also took pressure off his physicians.

That said, treaters can do much to help the person who deals with challenging pain. Melzack and Wall write,

> The essential ingredient is providing the patient with skills to cope with the pain and anxiety—at the very least, to provide the patient with a sense of control. . . . [W]hen the patients are taught skills to cope with their pain, such as relaxation or distraction strategies, the pain is less severe.[46]

It might be said that in discussing such matters, I am wandering from a phenomenological focus on the original pain experience to "second-order" issues of pain management. Yet, as the quote above suggests, such distinctions are far from absolute. In my own case, I found that merely learning a technique that could help diminish pain itself diminished it. That is, the pain came to feel less sinister, severe, and overpowering. Knowing "there is *something* I can do" made a real difference.

I must say that I received little in the way of skills (as opposed to pills) from the clinical "pain expert" I saw. However, in general I did access state-of-the-art medical care, including alternative approaches, provided through excellent insurance coverage supplemented by my own resources. Many are in a far less fortunate position. As Kleinman writes,

> The experience of pain in a world without security (in family, job, finances, or neighborhood) is what distinguishes chronic pain among the poor and the oppressed. When one cannot marshal resources, symbolic and instrumental, because they do not exist or one's access to them is obstructed, the very ideal of control becomes untenable.[47]

Achieving greater control over pain is clearly better, and functional and caring social systems, along with well-trained treaters, are crucial to support that goal. We still live in a time and society where many are without reliable access to high-quality health care, significantly augmenting the painfulness of pain.

Yet even in a supportive context, chronic pain can remain paradoxical, ambiguous. The sufferer both feels the lack of agency and a call to hyper-agency, that is, the rigorous monitoring and micromanagement of activity. The "pain control" achieved often remains partial and uncertain. It is not even clear when it is better to assert personal control, give it over to treaters, or let go entirely of the project of control.

9. Productive and Destructive

Implicit in the above discussions is a last question, which can also be the first question for the person in pain: *Why?* That is, why me? Why this? The answers found are as diverse as those asking the questions and may shift over time for each individual. Yet again we can discern a paradoxical antinomy as pain acts to both generate and destroy the many responses.

We find this ingredient in even a brief pain experience. In the middle of an ordinary day, bending over to tie a shoelace, one's lower back goes into spasm. Immediately one experiences a destructive and distressing component—the world of outward involvements is disrupted. Yet the pain can also be productive, generating new questions and meanings. What is this about? How do I treat it? How do I prevent it in the future? Hopefully, the messages received are both beneficial and practicable. With proper rest, self-care, exercise, the back problem may resolve—lesson learned, and perhaps one's life has been improved.

Chronic pain is not only quantitatively but qualitatively different in its challenge. As Melzack and Wall write,

> Pain, which is normally associated with the search for treatment and optimal conditions for recovery, now becomes intractable. Patients are beset with a sense of helplessness, hopelessness and meaninglessness. The pain becomes evil—it is intolerable and serves no useful function.[48]

Stella Hoff, a biomedical researcher who still suffers severe pain four years after a car accident, elaborates on this theme in an interview:

> Suffering is an evil. I mean suffering that has no meaning, that brings nothing good with it. . . . My spirit is hurt, wounded. There is no transcendence. I have found no creativity, no meaning in this . . . this entirely horrible experience. There is no God in it. . . . It shatters all I took for granted and believed in.[49]

In this poignant quote, reminiscent of Philoctetes' plight before his *deus ex machina*, we see chronic pain's destructive power, and in two senses. First, pain comes to be associated with a series of negative meanings. It is "evil." It signifies failure and retribution;[50] we have seen this in the very etymology of the word "pain" from *poinē*, the Greek word for "punishment." Many chronic pain sufferers have a core conviction they have done something to deserve it. Such an interpretation, even when subconscious, can make it difficult to practice self-care and compassion.

Second, pain is associated not only with negative meanings but with the *meaningless*—in its sheer repetitive aversiveness, its senseless reiterations, chronic pain can destroy all our attempt to find any reason, purpose, or divine plan. In Hoff's words above, this is "suffering that has no meaning, that brings nothing good. . . . It shatters all I took for granted and believed in." Pain can be "world-destroying,"[51] overturning that which makes life enjoyable and purposeful. As Frank writes, illness in general can be a source of "narrative wreckage," disrupting the course of our life and the stories we have told about it.[52] For the religiously minded, a sense of inexplicable abandonment may follow. In the Gospel of Matthew, the last words of Jesus, nailed so painfully to the cross, are "My God, my God, why hast thou forsaken me?"[53]

Thankfully, devastation does not always have the last word. (Jesus's cry is itself a quote from Psalm 22, a verse that ends in celebration of God and his people.) Pain is productive as well as destructive on the level of meaning, and again in two ways.

First, as noted at the beginning of this chapter, pain is a bodily experience that naturally produces interpretation. Health allows for a pleasant obliviousness; not so pain, which provokes a search for its significance and remedy. In chronic pain this search also becomes chronic, ongoing over time, as different meanings arise and are abandoned or layered atop each other. Chronic pain can function like a Zen koan: a question repeated, permitting of no easy resolution but therefore provoking us to penetrate ever further.

Second, some of these meanings so produced are genuinely *productive* for the individual. In Proust's words, "Griefs, at the moment when they change into ideas, lose some of their power to injure our heart; the transformation itself, even, for an instant, releases suddenly a little joy."[54] Over time, the pain we have experienced can trigger specific insights, or the strengthening of character, or the realization of blessings. (That such positives are sometimes thrust too quickly at the sufferer does not mean they cannot come true.) In my own case, I found myself reexamining old family traumas, letting go of guilt that I might be somatizing through bodily pain. My leg pain also has given me precise messages about modes of stress and exhaustion I need to avoid. Perhaps in this way it can help me forestall future stress-induced system breakdown, even the fatal sort. Unable to stride busily about the world, I feel a permission to slow down—to begin to transition into the wisdom years of later life. I have experienced the power of family and community as many hands reach out to help. I have become more serious about certain meditative and spiritual practices. I listen more closely to my body. I must.

Yet pain remains "the gift nobody wants."[55] Mixed in with anything sweet, the pain has brought me much that was bitter: feelings of personal failure, prayers that seemed to go unanswered, sincere efforts rebuffed by an unfeeling universe, incompetent practitioners, and an untrustworthy body. Again, this is the paradoxical dialectic of chronic pain. Pain is productive/destructive. These go hand in hand, though one or the other may have the *upper hand* at a given time or for a given person.

Conclusions

There is much that this discussion, of necessity, has omitted. Many paradoxes were introduced but only briefly discussed. Any one of them might merit a fuller treatment on its own. Working with generalities, specifics were glossed over—the specificity of particular types of pain; of different disease and injury processes, each with its own patterns; of cultures that may view and process pain differently; and of individuals, each of whom travels a unique journey.

In focusing on experienced pain, this chapter also said only a little about treatment and healing. One need not attain full physical recovery to heal. Sharing the same root with the words "holy" and "whole," healing can involve developing coping strategies, deepening relationships, discovering positive meaning—that is, reintegrating one's self and world in a way that counteracts pain's more corrosive effects.[56] More will be said on this topic in future chapters, including the next one on the healing powers of touch, and chapter 5 on medical practice as reimagined.

What I have tried to establish here is that chronic pain has a "liminal" structure.[57] Borrowed from anthropological literature and now used across a variety of fields, the term "liminal" refers to that which is not contained within, and defined by, ordinary situations and structures. Instead it inhabits an in-between state, a kind of nether region characterized by "ambiguity, paradox, a confusion of all the customary categories."[58]

I have catalogued nine ways in which chronic pain is liminal: that is, ambiguous and paradoxical, involving in-between states. Pain manifests as both sensation and interpretation, certain and yet uncertain to the sufferer and others. It unfolds in both a present and projective time, exhibiting a never-changing and yet ever-changing pattern. It is seemingly located simultaneously in body and mind, self and other, the here and everywhere. Presenting as both in-control and out-of-control, pain unleashes productive and destructive forces in the realm of meaning.

If one is fortunate, the pain finally goes away. But in the face of ongoing pain one can still "heal" such that the tensions above—epistemological, existential, even metaphysical—can to some degree be re-solved or dis-solved. At least their capacity to bewilder, frustrate, disorient, and drain the sufferer diminish. Yet this is no easy accomplishment. Pain is more than an aversive physical sensation. It can trigger a series of experiential paradoxes that shock and destabilize one's world.

3

Rethinking Touch:
How Then Does It Heal?

Our exploration of illness and pain raises the question of what can be done to alleviate this suffering, not only by oneself but by clinicians. This question is huge. Answers vary depending on the specificities of disease structures, personality types, and social contexts. I will try to particularize the topic, yet in a way that yields some general principles, by focusing on one key but often overlooked and underrated therapeutic mode—that of touch.

In many cultures and historical periods, physical touch has played a central role in healing. Jesus is portrayed as curing fever, leprosy, and a child at the point of death through the medium of his touch; a woman's chronic hemorrhages ceased when she but touched his garment (Mark 1:30–31, 40–42; 5:25–42). Such biblical examples illustrate a power used in many societies by lay, spiritual, and professional healers alike. These have ranged from those of lowly status, such as the women healers persecuted during the European witch trials, to the kings of France and England whose magical touch was said to relieve scrofula, epilepsy, and a diversity of other ills.[1] Touch is so central in healing work that it comes metaphorically to stand for the whole enterprise. "She has the healing touch," we say. But what specifically does healing have to do with touch? What is it about human touch, ever poised between movement, expression, and sensing; empathy and objectification; the soothing, stimulating, and invasive; that makes this modality a powerful medium of healing?

The Objectifying Touch and the Absent Touch

Before turning to the touch that heals, I will reflect briefly on two variants all too common in contemporary medical practice—the objectifying touch and the absent touch. (My collaborator in the original versions of this and the following two chapters, Dr. Mitchell Krucoff, cardiologist at Duke University, functions in this high-tech world but is also dedicated to the healing touch.)

Since the late eighteenth century, *disease* classifications have become progressively less based on patient reports concerning their *illness* symptoms and more on the pathologic lesions and mechanistic processes exposed in the corpse or in the living by medical examination and diagnostic technologies.[2] Hence "dyspepsia"—digestive discomfort—comes to be replaced by "peptic ulcer disease" with its observable lesions. The cadaver, when opened and probed, reveals its hidden secrets. The dead body becomes medicine's epistemic touchstone, the "ideal patient" so to speak.

We see this "advance" reflected in the physical examination, which gained ascendancy in the nineteenth and twentieth century.[3] The patient largely assumes a corpse-like pose beneath the physician's probing eyes, ears, and fingers.[4] The practitioner's discerning touch seeks out pulses, nodules, inflamed tissue, abnormalities, while checking for size, warmth, hardness. From time to time, the patient may be asked "does *this* hurt?" But for the most part, he or she lies silent and inert beneath the objectifying touch.

Historically the physical examination came to be viewed as providing more objective and therefore reliable data than subjective patient accounts of symptoms. In more recent times, the physical examination has been even further superseded as a "gold standard" by diagnostic technologies such as X-rays, ultrasound images, MRIs, CT scans, electrocardiograms, and blood tests.[5] While medical schools still emphasize the importance of information derived from history and physical examination, actual practice patterns convey to doctors-in-training that information gathered at the bedside is limited and questionable. The clinician's senses cannot reach fully into the patient's interior and may miss or misinterpret surface features. Technological diagnostics seemingly overcome these limitations. They provide highly detailed information concerning visceral, microscopic, and biochemical bodily processes. They can often generate data in mathematical form, which, since the time of Galileo and Descartes, has been viewed as the true language through which science deciphers nature.[6] Laboratory values or the images produced by sophisticated devices can also be compared over time and across populations, examined by independent observers, and archived as medical records. Of course, such laboratory and imaging studies are also *well reimbursed*. I'll say more about the role of money in medicine in chapters 4 and 5.

Historically, then, we perceive a trend from an objectifying touch to the all-too-frequently "absent touch" of modern medicine. Direct doctor-patient contact gives way to a reliance on intermediate devices that help diagnose, and later treat, the patient technologically. These are often seen as improvements, even miracles, of health care. Archetypical scenes results: the doctor strides into the hospital room and, rather than move toward the patient, grabs the chart or stares at a screen. Physician-author Abraham Verghese comments:

> For the past two decades I've felt that in the United States we touch our pa-
> tients less and less: the physical exam, the skilled bedside examination of the
> patient, has diminished to where it is pure farce. . . . One student wrote to me
> recently, "Honestly, I feel when I am doing the physical that I am just going
> through the motions." The prevalent belief is that it's hardly worthwhile ex-
> amining the patient, as none of these findings matter. . . . An anthropologist
> walking through our hospitals in America wouldn't be blamed for concluding
> (on the basis of where physicians spend the most time) that the real patient is
> in the computer, while the individual in the bed is a mere placeholder for the
> real patient.[7]

When properly contextualized, the two types of touch we have been ex-amining—the "objectifying touch" of the impersonal exam and the "absent touch" provoked by technological intermediaries—both make important con-tributions to the healing arts. Most patients, when seriously ill, would surely want a careful physical exam and appropriate tests. I certainly did when struggling with my leg pain. Problems arise, however, when these modes of "touch" dominate the clinical encounter. They then have the power to exac-erbate, rather than heal, the dis-integrations provoked by pain and illness.

The objectifying touch, for example, can exaggerate the patient's sense of alienation from the ill body, as discussed in the first two chapters. He or she is asked to remove clothing; expose flesh to be probed, squeezed, poked, and measured; and all in search of pathology. While clinically revealing, this can be a personally disconcerting process. One's sense when ill of having a distress-ingly flawed body-object is seemingly confirmed by its medical treatment.

We have seen that sickness and pain provoke alienation not only from one's body but from others. In ordinary life, touch can serve to bridge the physical and emotional gap between us. A peck on the cheeks, a hug, a pat on the back, a gentle touch on the arm: we thereby *express* (press-outward) our compassion and connection. Chapter 1 said much about the importance of truthful speech to Philoctetes. But it also describes how no one will nurse him, place leaves on his bleeding sore, or even come near him. He longs for a compassionate touch. In exactly this regard, the objectifying touch of medicine can prove a disappointment. It is not primarily communicative or empathic but analytic. This touch does not represent what Buber terms the "I–Thou" moment, a dia-lectical contact between two subjects.[8] Rather, it exemplifies the "I–It" stance of the sort used when encountering a *thing*. Ironically, this comes at exactly the moment when the patient may feel particularly thing-like as a result of the disease.

Of course, a certain amount of objectification is necessary, even beneficial, in the clinical encounter. It is also important to avoid an inappropriate intimacy that can violate boundaries, damaging both clinical judgment and patient trust. We are aware that professionals can misuse their positions to engage in sexual abuse. At the same time, confining the professional to the purely objectifying touch can heighten the patient's sense of bodily and social estrangement.

The "absent touch" of purely technological medicine is little better.[9] Poked with needles, inserted into CT scans, hooked up to electrodes, the body is annexed to a world of machines. One of the things I have most disliked about my persistent physical problem is the way it forces me to inhabit a *medical world* of clinics, laboratories, surgical suites. The illness already renders the body something foreign, unpleasant; now "high-tech" medicine intensifies this experience. As Varela writes (in the aftermath of a liver transplant), "it is not the body-technology that introduces the alterity in my lived body as a radical innovation. That technology widens and slips into what is always already there."[10] The disease and the treatment thus operate synergistically to increase alienation. Just when one most longs for the "personal touch," it is least forthcoming.

The Phenomenology of Touch

How is it that compassionate touch has such a capacity to heal, or the absence thereof to worsen, the disruptions of illness? What, after all, *is* touch? Having sketched out a phenomenology of illness and pain in earlier chapters, I will similarly touch on some elements of touch.

Though viewed as one of the five senses, "touch" actually includes within it a great diversity of sensory modalities. It may be understood as incorporating internal proprioceptions of visceral and musculoskeletal systems, as well as the experience of external objects and settings, rendered available by heat, pressure, and vibratory patterns. At least, this is the scientific account. Unlike our specialized eyes and ears, we might say much of the body functions as a massive organ of touch, including both the skin surface and interior regions. There is a debate within the literature about to what degree internal proprioception can or should be distinguished from outer-directed tactility.[11]

However, I will not here attempt a comprehensive phenomenology of this rich subject. I will instead confine attention to the issue at hand (pun intended):

the sort of touch that a clinician might employ on the patient, often using the hands in a way designed to be exploratory and/or efficacious. This is not, then, simply a sensory modality but a *sensorimotor act*. I will briefly focus on three characteristics of this sort of touch: it is *gestural, impactful*, and *reciprocal*.

Calling touch *gestural* highlights a number of features. To see or hear something it can be sufficient to wait motionless, receiving incoming light and sound.[12] By contrast, touch, when used to explore the world, relies on active movement, a gesture. By reaching out, pushing, probing, and stroking, the hand solicits sensory information. Moreover, this action needs to be varied and renewed to keep touch alive; tactile-receptor response can "adapt" and "accommodate" to unchanging stimuli, diminishing the signal over time.

Touch is *gestural* in the sense not only that it implies activity and activation, but that it therefore also bears within it *expressive* content. When I probe an injury, finger a soft linen, stroke a cheek, or punch someone with a fist, these actions embody gestural significance, whether investigatory, amorous, or hostile in nature. The body manifests meaningful intentionality—though that meaning may not always be fully conscious or articulable.

Touch is not only gestural in such ways, but *impactful*. It depends on the physical impact of one body on another. As Jonas writes, "touch is the sense, and the only sense, in which the perception of quality is normally blended with the experience of force."[13] This makes its social use something to carefully regulate by codes of behavior.[14] For example, one would hardly stroke the leg of the stranger sitting next to you on the subway. The police might be called. The sexualized touch, the caring touch, the invasive or hostile touch all have potent physical-emotional impact. So much so that touch provides a general metaphor for affectively powerful events: "I was really touched by that," we say, or "I felt it deeply," or "that hit me like a ton of bricks."

By way of contrast, vision takes place across a distance. Sight tends toward the objective and theoretical consciousness.[15] Hence, it provides many of our metaphors for knowledge—gaining "insight," or "shedding light" on a matter, getting a needed "overview." While sight illuminates things, it also protects us. We see things across a spatial and even a temporal distance, such that we know what we will encounter before we get there. Our fields of both space and time are widened. Not so with touch, where sensation is contingent on immediate impact.

This leads us to a third characteristic: touch is *reciprocal*. To touch another is, in turn, to be touched back. Borrowing it from Husserl, Merleau-Ponty makes central to his analysis of embodiment the example of one of your hands touching the other.[16] Insofar as you consciously experience through one hand (say, the left) the hand it is touching (say, the right) appears as a fleshy object to be probed. However, you can reverse focus, now flowing awareness through the right hand, and using it to examine the left. In truth, the lived body is always "reversible," double-sided, in that it is both an experiencing subject and a material object in the world. These two aspects of the body never quite coincide. You cannot quite touch the act of touching itself or see your own power of sight. Yet the lived body always incorporates both dimensions. This two-sided reversibility also implies a reversible relationship between the embodied self and its world. To see, for example, we need ourselves to be installed in the material realm, and therefore to be visible.

While this reversibility is operative in a general way, touch is distinguished by its direct and reciprocal mode of impact. After all, you can watch someone through a hidden camera without being seen. You can listen to another's voice while yourself remaining inaudible, hidden and silent. But you cannot generally touch another without being touched back. If I jostle a subway rider, he feels it too. Lightly caressing another's skin, I feel them, but they also sense my touch. Even when I push on the surface of my desk I have the experience of it exerting a counterpressure, pushing back on me. There is not a sense of self and other as at a distance, as with sight. Ratcliffe writes, "Touch thus serves to illustrate something of our relationship with the world, which is a matter of belonging and connectedness, rather than of confrontation between body and object."[17]

That touch has a physical reciprocity, both giving and taking, makes it well suited for expressions of emotional mutuality like the hug or kiss. We see this even in metaphors of social connection: "I'm back in touch with her," we say, that is, once more "in contact." To mention "I hear (or see) she is doing well," conveys that information has been received, but does not imply the same reciprocity of contact.

As reciprocal, touch brings us into contact not only with others, but with our own embodiment. Taking place at or near our skin surface, touch (of the sort we are examining) reaches outward to sense the world. At the same time, physical impacts provoke a stream of proprioceptive sensations that can make us more aware of our own body in action. In an amorous caress, for example, we awaken not only to the other's body but to our own, with its erotic impulses and pleasurable sensations.

The multifaceted reciprocal nature of touch is present in the many related but subtly different usages of the word "feel." For example, saying "I feel your hair" implies an outward-directed exploration, whereas "I feel your pain" is empathically sensitive but also inward-turning. "I feel anxious about going"—is this a cognitive judgment, a social communicator, a reflection on inward states—or all three? Touch and "feeling" cross boundaries of sensation, emotion, and judgment; self and other; subject and object; the inner and outer world, thus showing their intimate reciprocity.

The Healer's Touch

We are now in a better position to understand the crucial roles touch can play within the clinical encounter. As discussed in the first two chapters, pain and illness bring about a series of dis-integrations. Using Heideggerian language, Svenaeus speaks of the ill person as feeling *"unhomelike"* in their skin and world.[18] I used Philoctetes' wound and my own bout with chronic pain as examples of such exile experiences. *Yet, the properties of touch can assist the sufferer in the journey of homecoming and healing.*

How so? We have seen that the connection between self and other can be broken not only by the pain, incapacities, and disfigurements of illness, but by dehumanizing medical practice with its objectifying or absent touch. But when a healing practitioner, whether allopathic or alternative, touches a patient with attention and care, this act has *gestural* and *impactful* meaning. Someone is literally reaching out. He or she is feeling for the source of my pain with the aim of relieving it. This caring *gesture* has *impact*—I experience its force on and within my body. I understand the *reciprocity* embodied in the gesture—that the practitioner is consenting to receive touch as well as to give it. I am no longer, like Philoctetes, abandoned on my private Lemnos of pain. Another has made contact. I am touched by this.

Of course, some of this can be true of the physician-scientist's objectifying touch. I appreciate the diagnostic acumen that animates the hands of the treater. Yet this touch runs the risk of failing to acknowledge the reversibility and reciprocity of the flesh. The patient is being approached as a body-object more than co-subject. As such, this sort of touch may not embody *compassion*—the ability to *feel-with* the other—but simply touches the other in the sense we do a thing, a collection of organs to be probed.

Having just been to the doctor's office this week, I was struck by what an intimate act it is to take off one's clothes and sit half-naked before another, waiting to be touched. The sense of uncomfortable exposure can be exaggerated when one has a physical feature—as so many of us do—for which one feels some sense of shame: a fat belly, for example, or wrinkly flesh. (We speak of people who "are not comfortable in their own skin.") Then, too, the area of injury may be ugly (think of Philoctetes' wound). The patient's acute vulnerability calls for a comparable sensitivity from the treater.

What might compassionate touch be like in action? Clearly, a practitioner cannot take on all the suffering of others or she would soon be overwhelmed. However, her touch conveys sensitivity to the living patient as a "Thou," not just an "It." The treater therefore is careful not to cause undue pain or humiliation when conducting a physical examination. She understands this is a human being in distress. Caring touch is enfolded in a communicative relationship wherein the practitioner may verbally explain what is being done, and why, and what the findings signify, even while eliciting comfort and confidence through the medium of touch itself. Touch as an *impactful gesture* is thus used to heal the distance between self and other.

I have been fortunate enough to meet many practitioners who have "the healing touch," literally and metaphorically, but most often those are trained in complementary body practices—massage, acupuncture, Alexander Technique, and the like. Yet Gadamer points out that in German the word used for medical treatment in general, *Behandlung*, has its origin in the German word for "hand."[19] Clinical diagnosis and treatment always involve a careful "handling" of the patient. The true healer never fully disconnects from this original act of touching the sick body.

Richard Selzer, the author-surgeon, expert at the art of cutting flesh, and writing about it, witnesses a particular powerful example of this when Yeshi Dhonden, personal physician to the Dalai Lama, is invited to Yale University to do Grand Rounds. Using the Tibetan technique of diagnosis largely through palpation,

> his eyes are closed as he feels for her pulse. In a moment he has found the spot, and for the next half-hour he remains thus, suspended above the patient like some exotic golden bird with folded wings, holding the pulse of the woman beneath his fingers, cradling her hand in his. . . . [I]t is as though he and the patient have entered a special place of isolation, of apartness, about which a vacancy hovers, and across which no violation is possible. . . . All at once, I am envious—not of him, not of Yeshi Dhonden for his gift of beauty and holiness, but of her. I want to be held like that, touched so, *received*. And I know that I, who have palpated a hundred thousand pulses, have felt not a single one.[20]

I will add to this lovely story a bit of my own. As a medical student at Yale I was fortunate enough to work under Dr. Selzer during my surgical clerkship. I was profoundly *touched* by the experience. He was gentle, warm, and funny with his patients, not always an attribute associated with surgeons. When I would repeatedly grow faint and have to break scrub in surgery (all that blood, the hot lights, my own anxiety!), he praised me for my acute sensitivity, lifting my burden of shame. Knowing of my interests in philosophy, he

encouraged me to follow that passion, as he had his own as a writer. He even
asked me to write the essay on *Philoctetes* which has become the basis for the
first chapter of this book. The qualities he describes in Yeshi Dhonden he
himself embodied, and they informed the way he would touch his patients.

We have said that touch can be an *impactful gesture*, lifting the patient's
sense of isolation through its expression of care and its recognition of the *reciprocity* of I and Thou. Reciprocity means that the toucher is always touched
back. Expanded, this implies that the treater can also open to being "touched"
by the encounter. Practitioners have much to learn about courage and resil-
ience from their patients, and conversely can draw on their own strengths, as
well as personal experiences of woundedness and vulnerability, to be of most
help. The result can be a mutually nourishing encounter. Verghese writes of
the importance of the touch-mediated physical exam for both participants:

> The exam then is about trust, about a sacred privilege. I can recall occasions
> when my visit with a difficult or aggrieved patient, or with a garrulous and hy-
> pochondriac patient, changed course as I performed a detailed examination.
> On those occasions, I had a sense that the exam had flowed, it had become
> almost a dance, one in which the patient was an active participant, and that
> it had quieted and reassured my patient, the exam itself bringing about this
> change. Indeed, in those moments, I became aware that I'd changed, too, as
> though both of us—doctor and patient—had entered some sacred space by
> virtue of this ritual and had been transformed.[21]

Of course, it is not enough that a treater's hands embody compassion. We
also want them to demonstrate skill and expertise. They should be capable of
searching out diagnostically relevant information—feeling for the edge of an
enlarged liver, or the tell-tale edema of heart disease. When possible these
hands should also facilitate the alleviation of symptoms. Touch, as an impactful sensorimotor gesture, is used in many modes of treatment in a way that
sight, hearing, smell, and taste cannot be. As the story of Yeshi Dhonden suggests, touch can also dissolve the very division between "diagnosis" and "treatment." Even taking a pulse with sensitivity becomes capable of altering the patient's bodily states.

Touch is thus used in a wide variety of alternative and complementary
healing practices, as well as more conventional medical therapies. For example, chiropractic, physical therapy, massage (of many different sorts), bodywork modalities such as Feldenkreis and Alexander Technique, acupuncture
and acupressure, energy therapies (which can also employ "touch at a distance") including Therapeutic Touch, Healing Touch, Reflexology, and Reiki,
are but a few practices in which touch plays a central role.

As a client I have been pleased to discover practitioners not only compassionately attentive to my sufferings but, in some cases, able to substantially lessen them. I would count among them a wonderfully skilled massage and energy healer and an acupuncturist—see my acknowledgments. Their various modes of touch, coupled with talk, have at times brought relief or helped me cope with my leg problem discussed in chapter 2, or chronic back pain which plagued me for many years.

Both situations, in some ways intractable or progressive, finally led to surgery—I offer praise as well to high-tech invasive medicine when necessary. I have also found that different treatment approaches can be necessary at different times but, in the long run, be complementary and synergistic—one need not ally oneself dogmatically to a single camp, but remain open to the many kinds of help offered by conventional and alternative forms of medicine. Even surgery is a way for another to reach deep into our body, with the compassionate goal of relieving our distress.

The sense of self-other distance begins to heal as the other's touch demonstrates this care in action. As important, the disruption between oneself and one's own body begins to heal. In illness, one's own body surfaces as something painful, uncontrollable, alien. Now the hands of the treater help forge a reconciliation.

Varela, following a liver transplant, describes how he feels fragmented by his illness, and also the medical treatment thereof, including the radiological focus on disseminated "image fragments" instead of his living flesh. But

> occasionally in one of the check-up visits the clinician asks me to lie down, and he touches my liver region. I experience it as a relief, as return to an embodied presence. The touch reestablishes an older intimacy through his touching hand, touching/being-touched the paradigm of oneness, me-ness.[22]

If even the straightforward palpations of a physician can restore one to embodied presence, how much more so the skill of those trained in healing touch? I have had this experience many times over. The expert fingers of the masseuse relax my tight muscles, easing my pain; the chiropractor realigns my contorted spine; the acupuncturist carefully takes pulses and places needles to get the *ch'i* flowing; the Alexander Technique teacher helps guide my body to habits of posture and movement that heal and prevent further injury.

Touch may thus assist the receiver to inhabit his or her body in new ways. Again, touch is *reciprocal* in the double sense that I feel not only the touch of the other but the sensations and responses that it elicits from within my own flesh. Through my bodywork experiences I have gained greater proprioceptive self-awareness and found I could influence my own states of musculoskeletal tension, the flow of energies, the characteristics of my posture, and even of visceral functioning. One could say I grew "more in touch" with myself, a statement midway between literal and metaphoric truth. Illness has at times robbed me of a sense of agency and reduced my body to a theater of pain. But I have also learned of powers, pleasures, and potentials of which I was hitherto unaware. Gradually, the effects of the other's healing touch thus become *incorporated*, that is, brought within my own embodiment as a series of new possibilities.[23]

As healing touch penetrates within, it can also expand one's outer world. When pain is relieved, I can go for a longer walk with my dog, appreciate the autumnal foliage, focus more easily on other people—that is, "get out of myself." One recovers not only a physical but existential "increased range of motion."

Healing touch can also present itself through nonhuman forms. Studies have suggested health benefits from having a pet *one can pet*.[24] Going for that long walk with my dog Maggie, stroking her, receiving an appreciative paw, are marvelously restorative. Even inanimate things like stretch bandages and flexible braces can provide structural and emotional support. It feels like one's painful ankle or knee is being held, *em-braced* so to speak, lending a sense of comfort and security.

But could healing equally well be performed linguistically instead of tactilely—that is, by giving a patient verbal explanations and directives? Sometimes, but not always. The body may have deep-set, preconscious modes of expression showing forth in habits of contraction, hypervigilance, or imbalance. Illness may be both the result of these patterns and that which further intensifies them, generating a cycle of dysfunction. Such are stress-related illnesses, building on themselves. Words can be difficult to process at times of distress and insufficient to alter preconscious patterns. The *gestural, impactful, reciprocal* nature of touch speaks in terms the body can often better grasp.

That was true from our very origins. We were held close within the womb. After birth, we long remained dependent on reciprocal body-to-body intimacy. (More on this in chapter 8.) Simms describes her time as a nursing mother: "Never have I been in such close contact with another being's skin, arms, and mouth than during those early weeks of continuous holding and feeding."[25] Skin-to-skin parent-child contact (so-called kangaroo care) and modes of massage have been shown to help infants and preterm newborns gain weight, decrease stress and heart rate, sleep better, and neurodevelopmentally mature.[26] Something of the intimacy of parent-child touching is preserved as the child reaches for "transitional objects"—for example, a stuffed animal or soft blanket.

But as life goes on many of us *lose touch*. This may be one of the causes of our endemic stress-related diseases, reminding us to get back in touch with one another and with ourselves.[27] As Hosey summarizes:

> Regular touch eases stress and anxiety, improves breathing and heart rate, hastens healing, and increases mental aptitude and productivity. The calming effect can be immediate and just lightly caressing someone's hand can lower blood pressure. Babies' physical, mental, and emotional development progresses better when they are routinely massaged, yet, compared to other cultures, Americans are touch starved.[28]

Particularly touch-starved is the sick patient, experiencing all the forms of exile we have discussed. Pain and illness also tend to bring about an emotional regression. When sick we are like that child we once were, needing to be held, have our bruises kissed and bandaged, our tears wiped away. To a degree we can do that for ourselves. We can gently stroke our own arm. We can snuggle under a warm blanket or wrap ourselves in a shawl (more on the use of prayer/comfort shawls in chapter 5). But we often long for the presence of the other, the impactful gesture of a caring touch. The objective or absent touch characteristic of modern medicine does not begin to respond to that deep yearning.

Receptivity to Healing

I have focused on the healer's touch as informed by compassion and expertise. But this risks underappreciating the active, reciprocal role of the patient. Here, the very term "patient" can both mislead and reveal. We have seen that it is derived from the Latin root *pati*, which can mean "to suffer, feel, or endure" and which is also the root of the word "passive." Hence some practitioners and theorists eschew this term; it seems to characterize the ill person as an inert object of treatment. However, the word "patient" has other resonances. "Patience" as a primary religious/cultural virtue suggests not so much passivity as an active ability to endure waiting, suffering, and challenge, based on a fundamental optimism concerning the processes unfolding and/or the overarching positive nature of the universe. "Patience," we say "will be rewarded."

This can point us toward attitudes that enhance the patient's receptivity to healing touch. Accompanying patience is hope. To open an injured body to the impactful touch of another involves a leap of faith, a hope that healing, if not cure, is possible. For those with chronic and seemingly intractable conditions, this is no easy matter but essential for treatment to proceed. Hope enables the patient *to be patient*, enduring the embarrassments of exposure, the potentially invasive touch of another, the pains and discomforts this might elicit, the length of time needed for the body to incorporate new habits, the inevitable setbacks one meets along the way. How important it is to "not lose hope"!

Hope also encourages active engagement with the treatment. We have said that touch is *gestural, impactful, reciprocal.* To be maximally effective, touch must be received in this spirit. The patient opens to the impact of the chosen mode of treatment and adopts the recommended gestures, whether these involve muscle relaxation, visualization, focused sensory awareness, or styles of movement. The body aligns reciprocally with the practitioner's touch and suggestions. The skillful healer is not simply impressing a change on the flesh from outside. He or she invites, releases, and supports an expression of the ill body's own potential for healing. The patient's lived commitment to this process is as important as the therapist's expertise.

In this relationship, the patient thus assumes what might paradoxically be termed "an engaged surrender." The client exercises active will, but not in an egoic style characterized by self-assertion. (That style can be associated with insecurities and rigidities that themselves cause stress-related illness.) To be fully present to another's touch involves a certain surrender. One consents to be open, guided, touched—literally and metaphorically—by the other's embodied gestures. Even the patient being wheeled into surgery opens in trust to the knife about to be wielded by the skillful hand. (I have found that the kind touch of the nurses guiding in the gurney and lifting the patient to the operating table can also be a great assist.)

Physiologically, this openness often manifests in a state of relaxation. (With muscles held tight, glands secreting fight-or-flight hormones, we are apt to startle and pull away from another's touch.) Relaxation is both a physiologic and an ontological position. It represents an embodied faith that the universe is not simply threatening but that to which we may open. In relaxation, we reclaim a sense, reaching back to prenatal experience, of being part of an embodied circuit of connection that would care for us, not do damage. (See chapter 8.) The word itself suggests this element of return: to "re-lax" etymologically means to "loosen back," or "loosen again." The state of relaxation represents our body's felt reintegration with others, oneself, and the surrounding world.

Given the level of openness solicited by another's healing touch, the patient does well to proceed judiciously. Patience, hope, engaged surrender are all to the good, but only if exercised with proper discernment. Intellectually, we can explore the different treatments available and their potential efficacy given our particular ailment. Intuitively, our bodies may come to know whose hands have the "magic touch," those persons or practices with which we feel most suited. We need to be in touch with ourselves to decide who else shall touch us. Our body may tell us as it reflexively relaxes or recoils.

This is not the old-fashioned ideal of the "good patient" who submits passively to whatever the doctor prescribes. Nor is it the newer model of the patient as assertive consumer and decision maker, managing treatment step by step. While such may be of benefit when negotiating the overspecialized and financially driven world of modern medicine, an aggressive, egoic stance armors us against receiving the healer's touch. In the right situation, with the right person, judiciously chosen, we can reclaim the capacity to trust, surrender to, and participate in an intimate embodied dialogue. Ultimately, healing touch is not something the clinician does or the patient. Touch unfolds in the reciprocal space between, embodying the I-Thou relationship.

4

Rethinking Pills:
Fantasies, Realities, Possibilities

We have pondered the therapeutic modality of healing touch. This involves intimate and skillful person-to-person contact. However, to better understand the structure of modern medicine, touch can be counterpoised with another form of treatment now in ascendency—the use of pills. This seems on the opposite end of the therapeutic spectrum. But it would be too simplistic to contrast "good" holistic treatment with "bad" pharmaceuticals or "embodied" touch with "disembodied" pill popping. The latter is also embodied, although in a different and unusual way that calls for its own investigation.

Pills undeniably play a central role in modern medicine. The media is saturated with advertisements for over-the-counter and prescription medications. The training, licensure, and stature of physicians are tied to their ability to prescribe. Patients often arrive hoping to be given (or to suggest themselves) a pill to relieve an ill, ideally one that combines maximal effectiveness with minimal adverse effects, costs, and the need for time and effort invested in lifestyle changes.

Whether such a pill can truly be found, the clinician and patient often seal their contract at some point with a scribbled prescription. This validates a mutual desire that "something be done" to ritually and therapeutically justify the visit. (Simply touching and talking to the patient, or recommending behavioral changes, seems insufficient.) For many patients, the consequent attempts to order and take their medications on time, and to find a way to pay for them out-of-pocket or through insurance, restructure their lives. So too do the therapeutic or adverse effects of the ever-growing portfolio of pills produced by cutting-edge medical research and a profit-hungry pharmaceutical industry.

Nor are these pills prescribed only to the ill. Asymptomatic individuals may take pills for a lifetime, treating chemical abnormalities (which are not really diseases), such as hypercholesterolemia.[1] A large number of people take megavitamins and other supplements to protect health. Then there are pills for lifestyle enhancement—for example, sexual activity into the later years—where the "disease" treated, erectile dysfunction, may be as much defined and created by the existence of the pills as vice versa.[2]

Worldwide sales of prescription drugs are projected shortly to reach $1 trillion.[3] More than half of North Americans take at least one such medicine.[4] Twenty-first century medical practice has many characteristic features: its use of high-tech diagnostics, for example, and of dramatic surgical interventions, including organ transplantation, the topic of chapter 8. Nonetheless, the genius and potency of modern medicine, as well as its more alienating qualities, are most iconically captured by the diminutive pill—and the enormous industry that produces it. We say "take your medicine," referring to a pill. Yet when we swallow it, we also "take our medicine" in a broader sense, swallowing the modern paradigm of disease and treatment.

Again, my interest in the topic has a personal side. As I have aged and accumulated a number of physical problems—and practitioners, both conventional and alternative—I find myself taking an ever greater number of pills and supplements. For example, for the leg problem mentioned in chapter 2 I take a strong nerve medicine and a nonsteroidal anti-inflammatory drug. As an aging American man with some borderline values, I started taking blood pressure medicine and a statin to lower cholesterol (though I've recently discontinued that one). Then there are vitamins to energize me, sleeping pills to calm me down, and alternative herbal medicines—why put all your eggs in one basket? I observe with wonder the sheer quantity and variety as I fill my weekly pill container. Grateful for the good insurance that pays most of the enormous bills, I am also uncertain, even a bit guilty. Is this necessary? Healthy? It is certainly expensive for me, and the larger society. What is this all about? Dr. Mitchell Krucoff, my collaborator in the original version of this chapter, also encounters such issues from the other, professionalized side. As a cardiologist, he continually confronts the question of when and what to prescribe—and how to embed the use of pharmaceuticals within his practice of holistic care.

Many experts have looked at the sociology, history, science, politics, and economics behind the rapid rise of pill use. They include narratives of the twentieth-century pharmaceutical industry and its more dubious practices, and conceptual critiques of the "medicalization" and "pharmaceuticalization" of ever-more dimensions of life.[5] However, I will necessarily limit my scope. Again, I will use a style of phenomenological analysis that seeks to clarify the fundamental characteristics that define a region of the world *as experienced*. We have seen that for continental philosophers such as Merleau-Ponty and others, body and mind, materiality and subjective meaning, are not dualistically opposed as for Descartes, but ever interwoven in the experienced lifeworld.[6] I will thus discuss characteristic features of the pill first as a material entity and then as the object of a psychocultural fantasy that both builds on and distorts its material properties. Hopefully, we can learn to apply greater wisdom in "taking our pills" (or at times, *not* taking them) as assists to healing.

Characteristics of a Pill

Four attributes set apart the pill from an indefinite array of other therapeutic interventions, be they surgical, radiologic, psychotherapeutic, or alternative (for example, the modes of body and energy work I earlier mentioned). The pill is ingestible, potent, reproducible, and miniaturizable. Let's take each of these characteristics in turn.

INGESTIBILITY

The pill is an element of the external world that can be incorporated, that is, brought within the body, typically through the act of oral ingestion or buccal absorption. Once inside, it uses the body's digestive, respiratory, and circulatory systems to reach and alter various physiologic functions. Hence the pill manifests as an interface between the outside and inside, the world and body, serving as a transport system for healing chemicals. In the words of a 1954 ad, "Down, down, down the stomach through / Round, round, round the system too / With Alka-Seltzer you're sure to say / Relief is just a swallow away."[7]

This style of "incorporation" is different from that discussed in the chapter on healing touch. In that case, the patient receives something, often through the body's surface, that can transform kinesthetic and visceral functioning as well as proprioceptive awareness—for example, changing a habit of muscle clenching to one of relaxation as the result of massage or energy work. The patient responsively develops new styles of breathing, posture, and movement that transform the lived body's way of being-in-the-world. We have seen the impactful and reciprocal nature of healing touch. But all this can be displaced in favor of taking a pill. Here, the promise is that "relief is just a swallow away," vectored automatically through chemical alterations in the visceral body.

POTENCY

At least, that "swallowed relief" is the ideal toward which pills strive. A new medicine is developed, tested, marketed, and used in the hope that it will embody a healing potency (from the Latin word *potentia*, meaning "power"). The pill is like a genie in a bottle, containing vast power in an undersized package. This power is not only chemical but historical in origin. It relies on a medical knowledge base whose philosophical foundations were laid in the seventeenth century but that has dramatically increased in the last hundred years through advances in biochemistry and genetics.[8] This, in turn, depends on the power of the scientific method. Epidemiologic studies, and protocols such as the double-blind controlled experiment, enhance our understanding of disease causation and treatment, leading to pharmaceutical advances.

REPRODUCIBILITY

The pill is a distilled product not only of such knowledge power but of the technological power embodied in an industrial manufacturing system. The pill lends itself to being reproducible on a large scale. This is not true of healing touch, performed once at a time in a way adapted to the individual client. Nor, to take an example from other cultures, is this true of a shaman's brew delivered with ceremonial gesture and incantation. Rather, what supports the commercial value of a pill is its standardization and mass deliverability. We demand invariant contents and dosage, adjusted at most to body weight or kidney function. As such, each pill is homogenous, replaceable with the next, and the next. This assures reliability for the consumer and large-scale access to the treatment, as well as potentially vast profits to the manufacturer. Fabricated by high-speed precision equipment, approved by product-control inspectors, pills are then packaged and transported—under protected conditions and with expiration limits—for distant consumers to purchase and swallow.[9]

MINIATURIZATION

All of the above characteristics of the pill relate to another feature so obvious it might be overlooked: a pill is small. The word "pill" itself comes from the Latin *pilula*, literally meaning "little ball." This littleness has big ramifications. It is what allows for the ease of packaging, transportation, and selling of pills, making them an ideal consumer item. This also is what allows them literally to be consumed, operating as a delivery system for chemicals that, in turn, catalyze chains of bodily reactions.

Albert Borgmann, a contemporary philosopher of technology, discusses how our modern age is guided by the paradigm of the "device."[10] An ideal device disburdens us by making a commodity instantaneously, easily, and ubiquitously available. For example, rather than heat our house by having to chop and gather wood, which demands time, skill, and effort and then communal clustering around the wood-burning stove, we prefer to flick a thermostat. The warmth of a central heating system becomes available to us through a small, easy-to-use trigger. Such devices serve as portals into a life-world where long and difficult tasks become quick and simple. In this sense, the pill is an advanced device. For example, rather than losing weight through a regimen of careful eating and exercise, we might simply take a couple of pills a day, seeking disburdenment through pharmaceuticals.

As a technology progresses, its mechanical interface tends to miniaturize in size and demands. For example, many have replaced cumbersome LP record, and then CD, collections by downloading or accessing music in electronic formats through devices like a smartphone. What was once a huge music library now sits in your pocket.

Similarly, the tiny pill, when ingested, promises to "download" into our body the vast potency of medical science and therapeutics. Just as music can be made easily and instantaneously available through electronics, pills seem to offer renewed health, prolonged life, and relief from pain and restriction. The flipside of such promises are complementary fears. Pills may poison or hook us: beware the pill peddler or the pill-popping addict! We declare a "war on drugs" while simultaneously supporting a vast expansion of the drug industry.

The Cultural Fantasy of the Pill

Whether seen as technological savior or threat, the pill takes on layers of meaning that lead one author to call it "the quintessential icon of Western Civilization."[11] Other icons of our society invoke fantasy projections: for example, that wealth or celebrity is key to personal fulfillment. However, these attributes are often beyond our reach. With the medicalization of our self-understanding, happiness becomes associated with finding the "right pill."

By prescription or over-the-counter, legally or illegally, effectively or mistakenly, people thus take pills to supplement their diets, pills to sleep, pills to wake up, pills to kill bacteria or support bacterial growth, pills to quell heartburn after an injudicious meal, pills for erectile control and birth control. They take pills to lose weight, enhance athletic performance, lessen pain, lift mood, cope with stress, prevent possible future diseases (even while currently symptom-free), and, increasingly, to mitigate the adverse effects of other pills. A new generation of psychoactive drugs even promises to change our identity from the inside out. An ad for Paxil recommends the use of this antidepressant and antianxiety agent, "So you can see someone you haven't seen in a while. Yourself."[12] You might even be "better than well" through the miracle of Prozac.[13]

Many years ago, Janet Woodcock, then director of the US Food and Drug Administration's Center for Drug Evaluation and Research, raised concerns about notions "that the many common and relatively minor complaints of daily life represent diseases" and "that all life complaints can and perhaps should be treated with a pill."[14] This is an era "when there is a pill for every ill, but perhaps more significantly an ill for every pill."[15] A drug needs to be sold, so a correlative "disease" is labeled and coded such that it can become reimbursable. For example, in 2007 a drug company engaged in a vigorous "Is it Low-T?" ad campaign, designed to promote the notion that the low testosterone of aging men was a diagnosable and treatable disease. Two professors of medicine comment, "Unfortunately, 'Is It Low-T?' is not unique. It's just a particularly bulked-up example of what has become standard operating procedure for drug companies."[16] The astronomic growth of pharmaceutical sales and profits, driven by industry inducements to researchers and doctors, media coverage, and direct-to-consumer advertising, encourages us to medicalize life's diverse problems, seeking relief in pill form.

However, there is much that this cultural fantasy obscures. We have seen that the pill is a miniaturized, potent, and ingestible device, altering body functioning. However, this does not mean that therapeutic efficacy resides simply in the pill. Rather, it often potentiates the body's own biochemical and physiologic processes, which are constructed by evolutionary genius to restore and maintain a healthy homeostasis whenever possible. Most pills assist the body, providing a catalyst, a missing element, or a modification that allows the body's physiology to recover a more optimal balance. In this sense, pills, like healing touch, are actually in dialogue with the body, empowering its own capacities for self-healing.

This relationship is also illustrated by the well-known "placebo effect" elicited by our belief in pills.[17] Physiologically, this has been ascribed to the endorphin-release system, the immune response, changes in vascular tone and brain activation, or other neurochemical and hormonal shifts. Psychologically, the placebo effect can be understood in terms of the beneficial effects of hope, expectancy, and relaxation; interpersonally, as a benefit of the effective treater-patient relationship; or even spiritually, as faith in action. During double-blind clinical trials, one tries to monitor and "subtract" the placebo effect because it may help a substantial proportion of patients to get better even when taking an inert compound. But in actual clinical practice this is not a "subtractive" but an "additive" element, contributed by the patient's lived body and triggered by belief in the pill's efficacy.

However, it is the very characteristics of the pill, as earlier discussed, that lead us to overlook the role of the individual who takes it. As *ingested*, the pill is perceived as a power entering from outside. *Reproducible* and *miniaturized*, it becomes a ubiquitously available device that promises commodity delivery. Relief follows from swallowing an agent whose *potency* is often testified to by its exorbitant cost or bitter taste, the respect accorded to medical science, and the professional sanction needed to secure it. It is natural, then, to understand and misunderstand the power and healing as residing fully in the tiny pill, the deficiency within oneself. For an athlete taking steroids, an insomniac reaching for sleeping pills, a patient with pain who relies on analgesics, the pill seems an external remedy that confirms one's own sense of psychophysical lack. This misunderstanding is key to the fantasy aura surrounding the pill.

As well, the pill seems to hover in a liminal space: while a physical thing, it seems *almost immaterial* in the way it condenses our scientific, technological, and clinical power into the smallest packet imaginable. It even condenses time as therapeutic effects released in the present moment set the stage for long-term outcomes. The materiality of the pill, and of the act of ingesting it, seems minimal, marginal, as if on the verge of disappearance.[18]

Many studies have addressed how material characteristics unleash the placebo effect—how a blue pill may induce sleep better than a red pill, or an inert pill with brand markings has more analgesic effect than one without.[19] The pill's material presence—its color, shape, size, and cost—is a repository for projected meanings, as is the pill's name, carefully selected for its phonemes and verbal associations.[20] However, I would suggest that it is not only the materiality of the pill but its material *self-effacement*, a presence verging on absence, that adds to its mystical aura.

Earlier I discussed how self-effacement is characteristic of the evolved device, such as the smartphone, which condenses a vast music library, along with many other applications. Most of us do not quite know how this technology works but accept the new "magic" appropriate to our secularized age. The pill, too, operates like a secular version of a holy object. It belongs to the material world, but barely, seeming to point beyond, like a Eucharistic wafer. We do not expect the communion wafer to fill us up, taste delicious, transfix us with physical pleasure. This would distract from and diminish its spiritual efficacy. Like a work of sacred art, the scent of incense, or the flicker of candlelight, the wafer refers beyond itself to an extra-material potency.[21] So, too, the pill. We swallow it, but not in search of the pleasures and satiety provided by delicious food. Rather we are inviting the pill to melt and disappear and, in doing so, effect its quasi-magical transformations. We may not fully comprehend why the medication works or how something so small can contain such potency. Yet we have faith in the drugs and the doctor-priests who offer them, and collectively pay for and swallow hundreds of millions of pills seeking the power to transcend life's limitations.

Adverse Effects of the Cultural Fantasy of the Pill

Pills have been part of a revolution in medical science that has yielded for many great benefits. Before the advent of antibiotics, infectious diseases that are now routinely cured were often fatal. There is indeed something quasi-magical about entering a new therapeutic era. Other conditions that might have demanded invasive surgery or condemned a sufferer to lifelong impairment are now kept in check by a daily pill. Increasingly, chronic diseases may be prevented entirely from developing by early treatment. This is a blessing for public health, as for individuals and families. Furthermore, in the development of new pills, detailed research often identifies precise guidelines for optimal use and heightens awareness of potential safety concerns for vulnerable patients. It would be as big a mistake to demonize the pill as to angelify it, and these polarities of response share certain fantasy elements.

However, before turning to the beneficial uses of pills and how best to potentiate these in clinical practice, we need to acknowledge that not only pills but the cultural fantasies that accompany them have many deleterious side effects. Since this is the subject of numerous treatises, I will but briefly survey some central themes.

Many of these "side effects" result from the role played by pills, at least in the United States, within a consumerist and capitalist context.[22] The attributes of the pill earlier discussed make it an ideal consumer product. As miniaturized and highly reproducible, it can be mass-manufactured, transported, and sold through outlets ranging from the local pharmacy to distant countries, personal exchanges to Internet-facilitated shipping. Equally diverse is the number of pill applications given the reality and/or fantasy of its potency. Unlike a long-term one-use consumer item such as a toaster, we may purchase half a dozen pills a day for as many different uses. Pill potency is also used to justify exorbitant charges. We communally have come to accept a price tag of hundreds of dollars a bottle given the powerful nature of medical need and pill promise (and the lobbying efforts of the pharmaceutical industry, along with the politicians it helps finance). Some evidence even suggests that pricing a pill expensively may potentiate the placebo effect. We believe we get what we pay for.[23] That pills are ingestible also assures that they must be immediately repurchased. Unlike a toaster, this consumer item is literally consumed in the usage—or reputedly loses its potency if it exceeds its shelf life—leading us to buy ever more.

All this makes pills highly profitable for manufacturers but a financial hardship for patients. Illness can force hard choices, as between purchasing a needed medication or paying the mortgage, at a time when the patient is already existentially challenged by disease. To provide a global perspective, although the overconsumption of expensive pills is a hazard in many first-world settings, in poorer countries the problem is often the opposite. Medications may be unaffordable, or unavailable to begin with, for potentially treatable acute diseases.[24] New antibiotics, if taken only for a short period to fight rarer infections, are unlikely to lead to the blockbuster sales that would justify the costs of development. Pharmaceutical companies tend to tilt research and development toward the chronic diseases of more affluent markets where the profits generated by a new drug can be great—even if it is just a "copycat" or subtle refinement of an existing drug—rather than to focus on more urgent and unmet needs of less-resourced populations.[25]

Even in a first-world context, the role of the pill as profit generator tilts the playing field in multiple ways. Much data have suggested that physicians, more than they realize, are influenced to write prescriptions by the financial and personal inducements offered by pharmaceutical companies: giveaways, advertisements, drug-rep visits, travel junkets, lucrative contracts, and conference speakerships. Increasingly it has become clear that even the medical research and publications that validate a drug's efficacy can be shaped and distorted by pharmaceutical funding. Corporate money, more often than public funding, determines what studies are run and how the results are presented (or buried, if unfavorable). This can undermine the contemporary holy grail of "data-driven" medical practice.[26] For example, it is more likely that expensive research will be done on a new antihypertensive drug than on the effects of diet, exercise, yoga, and meditation on lowering blood pressure.

It is also not unusual that new drugs are approved for consumer use, only later to be found to have dangerous adverse effects or to be no more effective than earlier, cheaper treatments. Hogshire refers to a "therapeutic life cycle" with initial glorification of a drug, demonization when adverse effects become clear, followed eventually by normalization.[27] Yet the fantasy of the "new miracle drug," the media attention it receives, and the time limits set by drug patent laws combine to assure an often-exaggerated focus on the latest, costliest pill to hit the market.

Many problems and questions ensue from the sheer number of pills now ingested. Some pills are expensive but ineffective. Some, like statins, are taken to prevent future diseases that the individual will never know whether he or she would have developed if left untreated. Many medicines are clearly potent, but not always in the right ways. People suffer from the unpleasant or clinically serious adverse effects of individual pills or interactions between medications. Patients and physicians alike can lose track of the complex regimens many people are placed on, especially as they age, causing difficulty in patient adherence and in the monitoring of drug responses and interactions. It has been estimated that, in the United States, medication-related reactions are the fourth leading cause of death.[28] Potent pills can also cause mental and physical addiction. We grow dependent on this extrinsic chemical—to relax, sleep, lose weight, sexually perform—and other health skills atrophy in favor of taking a drug. This is the opposite of what we said about healing touch: that it can awaken a sense of self-mastery as we learn how to skillfully inhabit our own body.

Pills can even cause problems after they have left the body through excretion. Before decomposing, drug residues from humans and livestock contaminate waterways, posing potential health threats to aquatic creatures and to drinking water. The European Union and the US Environmental Protection Agency have begun to take note of this problem, though much remains unknown and unregulated.[29]

The cultural fantasy surrounding the pill thus contributes in a wide variety of ways to social and physical ills, even while promising to solve them. Some of the dis-eases pills are designed to fix—aging, fatigue, imperfect bodies, aches and pains—are things we may need to accept and learn from as aspects of our fragile, mortal being. Yet pills, and the advertising that surrounds them, create the opposite mentality: nonacceptance, with consequent distress. (Then, better take a pill for that.) We are also distracted from more holistic understandings of the causation, prevention, and treatment of genuine diseases. The miniaturized pill implies a highly localized problem and solution confined to an individual body. The ideal "magic bullet" targets a single organ, pathogen, or biochemical process—for example, the antibiotic that eradicates an invading organism. But the site of illness and healing are rarely "local" in this way. They usually unfold in the complex interactions between different bodily sites and functions, and of the embodied self with its life-world. Focused on the pill, we may neglect other treatment modalities like healing touch and lifestyle changes involving diet, work, intoxicant use, exercise, sleep, and social and spiritual activities, which may be key to many of our mood and physical disorders.

In fact, pill reliance can justify *not* attending to needed changes. Greene invokes "the image of the overfed, underexercised American consumer who takes a statin with his cheeseburger . . . the cure for the latter-day ailments of excess consumption lies, cleverly, not in limiting consumption but in consuming additional products."[30]

The fantasy of the pill can lead us to neglect not only personal changes but also sociopolitical action. Environmental toxins and carcinogens, a food system slanted by government subsidies toward unhealthy calories, chronic unemployment, racism, the lack of accessible day care and health care—these causes of disease can be understood and addressed only on the collective level.[31] Taking a pill tends to individualize and internalize sickness and treatment. It promises private relief, but thereby obscures broader contexts.

Recontextualizing the "Pill" as Gift

In an influential essay, "Plato's Pharmacy," Derrida explores the many contradictory meanings of the Greek word *pharmakon*.[32] "Among these are included: a drug, a healing remedy or medicine, an enchanted potion or philter, a charm or spell, a poison. [33] In focusing on deleterious side effects we have explored the more poisonous sides of modern pharmaceuticals. In a sense, what is needed is a *pharmakon*-as-healing-remedy for our *pharmakon*-as-poison. Many specific remedies have been proposed by critics of the pharmaceutical industry. These include lowering the cost of medications and the overreliance on newer, more expensive brands; a variety of strategies to counter the distortions introduced by powerful drug companies into research, product development, and clinical practice; lessening the prescription of unnecessary medications, and better monitoring of multidrug regimens and interactions; and, in general, weaning us as individuals and a society from the fantasy of the all-purpose, almighty pill, thereby reopening more holistic approaches to illness and well-being.

However, to only demonize the pharmaceuticalization of Western medicine is to deny how pills have functioned in the other senses of *pharmakon*: as "a healing remedy" or even "an enchanted potion or philter," yielding dramatic relief. Again, antibiotics have given us mastery over many infectious diseases. Birth control pills have offered women and couples new securities and freedoms. Pills, even when noncurative, have provided symptomatic relief from a variety of pains and limitations. Their ameliorative, preventive, and sometimes lifesaving effects extend throughout the developmental span from early infancy to the chronic illnesses of old age. The result for many people is enhanced mood, function, or quality of life. There are numerous reasons we like our pills.

Moreover, as discussed, it is not only their biochemical properties that are healing but also the psychophysical benefits triggered by our *idea of the pill*. The "placebo effect," the positive results yielded by taking even an inert compound, is but a limit case of a broader phenomenon that Moerman calls the "meaning response."[34] We respond not to the treatment alone but to the *meanings* the treatment has for us. When positive belief is empowered by a reassuring treater-patient relationship, and by a faith in the medication itself, the healing response is potentiated. To fully defuse our cultural fantasy surrounding pills would risk lessening their effectiveness. This would be like the shaman who abandons talismanic objects and rituals, informing the patient that it is all hokum and might do more harm than good. Power would then drain from shamanic practice. So, too, a doctor stressing only the ineffectiveness or adverse side-effects of pills may contribute to a self-fulfilling prophecy.

This leaves us with a paradoxical dilemma. Pills, and the cultural fantasy thereof, can be both poison and remedy, in need of debunking and of being extolled. How to be properly circumspect about our overuse of pills, and yet honor pills from which we can genuinely benefit, thereby empowering the "meaning response"? And how do we honor meds without dishonoring ourselves, obscuring our lived body's own role in healing? How to bless the miniature pill, yet not lose sight of broader perspectives concerning illness and healing?

I will end this chapter with a few remarks about how we might rethink our relationship with pills. I would suggest that instead of viewing them as a commodity for consumption or a technological device, we might better call to mind the model of a *gift*. That is, taking a pill involves receiving into ourselves a gift that crystallizes possibilities for healing. Etymologically related to the word "whole" and "holy," "healing" involves a process of reintegration. We have seen, as with Philoctetes, that illness can create disruptions between oneself and one's own body, other people, and the cosmos.[35] Yet these ruptures can begin to heal *through the very way in which we take a pill*, not simply through its biochemical action. This can be a time to reconnect with the gifts of a generous universe.

Many spiritual traditions have fixed prayer times during the day, or at least recommend periodic pauses to return to one's center. Meditators, yogis, or practitioners of *qigong* may practice at dawn and dusk, or have prebedtime rituals. In this way, the day is anchored in healing and holy rhythms.

What if the modern-day rhythms of pill taking—for example, the morning and evening reach for the pill organizer—was not a heedless process or minor annoyance, but the occasion for contemplative reflection? We might call this our *medication-meditation*.

We are, or could be, reminded of the healing powers embodied in modern medicine, including the researchers who worked with such skill and energy; our caregiver who, in prescribing, was striving to help; the sources of economic support, private and public, that has made the pill available. In short, this can be a time of gratitude to the larger community that provides for us. The pill is their gift meant to relieve our distress. (This is especially true in a society—let us hope!—that makes medical resources available to the needy, not just the affluent.)

This is also a time for acknowledging the gifts—the skills and miraculous powers—of our own lived body. Insofar as the pill operates by supplementing or assisting a physiologic process and stimulating a "meaning response," we remember that much of what the pill unleashes is our own self-healing capacities.[36] This reminds us to make changes that support, and may ultimately supplant, the pill. That is, one aspect of our meditation may be a focus on avenues of healing that may in time even erase the need for this particular pill. Taking an antianxiety agent can remind us to do what we can to lower life stress and increase well-being. Swallowing a cholesterol-lowering statin, we think of what we can accomplish through diet and exercise to assist and potentiate this healing. A heart medicine can help us reflect on the miracle of our own heart, physical and spiritual, and how best to protect it. This process of thanking, appreciating, and reminding the self gives us tools to limit the dosage, or let go entirely of a pill when the time is right, and to "bounce back" if the pill has failed to fulfill every fantasy. We recognize medications as a bridge to our own self-healing.

As the pill reminds us of the gift of the community and of our own lived body, it can recall us as well to the gifts of a cosmos of which we are but a small part. In the words of sixteenth-century neo-Confucian philosopher Wang Yang-ming,

> Wind, rain, dew, thunder, sun and moon, stars, animals and plants, mountains and rivers, earth and stones are essentially of one body with man. It is for this reason that such things as the grains and animals can nourish man and that such things as medicine and minerals can heal diseases. Since they share the same material force, they enter into one another.[37]

Such thoughts may incline us toward choosing less toxic, more "natural" remedies. But whether a pill includes herbs or manufactured chemicals, it still embodies properties found in the material universe that are capable of being incorporated into our body to bless it with restored functioning. Gadamer writes, "We are ourselves a part of nature and it is this nature within us, together with the self-sustaining organic defense system of our bodies, which is capable of sustaining our 'inner' equilibrium." The pill is valuable insofar as it assists the restoration of a homeostasis that is part of nature and yet miraculous. [38]

For some, pill taking may be resonant with not only natural but supernatural blessings. Depending on one's spiritual beliefs, it may be a time to express gratitude for life and/or to remember death; to thank God, or Buddha Nature, or the Tao. As noted earlier, swallowing the pill is like a modern, secularized version of Eucharistic communion. Rather than simply mocking or demystifying this impulse, we can recognize here the possibility for a holy and healing moment. Instead of remaining in its mass-produced plastic bottle or weekly pill organizer, medicines might be placed, for example, in a special box residing on a sacred altar and taken with appropriate ceremony.[39]

Such practices recontextualize the pill as a multidimensional gift. (In chapter 8, I will pursue a similar point in relation to organ transplantation.) Might this provide a holistic way to enhance the "meaning response" and thereby the therapeutic efficacy of the drug? Might some "nonresponders" gain greater benefit from their medications? Might others be less prone to suffering adverse side effects, having been prepared by rituals of receiving? Might this even reshape our scientific investigation of pill efficacy and toxicity, since these may be influenced by the context in which the patient ingests them?

In any case, our relationship to pharmaceuticals could take on richer, more redemptive meanings than our consumerist culture currently offers. Rather than grabbing more pills as a result, we might take fewer, but with greater care, gratitude, and even effectiveness. This would indeed be a novel way for us to "take our medicine," yet one that draws on ancient wisdom.

Rethinking Clinical Practice:
Toward a *More Materialistic* Medicine

We have been looking at a phenomenology of illness and pain, along with some clinical responses. In examining healing touch and pills, we were also reflecting on the larger topic of embodied (or dis-embodied) practices in modern medicine. I will now try to systematize the discussion within an overarching framework. Again, this will connect up with personal experiences as well as therapeutic examples. Some of these are drawn from the practice of my collaborator in this and the preceding two chapters—Dr. Mitchell Krucoff—Duke cardiologist with a holistic and world-traveling bent.

"Holism" is often counterposed to the "reductionism" and "materialism" characteristic of Western medicine. "Too materialistic"—medicine is thereby accused of having drifted from its primary concern with human suffering into the world of technology and billable pills and services, as indeed we have been exploring. This charge is brought by many critics including alienated patients, disgruntled health-care practitioners, sociologists, policy-oriented progressives, and alternative therapists, who collectively call for medicine to supplement or transform its reigning materialist paradigm.

Yet this critique is problematic if taken to imply that medicine should retreat from the therapeutic breakthroughs of the modern scientific era. "High-tech" diagnosis and treatment have proven to be potent instruments of healing. They can, for example, save a limb or save a life when prescientific interventions would be futile. The last chapter discussed not simply the problems but the efficacies associated with our use of pills. The task for medicine is not to go backward but to better integrate new discoveries with an age-old awareness of humanistic care, spiritual meaning, and healing environments. I would suggest this calls for a new paradigm of medicine that is *more*, not less, materialistic.

How so? Much depends on what the term "materialism" means. I will distinguish between two of its customary uses, independent in logic though often interlocking in practice: monetary materialism and mechanistic materialism. I will propose a third form—an "authentic" materialism. This is at play in the healer's touch. We have seen how even the act of taking a pill can be recontextualized and enriched. This chapter will explore further examples of authentic materialism at play. However, this also exposes deficiencies in modern medicine. It is not, I contend, materialist enough, but suffers from a series of alienating abstractions.

Monetary Materialism

A person focused on profit and possessions is often called "materialistic." According to this meaning, it is hard to deny that the US health-care system is strongly so—driven by finances, resources, and profits.[1] Money influences virtually every aspect of the medical world, at least in standard practice settings. Medical time is divided up into "billable" hours. Medical space is allotted into hospital wards, intensive care beds, clinic rooms, laboratories, radiologic units, and the like, each generating its levels of reimbursement. Monetary issues influence access to health care, choice of treatments, the development and marketing of new pharmaceuticals, and the dependence on powerful, costly, profitable technologies including pills, surgeries, and diagnostic tools. The training and licensing of health-care practitioners is largely market-structured and driven.[2] Some people would argue that even the taxonomy of medical diseases has been financially distorted[3]—we have explored the notion that there is "an ill for every pill." A sub-profession now exists that codes medical diagnoses and procedures to systematically drive reimbursement levels.

But is all this really "materialism"? Alfred North Whitehead, a twentieth-century philosopher and mathematician, identified what he termed the "fallacy of misplaced concreteness."[4] This is operative when one takes a theoretical abstraction and misunderstands it as concrete reality. For example, Whitehead critiqued the "concept of simple location" used in Newtonian physics. Separate bits of matter, localized to a discrete region of space and time, come to be viewed as the fundamental constituents of reality. Whitehead reminds us that these are actually high-level abstractions. All things exist and are experienced through their interactions with other objects, subjects, and fields. The "isolable thing" is a theoretical simplification, useful for scientific practice but deceptive if misidentified as "concrete reality."

Much the same can be said about money. "Monetary materialism" is really based on abstractions. As Loy, the Buddhist author, points out, money is the *least* concrete of entities. "[A dollar bill] can't shelter you when it rains, or warm you when you're cold, or heal you when you're ill, or comfort you when you're lonely. . . . Money is a social construction that we tend to forget is only a construct—a kind of group fantasy."[5] Medical financing rarely attains even the thin materiality of a dollar bill, instantiated in credit card swipes, electronic transfers, photons on a computer screen.

In his famous work, *Das Kapital*, Marx highlights the abstractions at the heart of capitalism.[6] Concrete objects have "use values"—a piece of bread can be eaten or a bed slept in. However, in a capitalist market, objects become commodities for sale.[7] The thing's actual "use-value" becomes subordinated to its abstract "exchange value," translatable into a price. In this "fetishism of commodities," "the existence of the things *qua* commodities, and the value relation between the products of labour which stamps them as commodities, have absolutely no connexion with their physical properties and with the material relations arising therefrom."[8] An entrepreneur may buy and sell soybean futures, gold, mutual funds, shares in a mining, manufacturing, or medical company, with little regard to the material objects at play.

Something like this can occur in a medical system in which sick people and their body parts, practitioners and their services, technologies of diagnosis and treatment, all become commodities. Patients are abstracted into billable visits and bed-stays. Their illnesses are translated into International Classification of Disease (ICD) codes, which invoke and justify Current Procedural Terminology (CPT)-coded treatments, which trigger predetermined reimbursement schedules. Administrators keep a careful watch over disposable resources, profit margins, patient flow, bed utilization, and the marketing potential, as much as the healing potential, of new technologies.

The key point here is to recognize that this is not medical materialism at work but rather *abstractions*. The ill person, as we have seen, comes to the practitioner with very concrete symptoms: pain, anxiety, impairment, dislocation, disability, disfigurement. The practitioner's desires and actions may be similarly concrete, as he or she probes for remedies. However, the "fallacy of misplaced concreteness" threatens to displace this encounter in favor of the primacy of abstract profit and productivity goals. The patient suffers from this, experiencing depersonalized care. Meanwhile, the physician, struggling under the weight of time and performance measures, may feel equally depersonalized.

Mechanistic Materialism

Another meaning of "materialism" is more philosophical, as in this common dictionary definition: "The theory that physical matter is the only reality and that everything, including thought, feeling, mind, and will, can be explained in terms of matter and physical phenomena."[9]

This sort of materialist metaphysics dates back in the West to ancient Greek atomism. Its current incarnation can be traced to the seventeenth-century rise of modern science. Experimenters and theorists, such as Galileo and Descartes, reconceived the natural world according to the new physics and mathematics of mechanics.[10] Descartes envisioned, as he wrote in the *Discourse on Method*, that this new mechanical science would make it "possible to attain knowledge which is very useful in life . . . and thus render ourselves the masters and possessors of nature." This was desirable, "principally because it brings about the preservation of health, which is without doubt the chief blessing and the foundation of all other blessings in this life."[11] The key to this science was reconceiving the body as machine. Like a watch or other automaton, the body functions through internal mechanics that can, when necessary, be repaired or replaced.[12]

The consequent ascent of scientific medicine, and the type of diagnostics and treatments it makes possible, have in many ways fulfilled Descartes's dream. For example, since the heart has come to be understood as an electrically driven pump, medications can be prescribed to lower blood pressure, cholesterol, or clotting factors; blocked cardiac vessels can be opened or bypassed; leaking valves can be replaced with artificial or animal analogues; pacemakers and defibrillators can sustain life-giving heart rhythm; even an entirely artificial heart can be implanted.

Again, these "material" treatments actually arise from—and are associated with—a series of *abstractions*. The living patient, embedded within a world of involvement and grappling with modes of suffering and concern, is reconceived on the model of a mechanical device. One piece of this complexity (for example, the heart) is isolated as a primary focus. This is a form of what Whitehead called "the concept of simple location" wherein we set aside larger contexts of relational interdependence. From the heart, we may narrow attention further to a cardiac vessel or a single biochemical parameter measured through a specialized test. For Descartes, as for Galileo, nature spoke the language of numbers: only the mathematizeable was objectively real.[13] This is an attitude that finds its place in the statistics and metrics of medical diagnostics and research. Modern medicine thus abstracts progressively away from social context, lived experience, immediate sensory perception, healing touch, and even human language.

Such abstractions, while key to modern medicine's efficacy, can also cause it to seem dehumanized. The physician spends time reviewing X-ray films and other test results, strides into a hospital room, grabs a chart, and prescribes specialized treatment in a time-determined "visit"—yet he or she may never truly encounter the suffering person lying in the bed. This can compromise patient trust and receptivity, undermine the "placebo effect" of positive clinical interactions, and impair understanding of the causes of illness and the best modes of treatment for this individual. We have arrived at what Svenaeus terms "the *crisis* of (late-)modern medicine."[14] I will say more on this subject in succeeding chapters.

How one conceptualizes the problem makes a difference in one's solution. If medicine is seen as "too materialistic," focusing just on the patient's "body," one might add psychospiritual counseling on top of standard treatment. But this leaves in place the core abstractions of Cartesian mind-body dualism. The mechanical body is treated by the scientist-physician, with "adjunct care" of the soul left to the social worker or chaplain.

Some critics of medicine turn thoroughly "antimaterialist." This approach too is problematic; it threatens to throw the baby out with the bathwater. Modern medicine has developed stunningly effective treatments for many acute and chronic ills. To simply abandon these in search of alternative "nonmaterialist" approaches may do patients a disservice. Some people too quickly place their lives in the hands of "alternative" unvalidated treatments when medical science may have produced a better result.

The key is not to forsake but to integrate scientifically developed and efficacious treatments into a more holistic framework. This need not be antimaterialist in spirit. On the contrary, it represents a deeper, more authentic form of materialism. To accomplish this, we need a greater attention to the embodied experience of the patient, the physical environments in which treatment unfolds, and the material things we use as agents of healing. We can be far more intentional about the symbolic resonances, esthetic beauty, and complex meanings of our medical materials. They then serve not as agents of depersonalization but as partners in the healing process. Chapter 3 focused on the therapeutic uses of touch, the physical contact between two bodies. Chapter 4, while critical of a culture of pill popping, suggested ways in which this miniature material thing could take on the resonances of a sacred gift. I will now broaden the discussion of the ways we might rehumanize and resacrilize medical practice.

The key may lie in harmonizing aspects of modern medicine with those drawn from age-old sources. Central to many indigenous traditions is the symbolic investment of material objects with spiritual significance and healing powers. At the same time, an "authentic materialism" is in harmony with contemporary philosophical advances. Twentieth- and twenty-first-century philosophers have proposed alternatives to Cartesian dualism in which mind and body, subject and object, experience and the concrete world, are not seen as opposed but ever intertwined.

As already suggested, and as will be discussed more later, phenomenologists such as Husserl[15] and Merleau-Ponty,[16] explored the notion of the "lived body." The person is not a dualistic "ghost in a machine." Rather, our living flesh is the vehicle whereby we perceive our surroundings, move toward desired goals, and interact with others, resonating with their moods and intentions.[17] Even the higher flights of the intellect—such as you are engaged in now—are mediated by embodiment, as you gaze at these words.[18]

We also see the material world reconceived in the "process philosophy" of Whitehead and his followers.[19] Drawing on influences as diverse as Platonism, quantum mechanics, and ordinary experience, Whitehead suggests that subjectivity is present all the way down to the fundamental building blocks of space, time, and matter.

Especially in Chapter 8 I will engage in a more sustained examination of the philosophical underpinnings of our notions of materiality and the human body. But rather than develop this now, I will turn right to concrete clinical examples. These are drawn from existing healing practices but also involve suggestions for the future. Together they serve to sketch the outlines of an authentic, holistic, medical materialism.

Shawls and Quilts

The "Prayer Shawl Ministry" was begun in 1998 by Janet Bristow and Victoria Cole-Galo, two graduates of the Women's Leadership Institute at the Hartford Seminary.[20] They were inspired to knit shawls for people experiencing illness, loss, and crisis, as well as for others seeking a tangible sign of divine care. The knitters establish a meditative environment and pray while making each knot. Materials, patterns, and colors are often chosen for symbolic meaning. After being blessed with special wishes and prayers, the shawl is gifted, sometimes in a ceremonial fashion, to the one in need. In a *New York Times* interview, Bristow explains, "It's an embrace. It's a hug. It's tangible. You're basically knitting your prayers, your good intentions and your thoughts into the shawl."[21] Sometimes referred to as prayer shawls, comfort shawls, or peace shawls, these are now being created by dozens of groups around the country with different denominational and spiritual affiliations. Annual national gatherings have had hundreds in attendance.

In a similar initiative, the "Quilts Are Love" organization, started by breast cancer survivor Susan Maddox, distributes quilts with panels on which friends and loved ones of a patient write personal messages.[22] Sick patients can then literally wrap themselves in the healing intentions of their loved ones. Such objects thus embody not only divine love but that of the community. Prayer shawls, for example, may be conditioned by the blessings of an entire congregation.

The *New York Times* article cited above supplies an example of a prayer shawl recipient, Jean Maddon, fifty-eight-years old, recovering from major abdominal surgery. She reported being very cold and wearing her shawl almost ceaselessly in the weeks following surgery. "I knew that people had prayed over it, and you can rationalize that, but somehow putting it on and wrapping it around you felt very peaceful. . . . I think it probably helped with my recovery."[23]

This object transcends any conventional Western division of body, mind, and spirit. While many patients experience the shawl as being imbued with spiritual energy, this is mediated by the garment's materiality. Care and healing are made tangible. This is one interesting form of the healer's touch discussed in chapter 3. Here the touch of the shawl or quilt re-presents—makes present, over and over—a communal embrace.

This shawl or quilt is in some ways reminiscent of the "healing objects" used in the shamanistic practices of many indigenous cultures. These are extensively documented in the literature of medical anthropology, which has increasingly taken up the theme of embodiment, and in sociologic texts on the mythic/magical worldview.[24]

For example, Sir James Frazer, in his groundbreaking work, *The Golden Bough*, talks of "sympathetic magic" as operating according to laws of "similarity" and "contact."[25] An object can harm or heal because it is *similar* to another (holding a doll might help an infertile woman become pregnant) and/or it has been in spatiotemporal contact with another (the garment of a pregnant woman might transmit fertility). The prayer/peace/comfort shawl embodies both principles in action. As something warm, sheltering, and beautiful, it is similar to, and expressive of, divine and communal love. The shawl has also been in contact with the special energies of the people who made and blessed it.

While such "magical" elements are frequently characterized as the antithesis of modern medicine, they need not imply the abandonment of the scientific worldview. We have discussed the power, demonstrated in medical practice and research, of the placebo effect—the *belief* in healing—to trigger real psychophysical changes. What Dossey called "intermediary objects" help us access this power: "We physicians are drowning in them. They range from white coats, stethoscopes, a mystifying vocabulary, and CT scanners, to thousands of pills and surgical procedures."[26] Many of these medical objects (for example, pills and surgeries) have mechanistic efficacy independent of the placebo effect, as validated through research protocols. However, the power of these medical objects can be enhanced by their symbolic resonances.[27] As suggested in the previous chapter, a pill's shape, color, and name make a difference. Studies show for example that blue placebo capsules induced drowsiness more frequently than pink ones, and that aspirin tablets scored with a "Bayer cross" had a more powerful effect than unmarked tablets.[28]

The material richness of the prayer shawl may be similar to—but also far transcends—that of a placebo pill. We have seen that illness can sever the patient's habitual trust in his or her own body, community, and universe of belief.[29] The prayer shawl helps "knit" these back together, regathering the world that illness has torn asunder.

To understand this, I again turn to the work of Borgmann, philosopher of technology. In the previous chapter I used his analysis of the *device*, which he distinguishes from a focal *thing*.[30] A *thing*—Borgmann takes this term from Heidegger[31]—is inseparable from its context, the modes of engagement that brought it into being and that it, in turn, makes possible. I mentioned Borgmann's example of a wood-burning stove. It gathers family around the hearth, providing the home with a center. The stove's workings demand engagement with the natural world and the rhythm of the seasons, the development of skills and strength, and the distribution of family tasks. This *focal thing* is thus associated with *focal practices* that orient life. Borgmann contrasts this world-gathering *thing* with the *device*: in his example, the central heating system. This device disburdens us of the work and limitations that characterize the wood-burning stove. Heat is immediately, effortlessly, and ubiquitously available. But disburdened by the device, we are also disengaged. We disconnect from the seasons; the family can scatter; prescribed tasks and purposes are dissolved. It is like the contrast between preparing and sharing a festive meal and ordering fast-food burgers, a kind of food-device. Much ease and freedom is gained through the latter, but also much is lost.

The medical world is filled with devices—the preceding chapter focused on the pill as paradigmatic example—that can serve healing functions but also trigger forms of alienation and dysfunction. Insofar as medical devices yield rapid, effortless symptom alleviation or cure, this is a clear good. However, such is not always possible, leading to disappointment. An overreliance on devices, such as pills, can also diminish our own engagements with good health practices. Finally, device-laden environments—think of the modern hospital—can exacerbate the modes of depersonalization and world-fragmentation that the disease initiated.

In such an environment, the rich materiality of the prayer shawl becomes a healing agent. Among alien devices, it serves as a world-gathering *thing*.

Its natural fibers reconnect the patient to sun and soil. Through form and color, and infused with blessings, the shawl helps a patient feel close to family, friends, and often a Higher Power. As noted, the word "healing" comes from the same root as "whole" and "holy." Such is not simply represented by the shawl, but embodied in it. Also, for those engaged in the acts of meditative knitting, quilting, blessing, and gifting, these become "focal practices" that help the helpers. Such acts allow a bodily/spiritual engagement with the loved one. Achterberg et al. explore how such "rituals of healing" reduce feelings of helplessness and knit together the ill person, community, and cosmos. "Rituals help us face together those things that are too painful, confusing, or awesome to face alone."[32]

Places of Healing: Hospital and Nursing Homes Reconceived

An authentic materialism calls us to reconsider not just an isolated *thing*, like a prayer shawl and its associated practices, but also the larger medical world in which the thing is embedded. The modern hospital, for example, not only contains devices but itself aspires to be a large device, battling disease through technology, sterility, and efficiency. But can we envision a hospital that, like the prayer shawl, itself serves as a world-gathering *thing*?

A suggestive example is provided by the Sri Sathya Sai Super Speciality Hospital located in Puttaparthi, India (a second has since opened outside of Bangalore). This is a tertiary care hospital with advanced specialty units, for example in cardiology, ophthalmology, orthopedics, oncology, and plastic surgery.[33] My coauthor here, Dr. Krucoff, has consulted on the design of cardiologic services for this hospital. State-of-the-art Western technology is used, but as we will see, this equipment comprises the tools, not the broader context, of care. Created under the auspices of internationally known (now deceased) guru/avatar Sri Sathya Sai Baba, and funded by his disciples, the hospital provides all of its services for free, making them available to India's poor irrespective of caste. This enables the hospital to provide a "medicine free of commercialization . . . which can be done only when it ceases to be a commodity bought and sold in the market."[34]

This hospital exemplifies what we have termed "authentic materialism," including the hospital's very brick and mortar architecture. This was designed by Professor Keith Critchlow, a renowned author and practitioner of "sacred architecture." When entering the main gate, one is greeted by figures of Hindu gods associated with life and healing. This leads to a prayer hall, topped by the central dome, which is 85 feet high and 80 feet in diameter, festooned with images of the Elephant, Peacock, and Lion, symbols of intelligence, skill, and courage, respectively. The dome is architecturally intended to represent a heart whose apex is pointed to God. The two main wings of the hospital wrap the front courtyard and entry, symbolizing God's arms reaching to embrace all who come to walk this path. The building itself is not referred to as a hospital but as a *mandir* (temple) of healing.

Hindu Gods, gurus—and free care—may seem very distant from our Western context. Yet the core principles are illustrative. The hospital speaks through its material symbolism to care, faith, beauty, integration as at the core of healing practice. This hospital truly offers *hospitality*. This assists the treatment of the ill person and family who may be struggling with the disintegrations caused by illness. In addition, this place is welcoming and focusing for those who work there—encouraging a spirit of awareness, compassion, and service to humanity. The powerful high-tech devices of Western medicine are not *displaced*, but rather *placed* within an enriched context. Heidegger, who first introduced the notion of the world-gathering "thing," pointed to the ancient Greek temple as a paradigmatic example: its site, architecture, and purpose disclose a world of meanings.[35] This is also true for the Sri Sathya Sai Super Speciality Hospital serving its patients, families, and practitioners. There are many principles here that could be incorporated into the redesign of Western hospitals.

Let me now turn to a closer-to-home example of authentic materialism at work. Harvard medical graduate, Dr. William H. Thomas, found himself questioning the design of an eighty-bed nursing home of which he had become medical director. Taking lessons from nature, he realized that elders needed a genuine habitat enriched with diverse social and natural engagements. In 1991 he created the prototype of what has come to be called the Eden Alternative.[36] Animals were introduced—dogs, cats, parakeets, rabbits, and chickens—providing opportunities for care and companionship. (In chapter 12, I will discuss the healing power of animals in *prison* environments.) Plants were brought inside the home, and an outside garden was created for the work, enjoyment, and fresh food it provided. Through starting an afterschool program and summer day camp, children were invited into the community. The nursing home came alive. As documented by the New York State Health Department, this switch of paradigm was accompanied by decreases in infections, daily drug costs, and staff turnover.[37]

This model has spread. When last I checked, some 17,000 "Eden Associates" have been trained, and 300 Eden Alternative homes registered around the world. Dr. Thomas's latest "Green House" initiative moves even further from the institutional model.[38] A Green House, built for ten to twelve residents, is thoroughly homelike. It includes a hearth, abundant sunlight, vibrant outdoor space, personal rooms, and communal living and dining rooms. Animals and plants, again, are welcome. In 2005, the Robert Wood Johnson Foundation initiated a five-year, $10 million-dollar grant to support the building of Green House projects across the country.[39] More than 100 are now operational.

Here, again, we see authentic materialism at play, not the abstractions of money and mechanism. The physical environment is redesigned to energize humane care and community. Rather than simply inhabiting an institutional device, the residents dwell with life-enriching focal things and practices.

The Implantable Cardioverter Defibrillator: Device and/or Thing?

Prayer shawls and Green Houses are wonderful things, yet they do not obviate the need for state-of-the-art technological care. In the last chapter we looked at how pills might be recontextualized. A final question for this chapter, then, is whether authentic materialism can lead us to reenvision even the highest of high-tech medical devices. I will close with a speculative example involving this sort of technology: an implantable cardioverter defibrillator.

Sudden cardiac death claims some 500,000 people each year in the United States. This defibrillator has become the treatment of choice for patients with life-threatening arrhythmias.[40] An almost ideal exemplar of what conventional medicine could wish for in a device, this defibrillator is small, surgically implanted, long-lasting, highly effective, lifesaving, and even relatively cost-efficient for the benefits provided. If a patient's heart fibrillates, the internal device automatically detects this and shocks it back into rhythm, often time and again defeating death itself.

Though by modern standards the benefits are great, and some patients report their sense of gratitude and enhanced security, many studies also suggest that implanting these devices provokes significant distress in patients. Aware that their hearts are so sick that their lives depend on the permanent implant of a battery-powered generator that might shock them at any time, and that itself requires a lifetime of specialized monitoring, a substantial proportion of patients experience anxiety, depression, and impaired quality of life.[41] Although research results are not consistent, attempts to isolate predisposing factors seem to point toward the individual patient's characterology—some persons cope better with this challenge than others—and the number of shocks received from the device.[42] Patients commonly have a fear of being shocked, which can be very painful. It has been described as "like being kicked by a donkey in the chest"[43] or being electrocuted from the inside.[44] One's inability to anticipate and control when this will occur is also trying: patients report their dread of being shocked in a public space or their fears concerning isolation, sexual activity, driving, and device failure.[45] Anxiety thus surrounds both the device working and not working. It can compound the sense of alienation from others, and from one's body, that serious illness itself provokes.

The defibrillator also provides continual reminders of mortality. It calls to mind the cardiac death one almost had, and the death that awaits the patient in the future, as well as the particular one that the device *prevents*. This technology's blessing can also be a curse: some patients feel they have "lost the easy death" associated with sudden cardiac fibrillation. Instead, they live the troubled half-life of a cyborg, part-human, part-machine, suffused by pain and uncertainty.[46]

Much has or can be done to alleviate such distress. Recommendations commonly involve patient education; support groups; adjusting the technology to reduce the number and pain of shocks; cognitive-behavioral therapy; relaxation and stress-management techniques; and psychoactive drugs. These are all potentially important palliative-treatment modalities. But they also largely adhere to Cartesian divisions, focusing on helping the "mind" or the mechanical "body."

What is almost never considered is working directly with the materiality of the defibrillator. What does it look like? How does the patient first "meet" it? Is there a way it can become more of a world-gathering *thing*—like the prayer shawl—and less of an offputting device?

Unlike a prayer shawl, a defibrillator has a mass-produced, synthetic physicality that does not bespeak beauty, comfort, and community. That is neither part of this device's form nor function. Although it will remain a palpable lump under the skin and trigger airport metal detectors, when used it will largely disappear from sight.

Yet what if the defibrillator's arrival were more like that of a prayer shawl? What if it was presented to patient and family as something truly to be given and received, perhaps blessed and prayed over, experienced as material friend and partner? How differently might this object then be accepted within the patient, that is, physically, psychologically, and spiritually?

Imagine, for example, that the patient had the opportunity to become familiar with the defibrillator prior to implantation, to see and touch it, even pray over it. If issues of sterility and security permitted, the actual device to be placed within the body could be ceremonially blessed. Friends, family, and/or a religious figure could endow it with healing energy as is done with the prayer shawl. The patient might be encouraged to create a poem or a painting to explore the meanings of the defibrillator and to create one's own symbology around it. (I will say more in chapter 7 about how personal narratives can facilitate healing.) The way would thus be prepared for this powerful object to be "accepted into one's heart."

In a personal communication, Dr. Kirsten Jacobson wrote that she once taught an earlier form of this chapter

> in a class on phenomenology and embodiment, and during a discussion students and I considered ways in which the defibrillators could be made more "friendly" and personalized for their "owners." It prompted me to think about the way in which Apple enables people to engrave their iPods and iPhones with messages of their choice. I suggested that someone might be given the opportunity to engrave his or her defibrillator before its placement in the body. Students and I then talked with great energy about phrases (often references to contemporary song lyrics) that might help a person to befriend this often surprising and literally shocking device—phrases such as "You light up my life!" or "Give it to me, baby, one more time!" or "Shock it to me!" or simply "I love you." I feel palpably that if I were to have a mechanical device in my body like this, it would help if my own words were inscribed on it rather than simply a serial number or other manufacturing indications.

Of course, all such preparations are unlikely to fully remove the pain and fear associated with defibrillator shocks. However, working with this device as a "focal thing" can also assist with the development of helpful focal practices. Jauhar wrote about a patient who struggled with severe anxiety around being shocked: "When the fear hit . . . she sang songs to herself that she learned when she was a girl. She chanted a Sanskrit mantra that she learned in her younger days as a yoga instructor. And she prayed."[47]

Focal practices can even help recontextualize the reminders of death associated with defibrillator shocks. Many spiritual traditions counsel using *memento mori*, the remembrance of one's mortality, to develop an authentic relationship with life, death, and the eternal. "Death meditations have been regarded as an indispensable element in a wide array of cultures: the Egyptian and Indian, the Chinese and Japanese, the Hellenic and Roman, the Hebrew and Islamic, in both their ancient and modem forms."[48] Defibrillator jolts present an embodied—literally shocking—*memento mori*. This can either lead to panic and depression or, through preparation, ritual, prayer, and the like, be made meaningful by a bodily/spiritual practice.

These comments are meant to be suggestive only. While using the defibrillator as an example, they open a window to reenvisioning the complex world of medical materials, including transplants (more on this in chapter 8), dialysis machines, surgical suites, monitors, ventilators, and other clinical devices and environments. Currently these are designed to be congruent with monetary and mechanistic "materialism." They do the job well of generating technologic interventions and revenues. However, these objects also can con-tribute to the abstract, depersonalized—even curiously *disembodied*—texture of modern medicine. What is needed is a medicine that does not abandon functionality but is attendant to the play of beauty, meaning, and the healing arts, embedded in an enriched materialism.

Words such as "material" and "matter" may ultimately derive from the Latin *mater* and the Indo-European root *ma*, meaning "origin" or "mother." It is that which nourishes, as in the word "maternal." What is the matter with modern medicine? Partly, it is that it does not pay enough attention to *what matters* to patients and family, including the material gestures, objects, and environments these people encounter when seeking help. Medicine need not apologize for being "too materialistic." It does need to rethink what material-ism means.

PART 2

Medicine and Bioethics:
Hermeneutical Reflections

Rethinking Diagnosis:
The Many Texts of Medicine

In previous chapters we have looked at health-care issues broadly construed and even re-conceived. Thinking through the phenomenology of illness and pain, and therapeutic approaches such as healing touch, pills, even prayer shawls and Hindu hospitals, we have considered the challenges faced by sick individuals, but as embedded within larger contexts of medical care.

In this second part, I want to make more explicit the significance of "texts" and "contexts" in health care and bioethics. To do so I will introduce some tools provided by continental philosophers who have focused on hermeneutical themes. In this chapter I will concentrate on the complex textual and interpretive structure that arises when even a single doctor and patient interact, seeking an illness diagnosis. In chapter 7 I will suggest how a hermeneutical approach can also help us critique and reenvision the field of bioethics. In chapter 8 I will then take an example of an emerging and complex area of medicine—organ transplantation—which itself raises a host of bioethical issues. This will further our inquiry into how we understand and treat distressed bodies.

However, in another sense, we now recommence the journey, this time looking at medicine through an epistemological lens. The *doing* in medicine is supposed to arise from its modes of *knowing*. But of what sort? Modern medicine is commonly said to rely on a scientific knowledge base supported by an edifice of conceptual schemata, technological instrumentation, and research protocols. A popular conception of doctors is that of trained, impartial investigators who arrive at differential diagnoses through induction from evidence, followed by stages of eliminating false hypotheses and verifying true ones.

Yet this model does not accurately capture how medicine proceeds. First, the very vision of science articulated above has come under powerful criticism.

Post-empiricist philosophers, drawing on the work of Kuhn and others, challenge the myth of scientific investigation as value-free and ahistorical.[1] These thinkers have argued that the "facts" scientists collect are preshaped by their theories, these theories in turn vectored by social values and forces. Even if medicine were but a branch of natural science, this might not expunge subjectivity on the individual and collective level.

Second, medicine surely incorporates extra-scientific elements. McWhinney, referring to the doctor's personal mastery of skills and tools, regards clinical medicine primarily as "craft."[2] For Munson, medicine is distinguished from the sciences by virtue of its practical and moral telos. Medicine seeks to promote the health of people rather than simply to acquire knowledge.[3] Similarly, Gadamer speaks of the art of medicine as a kind of doing or making that does not create an external product, but instead inserts itself into the processes of nature to try to restore the natural equilibrium of health.[4] Toulmin describes the physician as having a multiplicity of roles: scientist, but also biographer, historian, priest, personal adviser.[5]

Any integrated model of clinical understanding must be broad enough to address all these aspects of medicine while maintaining conceptual coherence and practical relevance. Authors such as Daniel,[6] Gatens-Robinson,[7] Gogel and Terry,[8] Good and Good,[9] and Svenaeus[10] suggest the model of medicine as *hermeneutical*. Let's now see what that means—with my apologies to those who already know it well and perhaps with a level of detail that will exceed this treatment.

"Hermeneutics" refers to the practice or study of *interpretation*. The term was first employed within a seventeenth-century theological context. Rules and principles were sought for interpreting sacred scripture, giving rise to a biblical hermeneutics.[11] Hermeneutics has since acquired a cross-disciplinary significance, encompassing any sort of textual interpretation. A literary work is interpreted to uncover its meaning and rhetorical structures; a juridical code, to determine the application of law; a set of scientific data, to find explanatory regularities. Similarly, medicine is a hermeneutical enterprise par excellence. Most simply, the practitioner interprets the patient's signs and symptoms to ferret out their meaning, the underlying disease.

In acknowledging the interpretive nature of clinical understanding, we leave behind the dream of a pure objectivity. Where there is interpretation there is subjectivity, ambiguity, room for disagreement. The personal and provisional character of clinical judgment cannot be expunged. However, this model need not lead us down a path of pure relativism.[12] Hermeneutics, as developed in literary theory, biblical scholarship, and a variety of other fields can serve as a structured discipline with teachable methods, canons of good and bad exegesis, ways of arriving at consensual validation. Such is surely the case with medical diagnosis.

To simply label medicine as hermeneutical, however, borders on the vacuous. As Heidegger discusses, human understanding in general is hermeneutical.[13] Upon awakening I interpret the hands of a clock face as signifying the time, the dark shape in the corner as the profile of my bathrobe, the clouds outside my window as suggestive of rain. Only via ceaseless acts of interpretation do I have a world, one charged with form and meaning.

The key question, then, is not *whether* medicine is hermeneutical but *how*. What sorts of texts define the clinical encounter? Who are the "authors," who the "readers"? How did this interpretive field take shape historically? What is the goal of medical interpretation? What problems exist with medicine's usual interpretive strategies? To such questions I devote the rest of this chapter.

The Medical Text

The notion of the text, while traditionally identified with a written work, can be expanded. Drawing on Daniel's definition, I will simply regard as a text any set of elements that take on meaning through interpretation.[14] In this sense, a dream, a perceptual panorama, a map, a kinship structure, a historical sequence all constitute texts open to interpretation.

What, then, is the text that defines the clinical encounter? In simplest terms, I will call this the *person-as-ill*. As we have seen in the first section of this book, the clinical text is never just a "disease" abstracted from the personality, life-history, existential concerns, of the sufferer. The clinician ultimately treats a person, not a set of symptoms or organs. However, neither is it simply a person-in-general who is thematized. Otherwise the clinical encounter would lose distinction from other human sciences or modes of communication. Doctor and patient alike focus on the person precisely *as-ill*, either in reality—as during the clinical visit—or potentially—as with the annual checkup meant to watch for and prevent medical problems. (In this chapter, as in previous ones, I will assume an alert person seeking care as opposed to, for example, the mentally impaired or comatose patient.) In the summarizing words of Svenaeus, "medicine is an interpretive meeting which takes place between two persons (the doctor or some other clinical professional and the patient) with the aim of understanding and healing the one who is ill and seeks help."[15]

Mol, in her study of clinical interpretation, says that diseases are not simply diagnosed but "enacted" through a variety of practices and materials.[16] In her book-length examination of atherosclerosis, she shows how there are actually many different sorts of "atheroscleroses." These are variously enacted through history taking, surgical investigation, microscopic examination, angiography, blood pressure cuffs, palpation, and on and on. She questions whether there is any single object or disease entity that all participants keep in view; hence her book title, *The Body Multiple.*

Mol's reading highlights the tensions and divergences present within the modern health-care system, with its wide variety of investigatory and therapeutic forms. Still, I think there is merit in beginning where I have with the *person-as-ill* as a kind of primary text. It seems to capture something *descriptively* true—the wide array of specialists, tests, and interventions are unified by a common concern with the ill patient. There is also a *prescriptive* element: when this focus is lost—for example, in favor of one on billable hours and profitability, or test results in and of themselves, or the jockeying for power among competing professionals—we sense the therapeutic project has gone awry.

While the person-as-ill may be considered the primary text situating the clinical encounter, the diagnostic question—"what is occurring here?"—can be pursued through a series of secondary texts. These I will call, respectively, the "experiential," "narrative," "physical," and "instrumental." The first of these texts corresponds to the experience of the ill patient—a central focus of earlier chapters. The latter three correlate with the traditional triadic structure of the medical workup: history, physical exam, and diagnostic testing.

Also traditional is the language I will use here of "doctor" and "patient." It may not simply be the patient but family members as well who present an account of illness symptoms and consult on treatment possibilities. It certainly is not only physicians, but many other sorts of staff, professionals, and clinical teams, who provide care. In this sense, referring to the "doctor-patient" relationship can be somewhat misleading. However, I stick to it because it provides a simplified model with which to begin and an ease of expression. Moreover, the concept of "doctor" and "patient" remains paradigmatic (rightly or wrongly), that is, understood as the heart of how we conceptualize, empower, practice, and reimburse professionalized medical care.

THE EXPERIENTIAL TEXT

By the time the patient arrives at the doctor's office, he or she has already gone through an interpretive process. This, we saw in chapter 2, is present even in the initial moments a pain is felt. More broadly, the text to be explained consists of any of a series of experiences that stand out to the person as significant and disruptive. These may be sensory in nature, encompassing a variety of aches, pains, chills. Alternatively, functional incapacities may arise—perhaps a loss of strength, digestive difficulties, or joint stiffness. The person might also note changes in physical appearance, such as an unusual lump or rash.[17] These experiences, by virtue of presenting a disturbing break with normal routine, initiate a search for meaning. Why is this happening? What does it signify? What caused it? Will it get better or worse? What should I now do?[18] In previous chapters, we've explored the disruptions, questions, even existential crises, with which the ill person may be confronted.

As Good and Good suggest, the symptoms of illness are always from the start *meaningful* in complex ways.[19] They are not simply biological indicators of underlying disease, but arise out of and are connected to cultural beliefs, personal history, one's explanatory models, work and family relationships, and so on. Something as simple as "back pain" is experienced very differently depending on the practical and symbolic meanings it has for the individual.

However, the initiation of a clinical encounter signals the achievement of one interpretive result: that this story is, in fact, a *medical* story. When reading a work of fiction, we may be uncertain as to which genre it belongs, whether comedy, romance, or murder mystery. Similarly, physical experience often exhibits genre ambiguity. A man plagued by exhaustion might interpret this as a job-related issue, the product of a moral or constitutional failing, an effect of the weather, or nothing special to worry about. Only when he comes to interpret this fatigue within a medical framework does he arrive at the doctor's office seeking help. As every physician knows, certain people are immediately inclined in this direction, while to others it is a matter of last resort.

This medical interpretation is a necessary but not sufficient precondition of the clinical encounter. The exhausted man might simply self-diagnose, decide that he is anemic and purchase iron tablets. His reading is, for the moment, closed. In contrast, medical help is often sought when there is a felt sense of hermeneutic incompletion. The patient contacts the doctor knowing the whole story—including within it diagnosis, prognosis, the proper course of treatment—has yet to be told. Hence the clinical encounter begins when the patient's interpretation has achieved enough closure to recognize its insufficiency.

This insufficiency may be related to a social division of labor. As opposed to the layperson, the doctor is perceived as commanding high-level expertise. She has been trained over the course of many years in a series of conceptual and technological frameworks that can be employed to "make sense" of the patient's symptoms. There is now a wider dissemination of health-related information, especially over the Internet, and the patient may engage in his own Google search and self-diagnosis. Still, for confirmation (or not) of one's suspicions, and access to a range of treatments, recourse to professionals often proves irreplaceable.

The ill person's hermeneutic insufficiency is also rooted in the structure of human embodiment itself. Most of the visceral functions on which one's life and health rest—digestion, circulation, metabolism—escape the province of personal command.[20] I cannot be considered the author of such anonymous processes: they proceed within me, yet without my help. As Lewis Thomas notes, if suddenly I were put in personal charge of my own liver, I would not know where to even begin.[21] Not only do these processes recede from my "authorship," but from myself as conscious "reader." I do not experience my microvilli absorbing molecules, my liver filtering toxins. The perceptual text available to me is radically incomplete when it comes to my own physiology. If I go to the doctor for abdominal problems, the intermittent cramps and acid reflux I experience are scraps of a page from which it is difficult to reconstruct a comprehensive plot. Hence the doctor is needed not only to interpret the text but to help *bring it into being*, to *enact* it, in Mol's usage. Via probing questions, fingers, and instruments, the physician assists the story to write itself more fully.

THE NARRATIVE TEXT

The first part of a diagnostic workup is traditionally the taking of a history. This gives rise to what I will term a "narrative text." This clinical narrative is, in a sense, the collaborative product of three different authors. The diseased body itself has provided the focal incidents of the story—the aches, blemishes, and incapacities. The patient gives these linguistic voice, but provoked by questions and guidance from the physician. In translating physical experiences into language, the patient may be asked to define their sequence and crucial features, to weave out of ambiguous events a continuous plot. This is not an exclusively "medical" story yet, but may also express existential fears and yearnings. Charon writes:

> As patient meets physician, a conversation ensues. A story—a state of affairs or a set of events—is recounted by the patient in his or her acts of narrating, resulting in a complicated narrative of illness told in words, gestures, physical findings, and silences and burdened not only with the objective information about the illness but also with the fears, hopes, and implications associated with it.[22]

As we have seen in earlier chapters, the very telling of this story may have therapeutic as well as diagnostic significance. It counteracts two primary features of illness previously discussed: the experience of senselessness and of isolation. We have examined how illness can involve the sudden disruption of life: one's routines, plans, and habitual identity are overturned by a collection of inchoate yet threatening symptoms, often manifesting no clear meaning or purpose. This is often accompanied by a feeling of isolation from others, who can neither experience nor fully relieve one's pain. The act of translating disease into language can begin to overcome this double alienation. What was private is now made public, what was senseless and random is woven into a meaningful tale. Hence, sharing the story can itself be healing.[23] We will revisit this theme in the next chapter.

Along with the patient, the doctor participates in authoring this text. From the start she is channeling discourse. She asks questions concerning the symptomatology and past medical, family, and social history, often filtered through interpretive hypotheses that may be formulated very early in the clinical encounter. Modes of expression are suggested to the patient: "Would you call it a burning pain or a crushing pain?" In history taking we see at play a collaborative coauthorship taking us beyond the simple division between "illness" and "disease" with which this book began.[24]

The doctor, however, assumes primary authorial voice when speech is converted into writing in the chart. The "chief complaint" is sometimes put in the precise words of the patient, but from then on the doctor selects and edits the discourse. While referred to as "the patient's chart," the patient is actually prohibited from writing in it, and often, even from reading it. This seems a crucial omission given that the chart is the central site in which clinical notes reside, specialists communicate with one another, key laboratory values are entered and interpreted, and the "case" as a whole is organized. Not only is the patient's voice effectively silenced, but so are those of family members. The wife of an ill man, the parent of a sick child: they may have witnessed a great deal, with rapt attention, over a long period, but still are not allowed to write in the chart. The right (or rite) of writing belongs to medical professionals alone.

THE PHYSICAL TEXT

At the beginning of an essay on medical phenomenology, Dr. Richard Baron describes a telling moment.[25] While carefully auscultating a patient's chest, the patient begins to ask him a question. His reply, which becomes part of the essay title, was: "Quiet, I can't hear you while I'm listening." (This is literally a *telling* moment, but not truly one of *listening* to the patient.) Here we see exemplified the textual shift when history taking gives way to physical examination. The doctor now interacts directly with the patient's body. Aside from responding to the occasional question ("does this hurt?"), the patient's voice is now largely silenced, allowing the ill body to reveal itself directly to medical perception.

But this body is not exactly the same one the patient experienced and described. We have seen that phenomenologists like Merleau-Ponty distinguish between the body-as-object, a thing that can be examined and measured like any other material entity, and the "lived body"[26]—that is, the embodied source of our perception, motility, desire, habits, and also of our vulnerability to wounds. Illness reminds us of the centrality of the lived body. However, it is the object body—that mass of structures and processes witnessed from outside—that is probed in the physical exam. Symptoms give way to physical signs, the "subjectivity" of the patient's experience and report to the "objectivity" of visible lesions. As discussed in chapter 3, the compassionate touch still preserves the patient as a Thou, not just an It, a real person like oneself. Yet during physical exam, for most doctors, the objectifying stance dominates.

A crucial point of commonality does remain between the body lived-from-within and objectified-from-without—its hermeneutical reticence. Just as the patient's perceptions of the inner body are fragmentary, so too are the doctor's. The barrier posed by the body wall, the microscopic nature of cellular processes, makes encounter with the illness often an indirect thing mediated through surface signs. "Tell-tale edema," "cyanosis," "angiomata" constitute signifiers whose meanings can be decrypted only by those who understand the code.

Here it is also worth noting a corporeal asymmetry. While the object body of the patient is being "read," it is the physician's lived body that does the reading. That is, while objectifying the patient, the doctor does not simultaneously objectify herself but lives out her motoric and perceptual capacities.[27] Through clinical training, the doctor's senses have been shaped into acute and knowledgeable instruments, enriched by practical experience. Just as music is heard differently by the educated listener, so the trained physician hears the murmur, feels the suprasternal thrill that are lost to the second-year medical student doing a physical. This interpretive process is not exclusively an intellectual achievement. As Merleau-Ponty points out, the knowledge resides right in the body.[28] The physician's fingers know just how to probe and have come to recognize the feel of a tumor, though she may have difficulty formulating this into the logic of principles and rules.[29] In chapter 3, we explored a little the skill and intelligence embodied in the physician's touch.

This capacity for perceptual interpretation is extended through the use of relevant technologies. Via stethoscope, otoscope, ophthalmoscope, the physician helps enact the physical text, sensing regions of the body that previously were inaccessible. As Ihde and Heelan note, such technologies function as if they were part of the user's lived body.[30] At first the medical student may look *at* the ophthalmoscope, and its fleeting images, as external things. However, with training the tool becomes a transparent medium *through* which she looks, an extension and enhancement of her own embodied gaze.[31]

In summary, then, the physical exam involves a largely noncollaborative perceptual hermeneutics wherein the lived body of the physician, expanded via the incorporation of relevant skills and tools, elicits and interprets the text constituted by the objectified body of the patient.

THE INSTRUMENTAL TEXT

We have seen the radical incompletion of the perceptually based texts available to the doctor and patient. Thus, machines are employed to coauthor a fuller story. The instrumental text corresponds to the third part of the traditional workup: the results of diagnostic testing. The body is assisted to speak forth in a variety of machine languages, its physiological processes translated into images, graphs, and numbers. The technologies used are *devices* in the sense discussed in chapters 4 and 5. They make available to us quickly and easily (depending on how evolved they are) information that would otherwise be burdensome, or perhaps impossible, to access.

Certain of these instrumental texts extend the perceptual hermeneutics just discussed. For example, the trained eye of the radiologist *sees* the fracture or pneumonia on X-ray, while the student still encounters a series of opaque blotches.[32] However, unlike the physical exam, this instrumentally derived text has now achieved the status of a separable artifact, detached from the body of the doctor and patient alike. The X-ray, MRI, or CT scan results are permanent, reproducible, open to inspection by anyone and everyone, and thus have come to seem the most authoritative elements of the workup.[33] (I will challenge this later.) In the physical exam, the patient's voice is quieted, but his living presence remains. Past a point, even this is no longer needed with the advent of the instrumental text. Diagnosis can be reached studying films in a remote location. The instrumental text is somewhat like a literary text in this detachability from its original authors and readers—the ill patient, the body, even the examining physician.

This text is recorded in a variety of "languages." Whereas some forms, like the CT scan, call for perceptual interpretation, others are based more in abstract representations or mathematical data.[34] Using blood chemistries to distinguish a respiratory from a metabolic acidosis is thus not a matter of educated senses but intellectual understanding. Here the "disembodiment" of the clinical text reaches its limit: the person-as-ill is translated into a series of numbers.

The Hermeneutic Telos

We have seen that a number of texts are constructed in the clinical encounter. But what are they for? When have they accomplished their goals? What, so to speak, is the hermeneutic telos of these texts? I will discuss three goals in turn: coherence, collaboration, and clinical effectiveness.

COHERENCE

We have seen the clinical encounter textualizes itself through a variety of forms—linguistic, perceptual, imagistic, mathematical. Achieving a coherent interpretation thus becomes a formidable task. The physician must interpret an X-ray shading in the context of the patient's self-reported symptoms, findings on physical exam, a relevant social history, and so on. In addition, though my discussion is based on the notion of a single treater, oftentimes multiple practitioners and technicians are involved in patient care, each with his or her own instruments and perspectives. Hence the need for, and at times the great difficulty of constructing, an integrative framework.[35]

On a material level, this framework is assisted through recording or stapling things in the patient's chart or posting to newer electronic versions thereof. The texts constructed during the diagnostic workup are collected within a single metatext, hopefully assisting a coherent narrative to emerge.

On a conceptual level, the nosology of diseases and syndromes provides the primary integrative tool. A set of discrete signs and symptoms—arthritis, a "butterfly" facial rash, proteinuria, anemia—can be unified via the single disease concept: "systemic lupus erythematosus" (SLE). The disease interpretation arrived at has multileveled significance. It not only clarifies the meaning and etiology of what is unfolding, but predelineates a future. A diagnosis of SLE triggers a prognosis, a plan for further tests, a program for appropriate therapy.

Diagnostic coherence does not come only at the end of the workup but guides it throughout. Heidegger notes that any confrontation with meaning presupposes a certain "fore-structure" of understanding.[36] That is, one's reading of a text is channeled from the start by interpretive assumptions and hypotheses, even if these later prove insufficient. This is true for the clinician. Almost from the moment the patient walks in, the doctor generates provisional diagnoses that determine which questions will be asked and what tests ordered.[37] The doctor must beware of conceptual inflexibility. Fixating too early on a judgment, which can trigger a "confirmation bias" to see only supportive evidence, may lead to a long-term misdiagnosis. So, too, can dislike for an individual ("she's a neurotic complainer") or assumptions about an entire patient population ("this emergency room is filled with alcoholics").[38] It is important to pursue information in an unhurried, open-minded way, though current time/money pressures make that a challenge. It is also important for the doctor to be honest about her limitations and learn from them. Groopman writes, "Studies show that expertise is largely acquired not only by sustained practice but by receiving feedback that helps you understand your technical errors and misguided decisions."[39]

Another phenomenon is referred to as "diagnosis momentum."[40] Once a diagnosis is formulated, even an incorrect one, it may be passed on to subordinates and associates and become difficult to question. When I was a medical student I examined a patient with a congenital polydactyly—she was having surgery to remove an extra toe. I conducted a physical exam and was expert enough to discover that her left foot indeed had six toes. When I went to record this in the chart, I found that the attending physician had written that she had six toes on her *right* foot. So, too, had recorded the resident. And so, too, the intern. Unsure of my skills, I went back and repeated my exam. Yes, in fact she had six toes on her *left* foot, not her right. Clearly, the attending physician had made a careless recording error, and the resident had gone by what the attending had written, without examining the patient, and so forth with the intern. This is a fairly innocuous, humorous example: the surgeon surely would never have operated on the wrong foot, leaving the poor woman with six and four toes each. But in how many other cases might "diagnosis momentum" lead to a case being seriously misconstrued and mistreated?

As one works through a differential diagnosis, it is thus important for the doctor to question initial intuitions. In Gadamer's terms, the text (in this case, the ill patient and the information from the medical workup) engages its reader in dialogue and may at any moment explode one's preexisting interpretations.[41] However, without a coherent set of hypotheses, generating queries and predictions, the reading is equally derailed. Many a doctor has ordered unnecessary and expensive tests on a random "fishing expedition."

Coherency can also be challenged by the sheer number of specialists, diagnostic tests, and therapeutic modalities through which a patient may process. Mol explores what happens when differing approaches to a case threaten to conflict and fragment.[42] One approach might "win out"—for example, the pathologist's report may be given pride of place or, in another situation, the clinician's assessment of symptoms. Translation terms may be found that mediate between different domains of evidence—the results of a duplex Doppler test may be correlated with what would be found on angiography, allowing physicians to understand one text in terms of the other. Finally, "composite" pictures may be used in which different modes of evidence (test results, symptom lists, social dysfunctions) are added together to yield a composite score that suggests whether treatment of a certain sort is warranted. Whatever strategy is employed, coherence remains a central hermeneutical goal. Central, but sometimes elusive, to the frustration of doctors and patients alike.

COLLABORATION

The achievement of coherence depends on effective collaboration among clinical and diagnostic team members. This depends on functional relationships, effective communication, and strategies for blending disparate kinds of information. But we must not forget about the patient. He probably initiated this quest for treatment. Its success depends on an effective patient-doctor collaboration. Here, as Svenaeus points out,[43] drawing on Gadamer's later work,[44] the model of textual reading and writing may not fully suffice. It may even be misleading if one imagines a passive object being interpreted by a subject. The "patient" is not truly "passive," though etymologically the words are related. Medicine involves a dialogical encounter between the patient and practitioner(s), which depends on mutual understanding and goal setting. In the next chapter, we will explore some of the impediments to this dialogue, which include power differences, time pressures, financial restraints, and the like. But much depends on the participants effectively working within, or overcoming, these structural problems. They should be able to talk frankly, listen attentively to one another, and employ discernment; that is, collaborate as active partners in the quest to clarify the patient's problems and achieve the patient's ends.

The groundwork for collaboration rests in structures held in common by the hermeneutic participants. The doctor, simply as a human being, can (hopefully) empathize with the patient's experience, knowing what it is to be in pain or disabled. Conversely the patient, as a member of our scientifically informed culture, usually participates to a degree in the physician's perspective. In chapter 2, I discussed how my own experience of pain changed dramatically depending on what I thought it medically signified—and this process began for me, as for many, before ever entering a doctor's office. The clinical encounter remains grounded in life-world concerns, but our life-world has also become saturated with medical meanings. Frank calls this typical of those who live in the "modern" experience, wherein the medical/technical understanding of disease has come to dominate, colonizing our language and self-understanding.[45]

However, there is still a divergence between our (at least two) collaborators. The patient continues to suffer the illness from within, which the doctor objectifies from outside. This divergence has a positive dimension. The very reason the patient seeks out the physician is for this "different point of view," more dispassionate and informed than his own. However, this divergence can also widen into an abyss if patient and doctor fail to communicate effectively. This problem can surface from the first moments of the encounter. The doctor strides in and may seem rushed or inattentive. It is well documented that physicians frequently interrupt patients as they try to tell the story of the illness in order to make history taking shorter and more efficient.[46] Yet this runs the risk that the patient may never feel *heard*.

Dialogic breakdowns can have very practical consequences. The physician who cannot participate in the patient's interpretive universe may miss crucial features of the case, fail to express empathy, squash the larger narrative structure that sustains the patient, or choose an inappropriate treatment for the person's mindset or lifestyle.

Even if the treatment prescribed is correct, it does little good if not successfully communicated to the patient. As Engelhardt writes:

> Until patients see themselves as, for example, hypertensives or diabetics, they tend to show failures of compliance. . . . They do not regularly do the things that hypertensives or diabetics ought to do, because their life-worlds are not yet structured by the relevances presumed by the physician's treatment plan.[47]

Both careful listening and explanation are thus crucial to the clinical encounter. Doctor and patient struggle to construct a discourse that successfully bridges their interpretive worlds.[48]

This is particularly true when the patient comes from a different cultural and linguistic tradition than the doctor. Fadiman's award-winning book, *The Spirit Catches You and You Fall Down: A Hmong Child, Her American Doctors, and the Collision of Two Cultures*, powerfully makes this point. From the Western doctors' point of view, infant Lia Lee suffers from epilepsy, a neurological disease based on damaged cells in the cerebral cortex. But her parents understand this as *qaug dab peg*, wherein a spirit has stolen the child's soul. From a Hmong perspective, this is dangerous but also gives the child a special sacred status. Barriers of language and belief lead to a slew of problems in diagnosis and treatment. The family is unable to understand, and at times unwilling to follow, the complicated and aggressive drug regimen the physicians prescribe.

Lia ultimately suffers a catastrophic seizure, resulting in a persistent vegetative state. Fadiman writes, "I have come to believe that her life was ruined not by septic shock or noncompliant parents but by cross-cultural misunderstanding."[49]

This dramatic example makes us wonder how often more subtle differences in culture, personality, and training undermine the doctor-patient relation.

CLINICAL EFFECTIVENESS

While interpretive coherence and effective collaboration are both essential to therapeutic success, they do not guarantee it. After all, the medical team could arrive at an agreed-on diagnosis and initiate treatment with the patient's understanding and approval, but it could be a misdiagnosis that leads to catastrophic results. Central to the hermeneutic telos is the ongoing quest for clinical effectiveness.

As Gadamer notes, any act of interpretation is closely wedded to *application*.[50] A work of art, even if centuries old, still speaks pragmatically to our situation, teaching us new ways to see and act in the world. A judge interprets law with practical ends in mind, attempting to apply it to a present case. (While Gadamer in his masterwork, *Truth and Method*, focuses on legal studies to illustrate the centrality of application, medical hermeneutics provides an equally apt example, which he did turn to later.)[51] The diagnosing physician is not primarily concerned with aesthetics or abstract truth: she seeks therapeutic results. This concern guides the diagnostic process from the start. The doctor looks not only for disease *per se* but especially for *treatable* diseases. Diagnostic categories themselves are often shaped by the modes of treatment available. For example, it became crucial to distinguish between schizophrenic, schizoaffective, and affective disorders once psychiatrists had available different classes of drugs. Chapter 4 suggested that not only is there "a pill for every ill," but "an ill for every pill." Sometimes this is driven by the search for profits, but sometimes by legitimate therapeutic advances.

In medicine, unlike most literary interpretation, the ultimate goal is an alteration in the primary text being studied—the person-as-ill. The doctor seeks not only to understand bodily events but to actively transform them. It is as if a reader studied a book with the goal of taking over its authorship. If doctor and patient can understand the principles of the malady, they can wrest the story from its anonymous malignant "author" and write a happier conclusion. At least this typifies the interventionist approach of a medicine that views the disease-as-enemy. Those holistically oriented often emphasize how the illness bears within it messages—for example, of a life that is unbalanced

and overstressed—that must be attended to in order to bring about true healing. In a certain sense, the illness arrives as your friend.

Whether consequent interventions are narrow or holistic, they can lead to a
sort of "hermeneutic circle."[52] This term commonly refers to the circular movement whereby a text is first encountered only through one's interpretive framework, although this framework is in turn modified as one continues through
the text. I may begin reading a book through a certain preunderstanding but
later discover elements of the text that change or supplement my original point
of view. Of course, in the case of a written work, a constancy underlies these
shifts. The text, for example, of *Pride and Prejudice* remains, for the most part, a
collection of fixed symbols as it passes down through the generations. The embodied textuality of medicine is different: it is actually, physically transformed
as a consequence of interpretation and application. That is, diagnosis leads to
treatment and thus to subsequent changes, for good or ill, in the sick person.
The patient's response to treatment feeds back to refine or transform the original diagnosis. This form of the hermeneutic circle need not be a vicious circle,
but one that leads to diagnostic and clinical progress.

Medical Objectivity: The Flight from Interpretation

This description of a threefold hermeneutic telos can help clarify what constitutes or impedes interpretive success. It can be applied not only to the individual doctor-patient encounter but to the structure of modern medicine at
large. That is, we can ask to what extent our medical system actually approximates these ideals of coherence, collaboration, and clinical effectiveness. Here
we return to themes from previous chapters in which we questioned the overreliance on pills, diagnostic technologies, and dehumanizing treatment and
environments, the dark shadow of modern medicine's shining achievements.

In the last chapter, I spoke of how medicine is not "authentically materialist." Nor does it authentically own up to the hermeneutical complexity
of the clinical encounter. To borrow a phrase from Marxists, a certain "false
consciousness" is at play. Clinical understanding, we have seen, involves mul-
tilayered texts and interpretations. Yet modern medicine has often been be-
witched by a different ideal—that of achieving an alloyed objectivity. The very
term "interpretation" suggests elements of subjectivity, ambiguity, opacity. In
trying to overcome these bars to absolute knowledge, medicine has sought to
escape its hermeneutical foundations and reconstitute itself as a pure science.
To explain, I will turn from synchronic to diachronic analysis, briefly tracing
the evolution of the modern medical text.

As Reiser recounts in *Medicine and the Reign of Technology*, the seventeenth century diagnostician relied heavily on the patient history, what I have termed the "narrative text."[53] The physical exam was superficial and ultimately dispensable—diagnosis was sometimes made through the mail, based on the patient's written account. Within this method personal interpretation plays an undeniably significant role. The patient, in telling his or her story, might exaggerate or minimize, misdescribe or entirely overlook key features of his case. By the end of the nineteenth century, this narrative had receded in the face of more "objective" diagnostic methods. These methods cannot be understood without reference to broader epistemological ideals sedimented in our culture determining what best counts as evidence and knowledge. I will briefly turn to two such ideals, one based in perception, the other, mathematics. This in some ways returns to but will deepen the analysis of the "absent touch" presented in chapter 3.

THE PERCEPTUAL IDEAL

Throughout Western history, knowing has been closely associated with sight.[54] Ideals of theoretical knowledge have drawn liberally on visual metaphors, from Plato's "eye of the soul" to Descartes's "light of nature." In the direct gaze, we seem to free ourselves from the vagaries of interpretation. Instead of decoding signs, inferring their meaning, we *see* the thing before us. In *The Birth of the Clinic*, Foucault recounts how this ideal of a pure gaze contributed to the rise of the pathoanatomical method.[55] Opening up a corpse, one seems to observe the disease itself. Gone is the dependency on the patient's rambling narrative or the painstaking interpretation of surface signs. A single look by the pathologist supplies the true answer—it was an aortic aneurysm! Here, in the corpse, the hermeneutical reticence of the body is apparently overcome. As Foucault paradoxically notes, "The living night is dissipated in the brightness of death."[56] This revelatory structure was to bring about a radical transformation in medical understanding. Diagnostic categories, previously organized around the patient's symptomatology, came now to be based on these visible lesions.[57]

The rise of diagnostic technology represents an attempt to achieve a similar gaze on the living. Via instruments such as the stethoscope, ophthalmoscope, and X-ray, the body interior becomes available to perception. As an eighteenth-century doctor said of the stethoscope, "We anatomise by auscultation (if I may say so), while the patient is yet alive."[58]

We thus attempt to replace the decoding of ambiguous symbols with the directness and indubitability of the gaze. I will call this a "flight from interpretation": the physician seeks an immediate perception free from hermeneutical subjectivity. But this project is doomed to fail. In opening a corpse, one does not, in fact, see the disease. One sees only marks of its former presence, whose relation to living processes must still be inferred. Nor do technologies yield a direct perception. As Ihde discusses, every instrument has an "amplification-reduction" structure that heightens certain sensory features while damping others.[59] The resulting image—the sounds heard with a stethoscope, for example—still requires interpretation. Indeed, this is true of "direct perception" itself. We early explored how even one's own pain, the very prototype of immediate sensation, is in fact mediated by one's interpretations of what the pain signifies and portends. Nor is the physician's outside gaze privileged. What she sees must be still interpreted as to its clinical meaning. Groopman discusses how MRIs and CT scans can be overwhelming in the amount of information supplied, ambiguous in what they show, subject to misinterpretation and false positives—MRIs, for example, can find abnormalities in almost everyone—and as such are an aid to, but no substitute for, clinical judgment.[60]

THE MATHEMATICAL IDEAL

Certain nineteenth-century physicians did recognize the interpretive subjectivity that always attends perceptual judgment.[61] This helped foster another epistemological ideal—that represented by quantitative data. This ideal, like the perceptual, has had a long cultural trajectory. Plato's concept of divine Forms was importantly modeled on mathematical truths that, unlike sense perceptions, seemed eternal, objective, immutable. The mathematical ideal also played a crucial role in the rise of modern science. The success of Galileo and Kepler in formulating quantitative laws of nature seemed to bespeak the privileged truth of numbers. According to Galileo's famous metaphor, nature is a book written in a mathematical language, employing the symbols of geometry. For him, as well as Descartes, only those features that could be described mathematically—height, breadth, velocity, and so on—were thought to represent true features of the object. The perceptual world, with its colors and odors, was regarded as a mere artifact of impacts on the subject's sensory organs.[62]

Imbued with this spirit of modern science, the nineteenth-century physician came increasingly to construct and value mathematical texts. An emphasis on the qualitative aspects of the pulse gave way to a focus on its count. The doctor no longer felt the patient's forehead but relied on numerical thermometry. Via the development of spirometer and sphygmomanometer, along with machines to measure electrolytes, hematocrits, and the like, ever more physiological processes could be translated into mathematical terms.[63]

Again, this textual tilt represents an attempted flight from interpretation. Physicians sought to free themselves from not only the patient's restricted perspective but also the subjectivity of their own perceptions. Only when translated into numbers did the illness seem to take a truly objective form.

Yet the search for a purified objectivity is once more doomed to fail. As Reiser argues, physicians' overreliance on such data has proved costly, both financially and relative to clinical effectiveness.[64] It has led to a neglect of the skills involved in history taking and physical examination. Quantitative data can also fall prey to problems with collecting and transporting materials, lab error, or simply individual differences and fluctuations in body chemistry that may have no clinical significance. Datasets, as much as any text, are mute without interpretation. The physician must engage in a hermeneutical process, making sense of the numbers within the context of an overarching clinical picture.

There is also a problem with the drive to "know everything there is to know" about a patient's body. It is true that technologies, both perceptually and mathematically based, can yield ever more detailed data of the interior body structure, biochemical processes, and genetic makeup. Yet an indiscriminate increase of knowledge is not necessarily a good thing. The MRI showing structural abnormalities in a spinal disk may or may not correlate with any clinical results, yet it can result in unnecessary surgery. Finding out that one has a genetic propensity for a certain disease could lead to a life lived in fear. It might have been better simply to treat the disease if it ever developed.

To personalize the topic, I recently found that I had a rising PSA (prostate-specific antigen), having followed my urologist's recommendation to take the test annually once I was past a certain age, which can help with the early detection of prostate cancer. However, is this necessarily best? PSA is a nonspecific test that can be elevated from a number of causes. Said Dr. Richard Hoffman, a general internist with a special interest in prostate disease, "Over time, evidence accumulated indicating that PSA testing could lead to overdiagnosis, thus unnecessarily subjecting men to the harms of treatment. . . . This led AUA [American Urological Association] and ACS [American College of Surgeons] to change their position away from mass screening towards informed decision making."[65] Of course, now I am anxious that I could have cancer; but also anxious that I have may have been swept by ambiguous numbers toward an invasive biopsy; and this could lead to radical surgery or chemotherapy for prostatic cancer cells that might, in fact, have been slow growing and well contained over the course of a lifetime—and thus may have been better left undiscovered. To paraphrase Aristotle's words about the virtuous mean (*Nicomachean Ethics* 2: vi), the key is not to know everything but to know the right amount about the right things for the right people in the right situation. Here enters truly "informed decision making" not only about what to do, *but what and how much to know*. Yet that which I have termed "medicine's flight from interpretation" involves an unconstrained push toward ever greater knowledge. Such may not always the path to greater wisdom.

This flight from interpretation has led to paradoxical results. Physicians have searched for an ideal of perfect presence—the immediate gaze, the unambiguous number. Yet, as explored in the last chapter, this has led medicine away from the very real presence on which it is founded: that of the living, embodied patient. The person-as-ill, what I called the primary text, tends to disappear from view when the focus is placed exclusively on privileged secondary texts. Lesions in a corpse, radiological images, numbers on a printout: these can displace our attention from the actual sick person. Such can happen not only for doctors but for patients as well, who may overfocus on a radiological finding or elevated cholesterol value.

Yet returning to threefold telos of clinical hermeneutics, a series of images and numbers do not serve well unless properly contextualized. Interpretive *coherence* is first grounded via the unity—existential and physiological—of the ill person. When the person dissolves into a collection of discrete findings, it can become difficult to form a *coherent* overview. Patients may become bewildered as they wander from office to office, each professional focused on his small part of the terrain. So, too, does doctor-patient *collaboration* suffer. The patient's own experience and concerns can seem irrelevant, even misleading, in the face of the latest set of lab results. Hermeneutic dialogue gives way to the sovereignty of doctor- and machine-speak. Such developments often then work against *clinical effectiveness*. Knowing too much and too uncritically can lead to false positives and overtreatment. Misdiagnosis and inappropriate treatment may result when the patient's perspective is not honored. So, too, can a loss of trust follow, and a refusal or inability to comply with medical recommendations. If not listened to, the patient may cease listening.

Modern medicine would do well to awaken from any dream of a purified objectivity. This dream has served a positive function, spurring medical science on to impressive conceptual and technological achievements. However, such achievements can best be employed within a context of hermeneutic humility. When it is recognized that interpretive diversity, limitation, and ambiguity cannot and should not be expunged, we can create a more effective collaboration between patients and doctors—not to mention family members, nurses, social workers, lab technicians, alternative healers, and all the other readers and writers of the complex texts of modern medicine.

Rethinking Bioethics:
Questioning Our Answers—and Our Questions

In the previous chapter, I suggested that the clinical encounter is a hermeneutical enterprise. Now I will apply this notion to bioethics, proposing that
it can modify or even transform our reading of certain cases and, to a degree,
of the discipline itself. It may be helpful to first recall and extend my brief introduction to the notion of hermeneutics.

The term first came into popular usage in the seventeenth and eighteenth
centuries. Invoking Hermes, the Greek messenger of the gods and mythical
discoverer of language and writing, "hermeneutics" was initially used to refer
to the principles of biblical interpretation.[1] Especially in the wake of the Prot-
estant revolution, clergy needed manuals of interpretation to assist them in
the exegesis of sacred scripture. Subsequently, the meaning of "hermeneutics"
was broadened to refer to the interpretation of secular as well as sacred literature, thus dovetailing with the classical discipline of philology.

Through the work of Friedrich Schleiermacher (1768–1834) and Wilhelm
Dilthey (1833–1911), hermeneutics took on an even more expansive meaning, seen as key to human understanding. For Dilthey, the human sciences
(Geisteswissenschaften) such as psychology, economics, literary criticism, and
jurisprudence involved with the subject matter of human beings, their activities and creations, employ a methodology distinct from that used in the natural sciences. Through a hermeneutical process of "understanding," one enters
into and comprehends living human experience, rather than simply "explain-
ing" a scientific object.[2]

Heidegger, as we have seen, goes even further: hermeneutics is not simply
a regional enterprise but one of ontological significance, for we interpretively
construct and experience the world in all its dimensions.[3] I interpret a visual

field as I form it preconsciously into background and foreground containing objects charged with meaning; I interpret the facial expressions of a friend during a conversation; I interpret the significance of traces on an oscilloscope, and other scientific data;[4] and so forth.

Heidegger's student, Gadamer, did much to thematize the far-reaching import of hermeneutics, especially in *Truth and Method*. Taking off from Heidegger's analysis of the "fore-structure" of understanding,[5] Gadamer suggested that all interpretation is necessarily "prejudiced."[6] This term need not be understood pejoratively. It indicates that we come to any text with a set of prejudgments shaped by our personal and cultural histories and our pragmatic interests. A contemporary individual seeking spiritual enlightenment cannot help but read the Bible differently from a fifteenth-century counterpart, or a widow coming to terms with her spouse's recent death, or a theologian gathering evidence for a scholarly paper, or a skeptic attending to the sexism of biblical images, and so on. The text opens itself up differently depending on the expectations and questions we bring. We can never find a "view from nowhere,"[7] detached from the situatedness of human life.

This bears on the notion of the "hermeneutic circle" previously discussed. In reading a text, one makes sense of a part through anticipating the meaning of the whole in which it is embedded. One has certain expectations of the story's unfolding genre, plot, and significance that shape the reading at each moment. This suggests the possibility of a circle rendering interpretation static and unscientific, for one may find in the text only what one came looking for. Yet Heidegger and Gadamer emphasize the *productivity* of the hermeneutic circle. Though one enters the circle through prejudgments, these always remain provisional and the text itself can modify or challenge them. It was written by its own authors, for its own readers, often of a different time and place. A sensitive reader permits the interpretive object its otherness. Rather than simply subsume the text within one's own categories, one engages it as a partner in respectful dialogue.[8]

We have seen the extension of this to the clinical encounter, where the doctor must remain dialogically present to the living patient, as well as responsive to the shifting nature of the diagnostic and clinical picture. (Gadamer did himself go on to write suggestive essays on medicine.)[9] I will now focus on how these ideas can apply to issues in bioethics. Throughout this chapter, I will use what I would call a "phenomenologically informed hermeneutics"—that is, one in which the embodied, contextualized situation of participants and practices, rather than abstract theory, remains the touchstone for bioethical reflection.

The Hermeneutic Structure of a Bioethical Case

Take, for example, the situation of a woman deciding whether to proceed with lifesaving surgery on her critically ill infant, born with serious birth defects. The unfolding bioethical case involves a variety of discursive elements. The deformity is imprinted on the child's body, its extent and prognosis to be interpreted by the physicians. There are technologically generated images and numbers that elucidate the clinical picture, verbal communications between the participants, medical charts in which findings are recorded, relevant legal statutes and decisions, standard procedures—whether written or secured by informal precedent—that are followed at the hospital, and so forth. Just as does a clinician, the bioethicist seeks to interpret and reconcile many texts.

This is also likely a situation involving multiple readers and writers, often with conflicting interpretations. Patients, family, and friends, the primary physician, consulting specialists, the hospital ethics committee, lawyers, sometimes even the courts or voting public, all may add perspective or render judgment. Each individual or group comes armed with a different set of prejudices (prejudgments). The mother of the defective newborn is concerned about the very real consequences—emotional, social, financial—for herself and family members of different courses of action. Her moral or religious background, economic situation, and social ties, all may influence her stance. The physician has been trained to diagnose medical pathology and, whenever possible, bring to bear the clinical armamentarium. The lawyer wishes to protect the hospital from possible liability, and so on. Different readings of the case will diverge, shaped by the disparate concerns and training people bring to bear.

That this case is perceived as posing a *bioethical quandary* also suggests that it invokes significant interpretive conflicts in the broader society. If there is a clear consensus about what is right in a given situation (for example, to treat insured and consenting pneumonic patients with the appropriate antibiotic), it becomes a simple clinical decision, not one that calls for thematized moral reflection. It is when consensus breaks down—must we provide lifesaving treatment even when a newborn is defective and critically ill and a parent wishes to halt treatment?—that we face a recognized bioethical dilemma.

Dispute arises not only about what we should do, but *what we are witnessing*—the nature of the main actors in the story, the structure of the unfolding plot, even to what narrative "genre" it belongs. Is this newborn a full-fledged person in danger of being discriminated against because of a handicap? Is this a dying child whose suffering may be prolonged by unnatural and misguided medical intervention? It is hard to agree on an appropriate end if we're not even sure what kind of a story we're reading.

Gadamer reminds us that interpretation involves questions of praxis and application.[10] This is true for the diagnosing physician, but also for the bioethicist. Bioethical interpretations are not simply free-floating theory but are bound up with recommendations for what to do. In this case, the practical consequences are of the utmost importance for the life of the child, the mother, and the larger society.

Again, we have a special kind of "hermeneutical circle," one involving living persons and unfolding in real time. The interpretations of key figures in the case give rise to real consequences that change the story: the "readers" take on authorial roles. For example, the newborn's status changes day to day based on what treatments she is or is not receiving. In a hermeneutical circle, though, the unfolding "text" is never fully subsumed, but may defy and alter one's interpretations. For example, the child may thrive in a surprising fashion even when certain therapies are withheld.

The issue of practical application is present not only in a living case but in the more theoretical discourse found within bioethics journals and textbooks. Though the issues they consider may be abstracted from any one case, this material still arises from, and responds to, real-life situations and decision making.

I have but briefly sketched out the hermeneutical structure of a bioethics issue. Perhaps of more interest is the question of how a hermeneutical sensitivity could challenge not only conventional ways of medicine but of doing bioethics. (As we shall see, advances have been made in the latter field, but in this discussion I will assume a bit the polemical tone of the reformer.) In the last chapter, I looked at how clinical medicine has engaged in a "flight from interpretation," seeking instead a purified perceptual or mathematical truth. The equivalent in bioethics would be a flight away from the phenomenological/hermeneutical richness of real-life situations, in favor of the abstractions of totalizing theory. Let me explain by turning to another case, one which builds on previous discussions.

Truth Telling and Autonomy:
A Hermeneutical Reconsideration

A patient is found to have a carcinoma with a very poor five-year survival rate. An issue arises: just how much is the physician obligated to tell the patient? We have reached a social and legal consensus that would prohibit the physician from entirely deceiving the patient about the diagnosis, though in an earlier era that might have seemed good practice. Still, we may wonder how much the doctor is obligated to detail, and whether revealing the "whole truth" is compatible with patient well-being.

A dominant tendency within bioethics is to approach such quandaries top-down by applying overarching theoretical principles. For example, a utilitarian calculus can be brought to bear, with concern for maximizing happiness and favorable outcome. This could tilt toward concealing aspects of the unfavorable prognosis that would trigger extreme anxiety or depression, perhaps even undermining compliance or clinical results. Conversely, and more commonly in contemporary bioethics, one can take a deontological approach. Whether the consequences are sanguine or not, truth telling may be viewed as an overriding obligation.

Immanuel Kant tends to be the go-to philosopher here. To deceive a patient by commission or significant omission seems to violate his "categorical imperative" on two grounds.[11] First, it fails the test of universalizability (could I will that *all* people deceive when it seems advantageous?) since the very possibility of effective discourse rests on the assumption of truth telling as the norm. Second, to conceal information fails to show respect for the rationality and autonomy of the person. If the doctor is less than fully truthful, she is manipulating the patient and depriving him of the ability to decide his course of treatment and future life in the light of true facts. The doctor is paternalistically abrogating liberty.

A general theory like this seems to supply a satisfactory method and answer. But in its abstraction from concrete particulars, much is concealed. On closer examination, "truth telling" is not a simple matter of transmitting data. The doctor uses certain tropes, metaphors, linguistic and bodily expressions that may be as important as any statistics quoted. Moreover, the patient is no passive receiver but will often indicate by questions, statements, or bodily habitus what he is ready to hear and how the information is being processed. Communication unfolds as a dialogue (again, from the Greek *logos*, "speech" or "knowledge," and *dia*, "between") in the space that both separates and connects the two participants.

Hermeneutics stresses that each of these participants will have operative prejudices (prejudgments) shaped by personal and cultural history. In this case, the physician draws on a set of experiences, values, and therapeutic philosophy that gives a personal cast to her clinical mindset. In addition to what sets her apart, she likely shares with her colleagues a communal system of understanding built up through years of training. When telling the patient he has a "cancerous tumor," she is not simply supplying "the truth"—she is telling a *medical story* about what is taking place. The patient, of course, has requested this. However, the medical story, unless carefully contextualized, may have the power to undermine or eradicate *other stories*—biographical, existential, spiritual—through which the patient interprets significant events of his life.

We have seen that illness can multiply disrupt a life, triggering a quest for meaning. The patient is a truth seeker about what is going on and why. The doctor offers one sort of truth, focused on diagnostic categories, cell types, stagings, and the like. But while reading the *person-as-ill* in this way, we have seen that other modes of interpretation may be neglected or suppressed. Leo Tolstoy's *The Death of Ivan Ilych* provides a famous example:

> To Ivan Ilych only one question was important: was his case serious or not? But the doctor ignored that inappropriate question. From his point of view it was not the one under consideration. The real question was to decide between a floating kidney, chronic catarrh, or appendicitis. It was not a question of Ivan Ilych's life or death, but one between a floating kidney and appendicitis. And that question the doctor solved brilliantly, as it seemed to Ivan Ilych. . . . All the way home [Ivan] was going over what the doctor had said, trying to translate those complicated, obscure, scientific phrases into plain language and find in them an answer to the question: "Is my condition bad? Is it very bad? Or is there nothing much wrong?"[12]

The physician's concerns and language here diverge from the patient's, shredding at the communicative tissue. Ivan goes home, distressed, confused, uncertain. All the doctor's diagnostic "brilliance" was like a gesture of power—over what has happened in Ilych's body, the questions that will and will not be answered, and the language that will be used. Frank writes of this tendency, comparing it to other modes of oppression: "Just as political and economic colonialism took over geographic areas, modernist medicine claimed the body of its patient as its territory, at least for the duration of the treatment."[13] Is this then truth telling or a kind of power play, one that nullifies or falsifies the patient's own truth?

In Kantian-style theory, truth telling is closely tied to autonomy. Only an individual armed with the facts is able to exercise the right of personal choice. But we can now turn our attention to what "autonomy" really means. Etymologically it refers to "self-rule," *auto-nomos*. But then we must ask what is this "self" and how does it exercise rulership? Hermeneutics draws attention to the role of narrativity in building one's life and self-identity into something resembling a coherent whole. This, in turn, depends on the rich legacy of available stories with which any culture is endowed.[14] These include stories of growing up; of journeys, physical or spiritual in nature; of heroes or religious figures and the exemplary way they behave; of great loves and battles; or simply the

inspiring way in which an ordinary person meets a challenge. From these stories we learn how to see ourselves, find meaning in the twist of events, and
construct worthy responses. This supports a capacity for *auto-nomos*, self-rule.

Just as we preconsciously unify a visual field into figure and ground, so
we intuitively seek the narrative coherence of our lives; when this is broken
we experience a deep loss. Serious illness can bring about such a fracturing.[15]
Career goals, love relationships, dreams of the future, suddenly thrown into
doubt, by what?—*a strange lump, a shadow on an X-ray*. As we have seen, the
shattering of our life's plot by something so absurd can be profoundly disempowering and disorienting.

Thus, lived "autonomy" is not simply something the patient *qua-rational-
subject* already possesses, as in Kantian theory. Rather, it is something the
illness has thrown into question, and perhaps diminished. For example, the
nerve problem discussed in chapter 2 that made me unsteady on my feet made
it harder to find my "footing in the world"—I lost a sense of strength, purpose,
and self-confidence, which I am still struggling to recover. As lived bodies,
our physical comportment, healthy or ill, affects our psychological and moral
capacities.

The word "text" comes from the Latin *texere*, meaning "to weave." Reclaiming an experience of autonomy can involve reweaving the text of one's life,
one that now incorporates the wounded body. The patient seeks to "make
sense" of events and to rewrite (or re-right) the story.[16] The literature debates
whether all patients do, can, or should build an illness narrative—some people
are more episodic and less "diachronic" in their way of experiencing life, and
here the physician may help best simply by offering responses to immediate
challenges.[17] But for many patients the reconstruction of long-term meaning
remains a central task.

When ill, one's life story takes a radically new turn, but it need not thereby
cease to be a coherent, even inspiring, story. The illness might be read as a
journey into the unknown, a hero's quest, a battleground, a cross to bear with
spiritual fortitude, an invitation to enhanced intimacy with others, or a call to
focus on what brings joy and lasting value.[18] As Frank writes:

> Stories have to repair the damage that illness has done to the ill person's sense
> of where she is in life, and where she may be going. Stories are a way of re-
> drawing maps and finding new destinations.[19]

It is not necessarily the job of the physician to paternalistically supply
this story. In fact, that can be dangerous. The tale that appeals to the doctor
("we're going to bring out the big guns and destroy these cancer cells") may be
inappropriate to the patient who does not want to be a bodily battleground.

The best story will usually evolve from within the patient's own interpretive framework.[20] Yet the treater can listen to and encourage this healing story, as well as grieve with the patient about illness elements that still seem random or inexplicable. (In chapter 2, we explored how chronic pain can destroy meaning.)

At times, metaphoric interpretations of illness can turn malignant: for example, blaming oneself for having a "cancer-prone personality."[21] The treater can challenge damaging elements of a narrative, such as an overemphasis on sin, guilt, and punishment, and assist a re-righting of the text.

Ideally, practitioners would be trained not only in the art of treating biomedical disease but also in treating the experiential *dis-ease* (loss of ease, security, narrative coherence) that accompanies serious illness. Charon thus calls for a revision in medical education and practice:

> A scientifically competent medicine alone cannot help a patient grapple with the loss of health or find meaning in suffering. Along with scientific ability, physicians need the ability to listen to the narratives of the patient, grasp and honor their meanings, and be moved to act on the patient's behalf. This is narrative competence, that is, the competence that human beings use to absorb, interpret, and respond to stories.[22]

In this regard, I received a lesson doing my surgery clerkship under physician-author Dr. Richard Selzer, whom I spoke of in chapter 3. I remember him introducing me to an unusual patient. The man had a skin rash, now faded, that he believed had spelled out a biblical verse on his flesh. (He was an ardent Christian.) What struck me most was the way Dr. Selzer treated this interpretation. He did not dismiss it or laugh with me about it behind the patient's back. He actually treated this story with the utmost respect—and communicated it to me with a sense of wonder, inviting me to come meet the patient and look at the faded version of the rash. I do not think for a minute Dr. Selzer himself bought this tale of divine inscription. But he knew that it provided meaning that helped the patient cope with his disease—actually, more than cope: find inspiration. And therefore Dr. Selzer delighted in this interpretation of the flesh-as-text.

In such ways, the patient's "truth" and autonomy can be supported within the clinical enconter. As Casado da Rocha and Etxeberria write, "Patient autonomy cannot be reduced to decisional autonomy: it is not so much a matter of what patients or proxies freely and knowledgeably decide at any given point, but rather an essentially conversational, dialogical process."[23] However, truth and autonomy can also be *disrupted.* The edict *primum non nocere* ("first do no harm") is often violated in the doctor's office. Many are the patients who, impaired by illness, feel more impaired once absorbed into the world of modern medicine, wherein objectification and technical jargon sets the stage for all to follow.

We have reanalyzed a clinical encounter, and issues of truth telling and autonomy, using phenomenological / hermeneutical tools rather than Kantian abstractions. But let's go further, acknowledging the multiplicity of *contexts* (from the Latin "to weave together") that are shaping the "texts" we are interpreting. For example, in a capitalist milieu, both physician and patient operate under economic constraints. Past a certain point, doctor-chat of the sort that might optimally support the patient's narrative construction is not reimbursable. A physician or hospital makes greater profits through seeing more patients for briefer times and ordering expensive tests and procedures. Another reality is that the patient's "autonomy" may be limited by economic factors. He may come to understand from the doctor the facts of his condition and the best available treatment, but discover his insurance company will not reimburse for it. Good clinical care remains an unaffordable luxury for many in our society. Do medical "truths" that the patient cannot act on still preserve his "autonomy"?

In other ways, the patient is disempowered from the first moments of the clinical encounter. The physician begins in a multiply determined position of authority.[24] The doctor, after all, is the healthy one; the patient, sick. The doctor has the medical expertise that the patient lacks, the ability to order tests, schedule procedures, and write prescriptions. Within the world of the clinic, the doctor governs time and space; that is, the patient is made to wait until the physician is ready (often long after the appointment time) and is then directed what to do. There the patient sits or lies half-naked, perhaps in a hospital gown embarrassingly open in the back. The well-dressed doctor strides in, maintaining the privileged upright posture,[25] often "speaking down" to the patient whom she probes.

Oliver Sacks, the renowned neurologist, encountered the world of medicine from the other side when he suffered a severe neurological injury. He discovered a dis-ability that was not only bodily and existential but

> was "moral"—not quite an adequate word—associated with the reduced stationless status of a patient, and, in particular, conflict with and surrender to "them"—"them" being the surgeon, the whole system, the institution—a conflict with hateful and even paranoid tones, which added to the severe, yet neutral, physical affliction a far less tolerable, because irresoluble, moral affliction. I had felt not only physically but morally prostrate—unable to stand up, stand morally before "them," in particular, before the surgeon.[26]

If the distinguished Dr. Sacks felt this, how much more so the ordinary patient, far less informed and perhaps also of a lower socioeconomic status than the doctor. Race and gender differences may reinforce this pattern: imagine, for example, a lower-income, elderly Latina under the treatment of a white male physician. Focusing on gender, Young describes how even healthy women are already conditioned by a sexist society to experience their bodies in ways that involve objectification and limitation; for example, they have learned to "throw like a girl" rather than to use and feel the full strength of their bodies.[27] Such a "preexisting condition" (being female in a sexist context) can be synergistically reinforced when a woman falls ill, and is objectified by the medical system.[28] This can increase the already present sense of bodily limitation.

Do such medical contexts, then, enhance autonomy, not as theorized about but *as truly lived*? The diagnosis pronounced, the esoteric terminology used, the treatment options recommended, can at times profoundly disempower the patient. Foucault has suggested that modern institutions enact power over individuals through a complex interweaving of language and practices, all of which promise to be liberatory—cooperate and you will be "cured," or "normal," or "forgiven," or "reformed."[29] So, too, medical language and practices promise healing, and sometimes deliver. Yet one must enter a world that is all too-often financially driven, bureaucratic, depersonalized, and at times invasive, painful, and humiliating. Truth telling? Autonomy? Deontological theory does not get at the dense context, and contestations, of the medical world.

What a Hermeneutical Bioethics Does and Does Not Do

Perhaps, though, an issue like "truth telling" seems too easy a place to make one's case for a hermeneutical bioethics. Is this sort of method applicable to a wide range of topics? I believe so. Consider standard bioethical issues involving euthanasia, abortion, informed consent for research, surrogacy, genetic testing, and so forth. In each case, our knowledge and praxis are deepened insofar as we are sensitive to the experience and viewpoints of multiple participants; the institutional settings involved; and the multiple contexts—social, economic, religious, political—that shape the emergence and interpretation of such bioethical quandaries. In the next chapter, I will use organ transplantation as an extended example of this approach.

In addition to enriching our understanding of canonical bioethics issues, a phenomenologically informed hermeneutics may introduce some new ones.[30] For example, Agich explores how the layout of a long-term care facility, and the infantilizing nature of the speech used with residents, tends to disempower and disorient in ways that can imitate or worsen senile dementia.[31] Similarly, Young focuses on the loss for many nursing home residents of the true experience of *having a home*—including privacy where one can be unobserved and the ability to arrange one's personal space in a way that supports one's identity and autonomy.[32] Similarly, for those receiving home care for chronic illnesses, the home can become a contested space, wavering between the private and the public, a place in which one is cared for and/or invaded.[33] As another example of a new kind of bioethical issue, Dyck traces out the particular challenges faced by women with multiple sclerosis and how they skillfully renegotiate their shrinking social and geographical worlds.[34]

After all, it is not simply the practitioner who is a moral actor but also the ill person (and loved ones). Though defined as *"patient,"* he is also an *agent* wrestling with profound existential challenges.[35] This is captured well by many personal stories of illness, so-called pathographies.[36] In the face of the disintegrations brought about by illness, the sick person still bears responsibility—that is, the "ability to respond." Depending on the qualities of this response, the individual can cave in to bitterness and despair, or forge a good life even in the face of suffering.[37]

Special virtues are called for in meeting well the challenges of illness—for example, humor, courage, patience, hope, humility, practical wisdom, generosity, and proper assertiveness. Alas, illness can also expose failures of character in sick people and those around them. Sacks describes a moment when, still impaired by his seriously injured leg, he gazes at school teams practicing rugby:

> I was surprised and appalled at a spasm of hate in myself. I hated their careless exuberance and freedom—their freedom from the limitations which I felt, so overwhelmingly, in myself. I looked at them with virulent envy, with the mean rancor, the poisonous spite of the invalid.[38]

Luckily Sacks recovers—morally as well as physically—but not all chronically patients do so. In retrospect, he reflects:

> If we have fame, fortune, favor, fulfillment, it is easy to be nice, to turn a warm heart to the world. But let us be disfavored, disfigured, incapacitated, injured; let us fall from health and strength, from fortune and favor; let us find ourselves ill, miserable and without clear hope of recovery—then our mettle, our moral character, will be tried to the limit.[39]

Sickness is an arena that calls us to question, test, and reforge who we really are and wish to be. We may meet our moral limits, but there is also a "pedagogy of suffering" that can enrich and deepen us, and give us something to gift to others.[40] *Yet this moral arena is often erased from medical ethics.* Just as the patient can be rendered passive, almost forgotten, within the clinical encounter, so too within bioethical discourse.

Remembering the experience and moral status of the patient can also lead to a correlative re-visioning of the practitioner. The most significant issue in one's career is often not "what action do I take here?" (the focus of utilitarian or deontological ethics) but "what kind of person and professional should I best be?" (the focus of virtue ethics). For example, the isolation and incapacity of the ill might call for the treater to exercise special virtues, such as compassion and trustworthiness.[41]

The customary bioethical focus on quandary cases can foreclose the modes of investigation with which we have been engaged—the subtle "micro-physics" of institutional power, and how to meet well the challenges of illness and old age. These topics are not as dramatic as those that make bioethics headlines, but certainly are as important, affecting us all.[42]

Bioethics is often operationalized within health-care settings by institutional committees. These too tend to concentrate on quandary cases: for example, those concerned with terminating life-sustaining treatment. These committees are largely made up by professionals. On the way to decision making, there is often little focus on patient complaints or attempts to include the narrative voices of the ill.[43] Nor do such committees usually consider the broader (but often subtler) "moral ecology" of their institutions: who is admitted, the quality of patient-staff interactions, the layout of particular wards, the treatment of family members, and all the other ingredients that make for a healing or disruptive environment. We can imagine a re-forming of such committees taking account of the sort of hermeneutical bioethics here outlined.

What other uses would such a bioethics have? Instead of employing ethical theory to generate the "right answer," hermeneutics tends to honor and help articulate the multiplicity of perspectives. In medicine, this may be especially useful in terms of giving voice to those who are silenced or excluded by institutional structures, be it the patient, family members, or others involved. As Charon writes, this alters power dynamics:

> With narrative competence, multiple sources of local—and possibly contradicting—authority replace master authorities; instead of being monolithic and hierarchically given, meaning is apprehended collaboratively, by the reader and the writer, the observer and the observed, the physician and the patient.[44]

Contradiction, and collaboration—the hermeneutical bioethicist is attentive to both and, when possible, a facilitator of dialogue even on contentious issues. For example, abortion calls forth some incommensurate narratives concerning "the woman's right to her own body" versus "the developing child's right to life." Yet advocates on both sides may share respect for human dignity (be that ascribed to the woman or the child); with safeguarding the rights of the disempowered (again, woman, or child); and a desire to minimize reliance on abortion as a mode of birth control, and to maximize social and financial support for raising children even under disadvantaged circumstances.[45] There thus may be an opportunity for communication and common cause even among traditional opponents.

The hermeneut not only helps articulate the experience and viewpoints of participants, and to facilitate dialogue, but also recollects contexts that may be systematically obscured even from the participants themselves. Ricoeur suggests we have entered an age characterized by the "hermeneutics of suspicion." Marx, Freud, and Nietzsche have taught us to look beneath the surface text to uncover hidden forces at play in shaping individuals and societies.[46] Whether as a result of ideological distortion (Marx), psychological repression (Freud), the will to power (Nietzsche)—or simply the difficulty of seeing structures in which one is immersed like a fish in water—it can be hard to understand the source of one's own positions. (Here I am taking up Gadamer's stance, contra Habermas, that hermeneutics can explore contexts that shape action in ways the actors themselves may be unaware of.)[47] In the next chapter, I will use organ transplantation to investigate such contexts—philosophic, historic, economic—that condition this practice. Being aware of these contexts, I will also suggest, can help free their hold upon us, allowing us to think anew.

I began this chapter with a meditation on "truth telling." Heidegger points out that the ancient Greek word for truth, *aletheia*, etymologically means something like "unhiddenness," "unconcealment," or "disclosure." For Heidegger, this originary sense of truth goes beyond the correspondence between a proposition and the thing represented. Truth in the sense of *aletheia* involves the disclosure, the bringing to light, of something hitherto concealed (although such presencing goes hand-in-hand with the concealment of other elements).[48]

This is a way of understanding the roles of the bioethicist here proposed. Disclosure is accomplished by allowing multiple perspectives to emerge, questioning taken-for-granted contexts and subtexts, and avoiding the closure provided by theory-driven claims to truth. Even the very questions of bioethics may thereby come into question. Why and how did we arrive at these specific dilemmas, and which other questions are being concealed? When we focus on specific quandaries, like end-of-life decisions, we often leave *unquestioned* many other practices and presumptions undergirding modern medicine and the larger society.

Of course, specific decisions still need to be made. Interpretation ever guides praxis. Do we pull the plug or not on the critically ill newborn? Give the liver transplant to the desperately sick alcoholic, or rather to an elderly humanitarian? At some point, hermeneutic explorations need to give rise to concrete choices. Hopefully, sensitivity to lived experience, and to the broader contexts that shape dilemmas, will eventuate in better decision-making processes and results—that is, ones that are more attentive, nuanced, and efficacious.

This can apply not only to an individual case but to social policy and legislation. For example, Dyck[49] explores a "caring space" (emotional, spatial, practical) that may develop between the often lower-income women who are both recipients and givers of home care. Yet this caring space can be undermined by governmental mandates and cuts. Dyck's work shows how costly such "cost savings" can be. We often wish social policy to be data-driven, but it should include *experiential data*, not simply mathematized measures.

Finally, this new bioethics suggests a need to refashion professional training. As Jacobson points out,[50] there has been encouraging movement in the last decade, particularly in the field of nursing, toward a phenomenologically rooted ethics education. A report, supported by a Carnegie Foundation grant, calls for a radical change in how nurses should approach ethics.[51] This goes hand-in-hand with increased attention in medicine to the lived experience of patients in hospital design, patient care, research studies, and medically relevant literature written for laypeople.[52]

More physician-training programs are offering courses in the medical humanities, for example, in a literature-based "narrative training" designed to help doctors be sensitive to their patients' stories, as well as their own stories and that of colleagues.[53] Some programs have even experimented with "virtual reality simulators" designed to give medical practitioners a taste of the diseases they treat. For example, strapping a thick belt around the chest can be used to stimulate angina pain (though probably not the full-blown panic that might accompany a true crisis).[54] Sacks[55] and other doctors testify that nothing fosters understanding and empathy so much as a taste of illness and "patienthood."

Sensitivity to the patient's story and experience, validation of multiple voices that the medical system tends to suppress, the disclosure of the workings of power and profit hidden beneath taken-for-granted practices: these are all elements of a phenomenological/hermeneutical bioethics. The result can be a more careful reading—and writing—of our biomedical world.

Rethinking Organ Transplants:
Whose Body, What Body?

For another, more sustained example of a phenomenologically sensitive hermeneutics at work, I now turn to the practice of organ transplantation. The previous two chapters focused on the individual doctor-patient relationship, including issues of truth telling and autonomy that arise within that encounter. Here I turn instead to an entire field of medicine, one relevant to a variety of diseases and specialties. I will look at specific bioethical issues raised by organ transplants. I will also suggest that organ transplantation takes us right to the heart (pun intended) of modern medicine, even modern culture in general, and their ways of viewing the body. Yet it also invites a deep *rethinking of embodiment*. As such, this will be our culminating chapter on matters medical.

Let's start with a brief survey of current practices. We now transplant hearts, kidneys, livers, lungs, corneas, bone marrow, spleens, pancreases, along with a multitude of soft tissues and fluids, such as blood, skin, and gametes.[1] Over time, transplantation has moved from the status of experimental procedure to routine therapy.[2] Both the demand and numbers performed are ever increasing. Novel methods for keeping the organs of the newly brain-dead suitable for transplantation, new immunosuppressive drugs that help prepare the host to receive the donor organ, advances in surgical technique, all are making transplantation a feasible option in a widening range of situations.

Whereas in 1978 there were fewer than 30 transplant centers in the United States, a check of state registries (2015) now shows more than 230. The possibilities for future growth of this industry are enormous. For example, the United States has about 1.25 million insulin-dependent diabetics who could benefit, in theory, from new pancreases.[3] Then, too, the morally controversial use of fetal tissue, which regenerates rapidly and is far less likely to provoke host rejection, if permitted could be the source of a multitude of clinical benefits. As with the fantasy of "the pill" discussed in chapter 4, the dream of "the organ transplant" as a solution for distressed bodies is a seductive one for the medical and general community. (It is also possible that eventually "tissue engineering"—in which parts of organs are grown from cells cultivated in the lab—may significantly displace transplantation technology, but this would bring its own clinical and bioethical issues.)

Increased demand has come into conflict with limitations of supply. Certain organs or organ parts, such as kidneys and pieces of liver or bone marrow, can be given while the donor is still alive. In recent years, living donations have also expanded to include parts of pancreases, intestines, and lungs. Other organs can be taken only from cadavers. In both cases, there are chronic shortages in the United States. The Uniform Anatomical Gift Act, drafted in 1968 and adopted in some form in all states by 1973, permits individuals to will their organs for scientific and medical usage after death, or permits their relatives to donate the deceased's cadavers. Updates of this act allow drivers' licenses to carry their owners' organ-donors status. The hope that demand for cadaver organs would be met by such voluntary contributions has proved a disappointment. For example, some 100,000 patients require a kidney donation, but the maximum number of deceased organ donors has been estimated at 15,000 or less, while living donations have fallen below 6,000.[4] Even "required request" legislation on the federal and state levels mandating that hospitals ask families for permission to donate organs from their recently deceased family members has done little to alleviate the problem: health-care workers are often loath to make such a request hard on the heels of a loved one's death. The waiting list for organs continues to grow, as many thousands of patients die while awaiting a needed organ. Bioethical debates arise around who should be saved under conditions of scarcity.

It is in this context that a cash market for organs has been proposed as one method for alleviating the shortage. The National Transplant Act of 1984 makes it a crime to buy, sell, or otherwise benefit from commerce in organs in the United States. At the time of writing, only Iran allows and supports a legal system for the selling of kidneys.[5] Certain countries, such as India, that used to permit such sales have now banned them; yet often they still allow thriving black markets, which hospitals and local governments tacitly tolerate.[6]

Is it clear such practices should be illegal? If individuals or their family members could sell organs during life or after death, the mechanisms of the marketplace might make organs available to tens of thousands in desperate need, while helping the sellers to climb out of poverty. Another less radical possibility is to inaugurate in the United States the sort of "presumed consent" system used in some European countries. That is, one is automatically classified as a potential organ donor unless one intentionally "opts out." I will later turn to such questions.

The range of its medical applications, and of the bioethical issues provoked by transplantation, makes it worthy of note. But as I said earlier, there is another reason to turn to this topic here: I believe it helps clarify the modern sociomedical way of viewing and treating *the distressed body*. As Dowie writes:

> Sometimes it is insufficient to examine a technology by itself, it being merely a symptom of a larger paradigm. Such may be the case with organ transplanting, which is surfacing as the clearest metaphor we have for contemporary Western healing. Transplantation must be regarded, therefore, as more than a stand-alone technology. It should, in fact, be observed as a window on modern medicine.[7]

Here we return to themes from the first section of this book. In chapter 4, I examined pills and how they, too, serve as a "window on modern medicine." I discussed alternatives such as healing touch (chapter 3) and other examples of an authentic medical materialism at play (chapter 5). In those chapters, the philosophical backdrop was briefly sketched, but the primary focus remained on clinical practice. Now, I will turn more sustained attention to the core paradigms that have shaped modern Western approaches to the body. I will first focus on Descartes and his metaphysics. Next, I query the body as subsumed within capitalism. These two systems, we will see, operate synergistically to undergird the practice of organ transplantation. The following chapter will examine similar forces at play in our treatment of animal bodies. In both cases, this hermeneutic will allow critique of current practices but also suggest possibilities for their reformation.

Cartesianism and the Body-Machine

Descartes, in a story often told, defined the human being as a compound of two very different substances. The true self was identified most closely with an immaterial mind or soul—"I can infer correctly that my essence consists solely in the fact that I am a thinking thing."[8] The body is more something I *have*, a material object with which I am intimately conjoined but without which I could continue to exist—hence his assertion of the immortality of the soul. Though Descartes at times recognized a depth of mind-body union that seemed to challenge his own dualist metaphysics and psychology,[9] it is this dualism that has had the most profound effects in the culture and that I will hereafter refer to as "Cartesian."

Within this paradigm, the human body is seen as a part of *res extensa*, a machine operating according to material principles. Impressed by the automata of his day, for example, the hydraulically powered machines in royal grottoes and fountains, Descartes suggested that the body could be thought of as a complex automaton motored by a variety of physical forces.

Material nature in general was viewed as devoid of intrinsic subjectivity and consciousness. This "death of nature," to use Merchant's phrase,[10] played a crucial role in subserving the modernist, mechanist project of mastery. Descartes writes in the *Discourse on Method* of a "practical philosophy" through which

> we could know the power and action of fire, water, air, the stars, the heavens and all the other bodies in our environment, as distinctly as we know the various crafts of our artisans; and we could use this knowledge—as the artisans use theirs—for all the purposes for which it is appropriate, and thus make ourselves, as it were, the lords and masters of nature.[11]

Descartes's dream of better living through science and technology has a general reach, but also a *medical* specificity. He continues:

> This is desirable not only for the invention of innumerable devices which would facilitate our enjoyment of the fruits of the earth and all the goods we find there, but also, and most importantly, for the maintenance of health, which is undoubtedly the chief good and the foundation of all the other goods in this life. . . . [W]e might free ourselves from innumerable diseases, both of the body and of the mind, and perhaps even from the infirmity of old age, if we had sufficient knowledge of their causes and of all the remedies that nature has provided.[12]

Descartes regarded this pursuit of medical knowledge and power as a cornerstone of his life's work. His goals may have been altruistic, but they were also rooted in personal concerns with aging and dying. For example, in 1637 he wrote to Huygens,

> The fact that my hair is turning gray warns me that I should spend all my time trying to set back the process. That is what I am working on now, and I hope my efforts will succeed even though I lack sufficient experimentation.[13]

Two months later, in another letter to Huygens, Descartes writes:

> I have never taken such pains to protect my health as now, and whereas I used to think that death might rob me of thirty or forty years at most, it could not now surprise me unless it threatened my hope of living for more than a hundred years.[14]

This biographical material relates to a broader cultural project. When compared to the religious medieval period, secularized modernity has suffered a collective crisis of faith. We fight desperately to stave off death, no longer as sure of having an eternal destiny. Though Descartes ostensibly sought to prove the existence of God and the immortality of the soul (there is some scholarly disagreement about whether this was sincere or a self-protective gesture), he also seeks to extend the power and longevity of the living body. As the protocol for an early computer conference proclaimed, "We are as gods and might as well get good at it."[15] Descartes's battle to protect and extend bodily life continues to be waged through new medical advances and the increasing proportion of our economy devoted to end-of-life health care. In Slatman's words, "The most characteristic strangeness of our time is not the bizarre nature of technological feats, but our sustained effort to defer death."[16]

Organ transplantation is a potent symbol and result of this cultural trajectory.[17] We see this not only in the goal of transplantation, its battle against illness, aging, and death, but also in the methodology it employs. The Cartesian mechanization of the material world helped overturn all prohibitions against tampering with nature. When the earth was thought of as sacred and ensouled certain invasive interventions, such as mining, were constrained—it was seen as an abortion, interfering with the gestation of metals in the earth's womb.[18] Similarly, there were often taboos against cutting up the live and dead human body. All these taboos can fall away, however, if natural bodies are simply mindless matter. The extracting and transplanting of organs becomes permissible. It would even be encouraged insofar as we are meant to defeat illness and aging, properly assuming the mantle of "lords and masters of nature."

Moreover, transplantation exemplifies the modus operandi of Cartesian science: to understand and control natural bodies by *analyzing* them into their component parts. Descartes rejected the essential holism of Aristotelian "substantial forms" in favor of a reductionist strategy. A thing is viewed as the sum of its parts and forces in interaction; we come to understand an object by "taking it apart" both in theory and practice. This analytic knowledge then yields power. As Jonas writes of modern science, "To know a thing means to know how it is or can be made and therefore means being able to repeat or vary or anticipate the process of making."[19] We see this scientific/technological power reflected in transplantation. The body is analyzed into its component organs, which can be replaced by machine analogues, or parts from living human donors, cadavers, or animals (or, in the future, from tissue cultures). We advance toward the Cartesian dream of remaking the body at will.

As I write these words, I have recently undergone a surgery seeking to resolve the peripheral neuropathy described in chapter 2. If necessary, the surgeon was simply going to cut the damaged nerve and deaden the region—though this can lead to subsequent problems. However, he found it possible to graft in a portion of a cadaver nerve tube that had been frozen until the time of use. This provides an acellular protein scaffold into which my own nerve, the damaged portion cut away, can regenerate at the rate of about a millimeter a day. I am happy to embrace this very new kind of transplant, which is already helping my leg to heal and my world to expand. Yesterday I took my dog on an hour-and-a-half walk in the woods. Bliss!

The Cartesian spirit of modern medicine has thus led to many powerful applications. They have contributed greatly to the successful treatment of disease and the extension of vigor and longevity that Descartes envisioned. We cannot dismiss his dream lightly, for it has spared us many a nightmare. However, the Cartesian worldview and its medicine has also given rise to nightmares of its own from which we are just beginning to awake.

The modernist attempt to overcome death proceeded from the start through its own strategics of death: the reconceptualization of the physical world as lifeless matter. This has brought about a kind of "death of nature," not only conceptually but in practice. A path has been cleared for massive technological manipulation with sometimes catastrophic outcomes. Pollution of the air and water, disruption of ecological systems, factory farming, species extinctions, depletion of the ozone layer, and global climate change are but a few phenomena that speak to us of the very real death of nature that threatens to consume us with it.

In the next chapter, I will explore more the conceptual/physical "death of animals." Insofar as animal bodies are treated as unconscious machines, without soul or meaningful subjectivity, we can mistreat them with impunity. This topic, in fact, is not unrelated to organ transplants. As Dowie writes, "An incalculable number of animals—mostly dogs, cats, pigs, horses, rabbits, calves, goats, rats, mice, chimpanzees, baboons or other simians—have died for the advancement of transplantation."[20]

As we can speak of the modernist "death of nature" and "death of animals," so too a sort of "death of the human body" has been brought about in the name of perpetuating bodily life. In Kimbrell's words:

> The body is not a machine. That is the "pathetic fallacy" in reverse. The original pathetic fallacy had the unruly passions of the human spirit inhabiting stones, trees, and rivers. Now we seem to believe that nothing has soul: We are all *inanimata*, analogous to machines or factories, and can be treated as such.[21]

If the modern doctor and hospital have often been criticized for delivering cold, depersonalized care, our hermeneutics of the body reveals the key role of Cartesian metaphysics. Once the body is understood according to the model of a machine, the rest follows logically. Does the mechanic explain matters compassionately to a car? He or she diagnoses and fixes it, then bills the owner. Though there are many humane practitioners (and I have been impressed by the caring attitude of the doctors who have treated me), the disease categories, technologies, treatment protocols, and institutions of medicine, all built on a Cartesian foundation, exert a powerful pull toward dehumanized care. We have explored such issues in part 1, and I will here say no more.

However, it is not surprising to find that organ transplants, as "a window on modern medicine," can open onto some troublesome vistas. Replacing part of one's body with another brings with it a slew of costs: not only the enormous price tag of the procedures and their sequelae but also the human costs associated with the chronic rejection syndrome, which leads to the failure of large numbers of organ transplants. (This was not an issue in my case since the cadaver nerve tube contained no living tissue.) Even for those who come to "accept" their organs using immunosuppressive drugs, there can be deep medico-experiential costs. Varela, in the aftermath of a liver transplant, describes how "a new lifestyle of masks, careful watching for the slightest sign of fever, and concern about opening windows, makes the body into a life of withdrawal, its proud movement and agency shrivelled down."[22] French philosopher Jean-Luc Nancy writes, after his heart transplant:

> The possibility of rejection establishes a strangeness that is two-fold: on the one hand, the foreignness of the grafted heart, which the host body identifies and attacks inasmuch as it is foreign; and, on the other, the foreignness of the state that the medical regimen produces in the host body, to protect the graft against rejection.[23]

In his case he was weakened and sickened by his immunosuppressive treatments, and eventually developed a related cancer.

In addition to the costs borne by individuals are hidden social prices we collectively pay. For example, the ever-growing popularity of transplantation and its metaphorical power within the public consciousness can serve to perpetuate many of the diseases that transplantation treats. The reasons behind this echo ones discussed in relation to our fantasy of the quasi-magical pill (chapter 4). We have seen that transplantation exemplifies the modern sense of body-as-machine and of disease as residing within a specific organ. This tends to discourage "holism" not only in medical treatment, but in understanding and addressing the etiology of disease. Thus, transplantation does little to encourage preventive approaches wherein individuals take responsibility for a healthy lifestyle and proper self-care. On the contrary, if one's diseased parts can be replaced, why worry so much? Nor need the broader causes of disease be tackled, such as air, food and water pollutants, occupational exposures, poverty, malnutrition, and stress-filled environments. Disease is not conceptualized as a product of the social field so much as confined within a replaceable organ. Meanwhile, the public monies allotted to transplantation represent resources that otherwise might have been used to address these social problems, or to foster preventive health care and education.

In addition to this problematic side of organ transplantation, there is something disquieting about its implicit reductionism vis-à-vis the human being. The Cartesian project is a kind of humanism, unlocking the potentials of our reason and praxis. Yet when we attempt to overmaster the natural world, we find that we ourselves are part of it and thus discover ourselves in a position of subjugation. We are so intimately one with our bodies that if the body is treated in a reductionist way, the self is also diminished. Hence the paradoxes of modern clinical treatment—the patient reaches out for all the powers of medicine, but feels degraded under the doctor's gaze; elders are promised the dream of near-immortality, but undergo needlessly prolonged deaths through high-tech care. The sense of vulnerability and suffering envelops even physicians, whose rates of suicide and substance abuse are inordinately high. Doctors labor under the specter of patient, bureaucratic, and self-imposed expectations, including the ever-present fear of failure and litigation. Even the most "powerful" within the system thus experience powerlessness.

We find this reduction of self most pronounced in regard to those whose selfhood is least established. In the area of transplantation, there has been a call to utilize the organs of newborn anencephalic babies who will shortly die or fetuses who are being electively aborted. Least person-like by standards of developed awareness and sociality, these beings can be most easily conceived of as *just* a body, a collection of organs qua valuable resource. At the other end of the lifespan, we can do the same with the corpse. Though almost all cultures recognize the inherent dignity, often sacredness, of the dead body so strongly identified with the once-living person, from the dualist perspective it is just meat and mechanics. Why not cut and extract its useful pieces?

This reductionism can be extended to others whose personhood is socially marginalized. Reports from the People's Republic of China suggest that the government has seized organs from live dissidents and executed prisoners. In third-world countries such as India, the sale of kidneys from the poor to those seeking transplants has developed into a multimillion dollar industry.[24] One can imagine further science fiction extensions wherein groups or entire societies are converted into organ farms to be harvested by the privileged.[25] Whatever possibilities actually play out, they are grounded in a Cartesian logic. When the body is viewed as a machine, our quest to be "lords and masters" of nature can also lead to practices of enslavement. Metaphysical issues intersect with those of a political-economic nature.

The Body within Capitalism

For such reasons, I will here make some general observations about the body within capitalism, the dominant economic system in many countries where transplantation has been most developed and utilized. For a time we will wander from the topic of organ transplantation, but only to return with fresh perspectives. We will see how Cartesian and capitalist paradigms intersect in the harvesting, sale, and distribution of organs.

First, the body surfaces within capitalism as an agent of *production*. The laborer uses muscle power and manual dexterity to produce a variety of goods and services. The more efficiently and productively the body can be employed, the more profitable the results. (In the next chapter, we will observe how this also applies to animal bodies.) Hence most of us receive training from early on concerning how to discipline our bodies and maximize their utility.[26] Even after the workday ends, we multitask, talking on the phone while simultaneously putting away dishes.

Undoubtedly, one reason the Cartesian machine-body has proved so popular in our culture is that it resonates with and supports the body appropriate to capitalism. If maximum productivity is the goal, employees should operate in a machine-like fashion—rapidly, dependably, efficiently, ideally requiring little maintenance or training, and easily replaceable. Though proponents of advanced technology have promised that devices will relieve humans of the most mechanical tasks, Garson argues in *The Electronic Sweatshop* that they have often done the reverse. The intelligence involved in running a McDonald's restaurant is located in sophisticated protocols, computer programs, electronic systems—but what's left for the people? As an ex-worker describes:

> You follow the beepers, you follow the buzzers and you turn your meat as fast as you can. It's like I told you, to work at McDonald's you don't need a face, you don't need a brain. You need to have two hands and two legs and move 'em as fast as you can.[27]

We are reminded of the Cartesian body-automaton, devoid of intentionality.

In fairness, it should be noted that it is not only capitalism but communism (as practiced, not as Marx envisioned it) that has embraced man-the-

machine. Aleksei Gastev, a Bolshevik engineer who headed the Central Institute of Labor in the 1920s, oversaw the mechanization of Soviet Russia.
His stated aim was to turn the worker into a sort of "human robot," imitating mechanized movement. "Hundreds of identically dressed trainees would
be marched in columns to their benches, and orders would be given out by
buzzes from machines."[28] Maximizing production holds a powerful allure
across different economic systems.

Within capitalism, the body is taken up not only as this producer-machine,
but also as property, a *commodity* for possible exchange. In the modern era,
the body has sometimes been considered the paradigmatic example of private
property, such that other forms of ownership are derivative, based on the
body's labor.[29] As property, the body can be exchanged on the open market.
In a sense this lies at the foundation of the wage-labor system: the worker sells
her labor-power (to use Marx's term) to the employer for a period of time.
It might be denied that this is selling the body per se, for labor is but one of
the body's renewable expressions. However, the distinction is tenuous. The
McDonald's worker is selling—or we might say renting— his "two hands and
two legs" to the corporation for its use. This body (to again use Marx's term) is
alienated from the self.

This style of body-regard diffuses into many domains. For example, in por-
nography and prostitution the intimate arena of sexuality gets commodified
through the sale of body images or services. In a generalized way, sexualized
imagery comes to pervade modern commerce, also shaping our private imag-
inings. Products are posed next to an alluring model. His or her (often *her*)
body image has been airbrushed into an unrealizable ideal of the human form,
illustrating a kind of erotic quasi-Platonism. Such practices are compatible with
capitalist economics. The visual image of the body is easier to detach and sell,
and use to sell products than, for example, the tactile elements discussed in
chapter 3.

In all cases, whether selling bodily labor, images, powers, or parts, the ability to commodify the body depends on being able to regard it as *other*, detachable from the essential self. As Marx writes, "A commodity is, in the first place,
an object outside us."[30] Again, we see why the Cartesian model is congenial to
capitalist structures. Descartes notes that I "have" or "possess" a body that is
essentially distinct from the thinking thing I am. We can regard our bodies
as alienable commodities insofar as we have been well prepared by dualistic
metaphysics.

In addition to the body as *producer* and *commodity*, it plays a crucial
role within capitalism as the *consumer* of goods. That is, the body is the locus of needs and desires that provoke purchases. We not only have physical

requirements to be satisfied—for food, clothing, shelter—but a virtually un-limited set of potential cravings that it is the business of advertising to stimu-late. We are called to ornament the body, give it pleasures and comforts, in-toxicate, transport, transform, or heal it. First, we are often reminded of bodily deficiencies. Bad breath may drive away potential consorts; cellulite is intoler-ably ugly. The strategics of body insecurity trigger the purchase of that which will make us whole. In chapter 4, we saw how the pill serves as such a com-modity, easily reproducible, transportable, purchased, and ingested—whereon another and another are soon needed.

But let us turn back to our topic of organ transplantation. I will suggest that here we see another kind of "ideal case" that even more clearly demon-strates the position of the body within capitalism. In fact, in the practices of organ transplantation we see bodies taken up as producers, commodities, and consumers all.

As discussed above, the productive-body is ideally something of an autom-aton, fashioning its product cheaply, reliably, mindlessly. One wants an indefi-nite supply of workers who require little training and are easily replaced. In the case where *the product is a transplantable body organ*, ideal conditions to a degree are fulfilled. Everyone can and does make one without training or talent. The supply of producers is virtually unlimited. Of course, each worker can produce only one or two of each key organ, and in many cases the donor must die appropriately (as through a youthful motorcycle accident) before the product can be "harvested."

Just as the production mode approximates a certain ideal, so the body organ is a kind of ideal commodity. One no longer need contrive a detachable image or service; body parts themselves become the product for exchange. Moreover, this commodity promises to satisfy the greatest need a consumer-body can have, that for continued health or life.

The potential market is almost indefinitely extensible. After all, everyone has a body, and all bodies ultimately run down and break. Most people would, if they could, choose to prolong life if this were compatible with a decent stan-dard of functioning. The promise of transplantation to fulfill this (potentially limitless) desire helps provoke an ever-growing demand that, rather than be-ing satiated, expands with each new technological breakthrough. In developed countries, we have seen that the demand for certain organs well outruns the supply. But this desire, we must remember, is not simply a natural fact but a cultural construction, built on the Cartesian dream of the scientifically elon-gated lifespan and the capitalist profit motive to sell a solution. We see this ex-emplified in many trends. The anti-aging industry now generates some $80 billion in the United States, and a series of multimillionaires have funded efforts to dramatically prolong the lifespan or even attain human immortality.[31]

From the point of view of consumerism and wealth, transplantation procedures and their pre- and after-care have proven immensely profitable to the health-care industry in ways likely to grow in the future. Far more than the low-cost, disbursed techniques of preventive medicine, organ transplantation is capital-intensive, can be centralized in the hands of an elite, and thus lends itself to the accumulation of large revenues. A common kidney transplant costs more than $300,000, a liver or lung, more than $700,000, and a heart transplant upwards of $1.2 million.[32] Again, we are reminded of the hegemony of the pill as a medical technology/commodity that generates huge profits—or expenses—depending which side of the transaction you're on.

A Market in Organ Parts?

So far I have looked at the "text" of organ transplantation through a hermeneutics of the *contexts* formed by Cartesian and capitalist constructions of the body. I have not directly focused on answering a specifically bioethical question, such as whether individuals should be allowed to sell their organs. Instead I have tried to suggest *how and why such a question arises.* That is, how we can come to see the body as (1) something *other* to the essential self; (2) that functions as a machine; (3) composed of a collection of potentially replaceable organs; (4) that could be obtained from others when ours have worn out; (5) through an exchange that generates revenue. Reflecting on how we have arrived at a "bioethical dilemma" (in this case, the sale of organs) can often be of greater import than the specific answer we supply.

Nonetheless, the answer counts too. It may be a life-and-death matter for some awaiting transplants. What if we permit the sale of organs from living donors and cadavers? The practical scenario has many alluring features. We surmise that the supply of organs might increase dramatically, though this is by no means certain.[33] This may lead to an improved system for matching up those in need with those in possession of the organs. The profit motive and market structures have often been a spur to ingenuity and efficiency. In such an exchange, the purchaser receives a lifesaving, life-extending, or life-enhancing organ. The seller or seller's relatives may also receive the ticket to a better life in return for an item of which they have little or no need. After all, for example, most of us can get by well on one kidney while alive, and the dead have exhausted their demand for viscera. This seems like a classic win-win market exchange.[34]

One can also construct a defense of the practice on theoretical grounds. Engelhardt[35] argues, along with MacIntyre[36] and others, that we live in a culture that no longer exhibits a moral consensus based on traditional metaphysical assumptions. While many of us hold onto fragments of the old morality—for example, the notion of the human body as having a sacred dignity—the religious worldview that once undergirded such notions is no longer universally shared or even necessarily dominant within our secularized social context. In this milieu, it is problematic to restrain individuals from exercising the freedom to contract with one another on matters of mutual agreement.[37] To prohibit organ sales could be seen as a not-so-benign form of paternalism.[38] In fact, the market serves a crucial function in our pluralistic society, allowing for exchanges to take place between individuals simply on the basis of mutual consent. No particular worldview or set of moral commitments is presumed or imposed on the people involved. They can contract with one another as they wish. In this reading, the marketplace is largely value-neutral and hence ideal for actualizing human freedom.

However, I would question this presumption. My own discussion of the body in capitalism has suggested that the marketplace comes laden with an implicit worldview that shapes our lives in morally contentful ways. Nature is taken up as a useable and improvable resource. The embodied self is constructed as a machine-like producer of value, a commodity for sale, and the locus of consumer desires. These are ways of valuing things, and therefore not "value-neutral." Nor is the way the market shapes social relations. Self-interest serves as the assumed engine running capitalist exchange. All parties are out to make the best deal, their interactions a form of mutual use. I want your product, you want my cash. The rule of market values is not only appropriate to a context where shared community and tradition have broken down, but can actively further this disintegration.

Moreover, where the market predominates, those with money and goods are in advantaged positions. The result is power inequalities, differential standards of living, and modes of dehumanization that particularly affect the materially poor. We often accept these features in the name of "justice" and "freedom." It seems unjust to encroach on basic rights of ownership and exchange or to punish those who have been successful in a market system. Moreover, this all depends on the liberty to enter contractual relations. The impoverished mother who sells her kidney to help feed her child can be seen as exercising, maybe even exercising well, a basic freedom.

But this reading of "justice" and "freedom" seems thin indeed. Especially those driven by financial need will find it hard to avoid self-objectification and the reduction of human dignity involved.[39] In the case just mentioned, the real-life context has left the woman to choose between highly limited options—for example, a malnourished baby or the sale of a body organ. The latter may in fact be her best option, and yet is hardly to be called "free." In a situation sometimes referred to by academics as "defective consent," she is coerced by circumstances. Social, even legal, pressures can come to bear, along with criticism for those who choose *not* to sell an organ.[40] This can be accompanied by inward guilt—*I selfishly chose to keep my extra kidney though it could have helped buy my child food.* We might well wish to avoid this new "freedom of choice."

The practices that could play out under conditions of social and economic inequality are thus disturbing. On the side of the seller, we have the specter of individuals being all but forced to offer up their body parts, or those of deceased relatives, to deal with financial hardship. On the side of the buyer, only those with enough money or proper insurance may be able to acquire these potentially lifesaving goods.[41] Others, with scarce resources, will have to live without or, in many cases, *die* without. The upshot is the possibility, already seen in third-world countries, of an impoverished class providing the organs to sustain the bodies of the well-to-do. Hence, May's criticism:

> A society that would exploit the penurious to sell a part of themselves demeans itself and its members and fails to solve its problems fittingly. The desperately ill ought not to solve their health care needs through the desperately poor.[42]

It is not even clear to what extent the poor end up benefiting from this exchange. Studies have suggested that those in India and Iran who have sold kidneys, often to repay debts, usually do not end up better off economically and are left with serious postoperative pain and physical problems.[43]

The conclusion might then seem simple: we should maintain the current legal ban on organ sales within the United States and hope that such a policy is universally adopted and respected.

But we would be wrong to stop here. This position is far from a "satisfactory solution" to the issues our hermeneutical investigation has disclosed. Why not? On the practical level, the poor would still remain poor. While I mentioned studies that suggest organ sales do not lift most out of poverty, there are counterexamples: people on occasion have made many times their average annual wage by selling a kidney and using the funds to buy a small farm, shop, or business.[44] The disadvantaged, deprived of this alternative, remain subject to the oppressive effects of poverty and to other forms of dehumanizing labor and treatment, some of which could be even worse than a kidney operation.

Moreover, it is questionable as to what extent legal bans ultimately work. They can be circumvented in third-world countries where sheer need and opportunity—and complicity by authorities—drive a thriving black market.[45] Even in the United States, it has been suggested that some economic benefit is being exchanged under the table in many organ donations between living relatives.

Whether such suspicions are true, stopping organ sales by itself does little to remove the entire business of transplantation from the logic of the market-place. As May writes:

> The problem of commercializing transplants does not hinge solely on whether we secure organs by purchase or gift. The organ itself may be a gift, but the system by which we extract, preserve, transport, and implant organs may be so expensive and market-driven as to pose serious questions of justice, not in their acquisition, but in their distribution.[46]

In this context, it can seem to heighten, rather than ameliorate, the in-justices of the marketplace to deny the donor any recompense. In the words of nephrologist and bioethicist Dr. John Dossetor, "I can't see why the only persons not to make a legitimate degree of financial advantage from trans-plantation are the people who give the organs. Everybody else is living by it, including myself."[47]

Just as saying no to organ sales fails substantially to challenge marketplace logic, so it does little to overturn the Cartesian paradigm. For example, the current shortage in human organs, perhaps traceable partially to prohibiting organ sales, heightens interest in alternatives such as animal xenografts, or-gans grown from laboratory tissue, or artificially built organs. Viewed as mere machine, the human body is essentially no different from that of an animal or something constructed in the laboratory. Parts of human and animal bod-ies, lab tissues, and devices can be interchanged because they share a meta-physical commonality.

What then *if it remains problematic to say yes to organ sales—and to say no?* A third option arises: *the refusal to resolve the question simply on these terms.* As I said in the last chapter, the bioethicist can serve as more than just the "an-swer person." He or she can also question the questions. How did we arrive at this quandary? What does it reveal about our cultural understanding, includ-ing its fractures, limitations, and injustices? Beyond the simple yes/no debates, a hermeneutical investigation may suggest responses that are more nuanced, creative, and responsive to on-the-ground realities than would be otherwise. Ways of approaching the issues may appear that were nowhere on the menu as first presented. Let me give an example of a way to rethink organ transplants, and let's see where it leads.

A Paradigm of Interconnection

In many of the problems addressed above, we see a recurring theme: that of *disconnection*. The self is understood as largely disconnected from its embodiment, which can be treated as mere machine and commodified. By much the same logic, the self is disconnected from the natural world, the latter viewed as passive matter. Moreover, selves are disconnected from one another. In the Cartesian epiphany of the *cogito*, we find knowledge grounded in a self-enclosed consciousness. This resonates with the self-interested individual of capitalism relating to others in attenuated modes. Commodity production and exchange displace fuller sorts of human communion. We find this in medicine, which, as Frank writes, encourages "monadic bodies."[48] Hospitals, administrators, payment systems, and clinicians all prefer to treat patients *one at a time*, detaching them as individuals from their meaningful relationships.

The modern self is thus disconnected from body, nature, and other people, and also and often from a sense of the sacred. This is not to deny a widespread belief in God and interest in matters spiritual. However, our public discourse and practices have become widely secularized, while the marketplace renders the sacred irrelevant or else something itself to be commodified. Surely the sacred dimension is little present in the medical system, which, as discussed in chapter 5, tends to worship a desiccated "materialism."

We might then think of organ transplantation not simply as a mode of treatment but as symptomatic of a *shared illness* endemic to our culture. In chapter 1, I discussed how illness creates a sense of lived exile from the body, others, the cosmos. But now we are seeing that our cultural contexts create much the same threefold exile: that is, we can feel disconnected from body, others, and the cosmos, by a reductively Cartesian/capitalist worldview.

What if we imagined an alternative metaphysics—one that stresses our profound *interconnection*? I will suggest that this model, in fact, is supported by clinical, phenomenological, and scientific evidence.

Within medicine there is an increasing realization of the complex intertwinings of the Cartesian "mental" and "physical" realms, to the point where these categories all but break down. A number of developments have suggested a far more integrated picture: research into the multisystem effects of stress; the study of "psychosomatic" diseases and disease-prone personality-types; attention to the import of the placebo effect in determining clinical and research outcomes; the burgeoning field of psychoneuroimmunology; the development of "behavioral medicine," including treatment techniques such as biofeedback, visualization, and meditation; research into the correlation between social stressors and subsequent disease or mortality; studies that showcase the import of the patient's attitudes, and relationship with her practitioner, as predictive of treatment outcomes; and so on. As I have explored in this book and previously,[49] it is the *embodied self* as a totality that falls ill and is healed. Sickness is not best understood as machine malfunction.

The work of twentieth-century phenomenologists here proves helpful. As noted, philosophers such as Edmund Husserl,[50] Maurice Merleau-Ponty,[51] Erwin Straus,[52] and Richard Zaner[53] developed the notion of the "lived body" as an alternative to the Cartesian "ghost in the machine."[54] Through my perceptual and motor abilities, my embodied needs and desires, I inhabit an experienced world charged with meaning. A bodily "I can" lies at the root of my competencies—I *can* sit down in the chair, *can* gaze out the window, *can* reach for my cup of tea. The lived body plays its part even in relation to higher-level cognition.[55] This book draws on my reading, experience, and cultural surroundings, my nervous system, my typing hands. Your lived body is receiving it as you sit and read.

Just as the notion of the lived body highlights the integration of mind and materiality, so it shows how the embodied self is integrated with its world. I am not locked inside my consciousness as an isolated *cogito* but "out there" in a nexus of involvements—with my computer, my tea, the other house I see through my window, the lunch I anticipate. I inhabit an experienced world that inhabits me.

Taking a scientific perspective, we again see the primacy of connection. While my skin forms a boundary, my very life depends on its constant transgression. In the act of breathing I continually exchange inner for outer and back again. Eating, I take the substance of other living things and fashion from them my flesh. The carbon-gift will be returned after my death. (Going further back, all of this shared carbon and other heavy elements were created and transported by exploding stars.) My "own" cells probably formed from prokaryotes enveloping each other in endosymbiotic relations, then reproducing and colonizing to form something like "me." And within each person are 100 trillion bacteria (collectively the "microbiome") that digest my food, assist with immunity, and ease childbirth, while one provides them with hospitable environs.[56] As Biss writes, "From birth onward, our bodies are a shared space. . . . We are not just 'tolerating' the nonself within us, we are dependent on it and protected by it."[57] The "I" is not disconnected from the world. This world is within us, and without, and we are one of its marvelous expressions.

The person reconceived as continuous with body and world is also intimately related to other people. The Cartesian/capitalist model begins with the self as an island of self-awareness and self-interest. But is this so? Biologically, one first comes to be from within the body of another, sustained in the months of formation by her blood and breath. Though upon birth we gain a measure of physical separation, our young life continues to depend on embodied connection: we need to be fed, clothed, touched, and nurtured to thrive. Throughout our lives we bear the genetic imprint of our biological parents and inhabit communal settings constructed by previous generations and our contemporaries. We, in turn, play our part in creating new life, but only through intimate coupling, bodies interpenetrating. The "separate self" is thus something of an abstraction from this rich structure of intertwining. "We are, in other words, continuous with everything here on earth. Including, and especially, each other."[58]

But do I not find my isolate self within my consciousness and thought? The long list of references contained within this book suggests otherwise. Our thinking is part of a communal conversation produced by our language, culture, teachers, books and other media. We think, as much as breathe or eat, through multiple membranes of exchange, including the *Internet*, or as it used to be called the *Worldwide Web* (www).

Interconnection and Transplantation

In closing, I will briefly suggest how this recognition of embodied connection might change our use and understanding of organ transplants.

First, it might diminish the focus on transplantation as emblematic of the "medicine of the future." Clearly transplantation can be a powerfully life-enhancing and lifesaving mode of treatment, sometimes in situations where no other good options exist. It is hard to imagine our society abandoning the procedure. However, organ transplants might not play as central a role, either practically or symbolically, in a medicine that emphasized connection. The notion of self as a fully integrated lived body is a reminder that thoughts, emotions, attitudes, and lifestyle all may lead to or prevent disease. Intervention is often more appropriate at this earlier and personalized level than at that of the end-stage diseased organ. Moreover, if the person is seen as integrated into a broader social and natural context, the locus of illness and treatment must be similarly broadened. We live in a world of financial and racial stressors, substandard public schools, difficult-to-access health care, unemployment, peddled alcohol and cigarettes, repetitive and hazardous work. We are surrounded by carcinogens in the air and water, and plied with unhealthy (but government-subsidized) foods loaded with starch, fat, sugar, and salt. As always, the materially poor bear the disproportionate brunt of these hazards. Organ failure and the need for transplantation may be the end result, but a medicine of interconnection would attend "upstream" to socially causative factors. Our current medicine often deals with consequences rather than causes, treating disease patterns one organ at a time.

Organ transplantation may be urgent (life-and-death!), dramatic (new breakthroughs!), and certainly lucrative (hundreds of thousands of dollars a pop!)—but is not necessarily the most efficient nor humane way to approach disease. While there is a place for high-tech interventions against end-stage organ failure, the costs must be counted as well. Communal resources poured into this kind of treatment can often be more profitably used elsewhere—for example, in preventive care and education or the amelioration of social ills.

It is also possible that a focus on—no, an *experience* of—interconnection would diminish the great fear of individual death that leads many to go to any lengths for life prolongation. We may be more accepting, when appropriate, that our time has reached its limits. Descartes, we saw earlier, wished to live to be at least one hundred and thought he should spend all his energy on retarding the aging process. This is a mindset appropriate for the isolated self—Descartes famously began with: "*I* think, therefore *I* am" (italics mine). Though he strived to prove the existence of other people, God, and the immortality of the soul, his work is haunted by a death anxiety.

Paradoxically, the fear of death that helps drive the demand for organ transplants may also diminish the number of donors. Carel, suffering from a rare pulmonary disease, realizes lung transplantation might be "the life-saving miracle restoring health and giving life." She wondered why so few friends and acquaintances had joined the organ donor registry. Though they say "I just never got around to it," she realizes that in truth "it was the squeamishness involved in thinking about their premature death."[59]

Carel's case (she was stricken in her thirties) gives an example of transplants as an invaluable mode of treatment. Could a paradigm of interconnection make a difference not only in the quantity but the quality of interventions—how we conceive of and conduct transplants?

As discussed, within the Cartesian/capitalist model, transplantation plays itself out as a battle for the preservation of the separate self. But we have challenged this notion of the "separate self" through noting the myriad of ways we arise from and flow into each other, emotionally, intellectually, biologically. In such ways, we are constantly "transplanting." For example, even as you read this sentence my ideas are transplanting into you, though of course I in turn received them from other donors.

Organ transplantation realizes this interpenetration on a deep visceral level. A piece of another's inner body enters right into mine, sustaining me from within. Dowie notes that this procedure can give "the human family" a whole new meaning: "By sharing organs and discovering ways to make them function in each others' bodies, we confirm our interdependence and expand our sense of community."[60]

The closest analogue in nature might be that of gestation and birth. Therein one's own body forms within the visceral organ of another. Conversely, in transplants another's organ enters into one's own body, granting new life. (With cadaver donation—I mentioned that I myself just received one—this new life can paradoxically be born through death.)

The visceral/emotional interpenetration does not end at the moment of birth. The child's body continues to intertwine with and depend on that of the parent, most strikingly through a mother's breastfeeding, for those who do. Simms writes of her experience:

> The skin as the boundary line between two bodies is breached again and again in the evocation and gift of milk. . . . I often looked at her and marveled that even though she had left my body, she still grew through it. Milk was the line that tied us together, the very special stuff that gave her life, growth, and contentment. Milk is the glory of our animal being, the need to give of ourselves and pour out our care and love because our body says "Thou shalt . . ." And the wonder is that for a brief time we are one with the world.[61]

Though technically not an "organ transplant," we might reconceive breastfeeding as the original postnatal prototype of the donor-recipient exchange. One body donates life from within to the other. In fact, the bodies and urges, the infant's hungry stomach and mouth, the mother's breast tissue and nipple are evolutionarily preshaped to fit one another.

Let us then reconceive transplantation as a continuation of this deep interconnection between embodied selves. Such might influence the ways in which we accomplish these procedures. For one thing, it would tend to lead away from the metaphors and practices of the marketplace. We have seen that organs can be thought of as simply body parts to be sold. A model of interconnection suggests a different approach. Our lived bodies are in interdependence from before we were born. This vital mutuality is ignored or reduced when transplants are treated as high-profit commodity transactions. The intense commercialization of transplantation, as well as the sale of organs themselves, would not seem the way to go. To quote May again, "The desperately ill ought not to solve their health care needs through the desperately poor."[62] This does not mean the plight of the materially poor should be neglected. Quite the contrary: this should be confronted through more humane and equalizing social policies. Poverty prevention, like disease prevention, is preferable to the "end-stage emergency treatment" of both through the sale of organs.

Ideally, better disease prevention, along with releasing on the fear of death and on the Cartesian dream of the ever-longer lifespan, would lessen demand for organs. Still, this is likely to continue to outrun supply in developed nations, especially ones without a presumed consent system (which I will discuss in a moment). Where are these organs to be found if we disable marketplace incentives?

It may be worth considering the notion of "gift," a topic first raised in the discussion of pills (chapter 4). Murray,[63] drawing on Mauss,[64] explores how certain societies distinguish the ceremonial exchange of gifts from commerce. Whereas the marketplace forges limited relationships designed to accomplish specific purposes, gifting is understood to sustain deeper modes of relatedness. Presenting a gift is a way of both recognizing and creating forms of moral obligation, dependency, and affective bonding. In this sense, the gifting of organs seems far truer to the model of interconnection than market practices. It has even been suggested that a system of organs for purchase could, paradoxically, lessen total supplies by discouraging the spirit of gifted donation.[65]

In response to the failure heretofore of voluntary gifting to provide all the organs needed, May suggests that our religious traditions and institutions can play an important part in encouraging the practice.[66] For example, organ donation deeply resonates with the message of the Christian gospel. Individuals are called to self-donative love. This is exemplified by Christ's gift of his body that others may be saved, a gift that is repeated sacramentally through the Eucharistic ritual. We see here unfolding on a religious plane the same elements identified with organ transplants: from death, new life; one self revitalized by the gift of another; body entering body.

May is doubtlessly right that our religious traditions help reveal the rich significance of organ donation as a mode of interdependence and care. One also sees this enacted among family members when, for example, one sibling donates a kidney to another. (This was the case for one of my colleagues in the philosophy department, relieving the need for lifelong dialysis.) Here the closeness of tissue-type is accompanied by an even deeper sense of kinship. Religion tends to universalize such ties: we are all called to be brothers and sisters to one another. Even if much organ donation remains anonymous, Varela, recipient of a liver transplant, speaks of the desire many feel to personally acknowledge and thank their benefactor: "They go to a cemetery and offer flowers to an unknown grave. Or to a wood and make an offering to the spirit of the deceased donor."[67] I, myself, feel a sense of deep thankfulness to the person who gifted the nerve tubule I now have in my body, helping me back to a fuller life.

However, relying on donative love to fulfill our collective organ needs can be dicey as a social policy. All depends on the exercise of personal initiative within a culture that emphasizes self-interested individualism. Even donations based on emotional and family relations can be problematic. For example, women tend to engage in more live kidney donations than do men. This may speak to gender-related dynamics that place pressure on women to do demanding forms of "care work." Zeiler writes of how organ donations in the name of "love" can sometimes be coercive and exploitative if proper procedures to safeguard justice are not in place.[68]

As mentioned, another way of securing organs, used, for example, in many European countries, is that of "presumed consent." Though an individual can opt out of participating, unless he or she explicitly declares this intent, it is presumed that cadaver organs can be used for transplant. At first glance this may seem to undermine the rich moral and affective resonances associated with gifting. Who can really give a gift if it has already been presumed? "Presumed consent" can be interpreted, as May does, as the final totalization of a coercive state exerting its control over the individual even postmortem.[69]

Within the contemporary Western paradigm of the separate self, "presumed consent" does indeed seem to signify state intrusion and the abrogation of personal freedom and dignity. *But might it have a different meaning in a context based on mutual connection?* Here it may be helpful to step briefly outside our contemporary circumstances, and even our Western heritage, for alternative worldviews. For example, in Neo-Confucian philosophy, a central idea was that we "form one body" with the universe.[70] I referred to this in chapter 4 and will now say a little more. Neo-Confucianism was a philosophical system developing out of Confucian, Taoist, and Buddhist strands that flourished in eleventh- to seventeenth-century China. That "we form one body" was there presented as an ontological fact. The human being is seen as composed of *ch'i* (or *qi*) a kind of nondualistic psychophysical power that also flowed through and animated other people, animals, plants, the earth, wind, water, and stars. However, it was not enough simply to know that we were part of this cosmic process: to lead a good life one must morally/spiritually actualize this interconnection through compassion and service to others.[71]

We find a similar sense of profound interconnectness in the worldviews of many indigenous peoples. The human being is seen as continuous with all of nature (more on this in the book's last chapter). Abram writes of this ontology:

> The "body"—whether human or otherwise—is not yet a mechanical object in such cultures, but a magical entity, the mind's own sensuous aspect, and at

death the body's decomposition into soil, worms, and dust can only signify the gradual reintegration of one's elders and ancestors into the living landscape, from which all, too, are born.[72]

Such cultures practice their own form of postmortem "organ transplantation," for example, dismembering the body and leaving parts in locations where they will be consumed by condors, leopards, or wolves, thus facilitating the rebirth of the individual into that animal realm.[73] At death, the individual who *emerged* from nature now *remerges* back into it, giving rise to new life.

While not quite the same, I have suggested that contemporary work in medicine, biology, phenomenology, and other disciplines has brought us to a deeper appreciation of such notions of interconnection. If we do form one body with each other, if life naturally regenerates itself from death, then the use of cadaver organs to give another renewed life is not a violation of individual dignity so much as a *celebration of the way things are.* Heidegger emphasizes how our mortality radically individualizes us—we always face death alone.[74] But need this be so? As Svenaeus writes, "organ donation might be the perfect example of dying (and avoiding dying) *together* with other people."[75] This can include people who are radically different from oneself in terms of race, socioeconomics, geography, gender—people with whom one would not ordinarily "mix," and yet with whom one might now mix in a profound way.

This mixing does not imply an easy unity. We referred earlier to how the foreignness of a grafted organ can provoke a rejection syndrome; one's immune system recognizes its biological otherness and will often attack, creating the need for immunosuppressive drugs. In Nancy's words, the grafted organ— and in a sense, one's own body—surfaces as "the intruder."[76] To a degree, we are always strangers to one another, and this dimension surfaces when we try to merge our bodies.

Yet this strangeness was already present within our own embodiment itself. Earlier in the book, we explored how the body is both the foundation of self and yet also *other* to it, especially when encountered in forms of heaviness, resistance, pain, or illness. I *am* this body but also *have* it, and *it has me*— sometimes uneasily—in its hold. Yet paradoxically the body's otherness-to-self also prepares me to accept the gift of a stranger's organ. As Slatman writes:

> Precisely because my experience of *me-ness* has always been based already on an experience of the thing-like nature of the body, it becomes possible that this experience of *me-ness* may also pertain to something thing-like that initially does not belong to my body at all, but was later added to it.[77]

That is, a piece of another body can be assimilated into my own corporeal schema.

More broadly, we can say that the other's alterity does not defeat attempts at interconnection but is their basis. After all, it is only through difference that we can encounter one another face-to-face in a shared world.[78] To perceive something or someone, we must be separate from them. To engage in discourse is already to presume this distance (again, the etymological meaning of *dia-logue* is speech *across* or *between*). We can relate to another only because he or she is *an other*, but also another one who in many ways is like myself. Thus we have the grounds to discover or forge commonalities, exhibit care, develop social bonds. The "presumed consent" system of organ donation can be a way not to eradicate all separation, but to acknowledge and strengthen our mutual ties.

However, much depends on what we are "presuming." If we are presuming the state's near-unlimited powers, then there is no true "consent" and organ harvesting may be enacted in insensitive and invasive ways. (Organs could even be snatched prior to a person's death, or this death hastened to make body parts available.) However, a society that teaches interconnection may be presuming something different: that "my body" was never only mine to begin with but an expression of a larger natural/social whole. Thus contextualized, the gifting of organs can be presumed because *such is our deep mutuality.* Therein, a transplant is not simply a technological procedure but an offering and receiving. As with the taking of pills, discussed in chapter 4, surrounding the act of transplantation with ceremony, celebration, and commemoration might help alleviate some aspects of transplant rejection syndrome, immunological and/or emotional.

Of course, this may sound highly idealistic. History has taught us to be suspicious of utopian ideals and vigilant about abuses conducted in their name. It is thus important that individuals should be able to "opt out" of any presumed consent system without fear of punishment or censure. Moreover, if presumed consent is based on a recognition of mutuality, it would be applicable only in situations where individuals are fully part of the circulation, givers and receivers alike. We could not, for example, employ the logic of mutuality to justify the appropriation of the organs of animals, especially those kept in inhumane conditions. (I will say more about animal mistreatment in the next chapter.) Moreover, in a human society filled with inequalities, presumed consent could not be applied to individuals who would not have an equal chance to be organ recipients if the need arose. When the rich are given a preferred status to receive transplants, the principle of mutuality is broken.

Yet when interconnection is embodied in equitable social policy, "presumed consent" need not undermine the resonances of the gift discussed before. Rather, it takes this practice to a different level. I am not simply giving "my" or "my family member's" organs away. (This still views the body as a personal possession, the Cartesian/capitalist premise.) Rather, *each person's body was a gift from the start*. I did not fashion my limbs nor weave together the intricate tapestry of vessels and nerves that sustains me. This was accomplished by an anonymous natural wisdom coursing through me (or Divine wisdom, to a believer), one that I neither fully understand nor control. I am a site wherein mysterious energies coalesce, and have been helped into existence by countless ancestors, benefactors, natural and/or supernatural powers.

Murray writes of the obligations that flow out of the reception of a gift: to accept it with gratitude, to use it well in the mode of stewardship, and in the appropriate way and time to reciprocate, giving back.[79] If one's body itself is seen as gift, organ donation becomes a way to graciously reciprocate.

PART 3

Discarded and Recovered Bodies: Animals and Prisoners

Rethinking Factory Farms:
Old McDonald's Had a *What?*

In the last chapters I have been engaged in a phenomenological hermeneutics of modern medicine and of bioethical issues, such as those involved with organ transplantation. We have examined our modern concepts of human bodies, and correlatively what we do with and to them. But humans are not the only one with bodies. We inhabit the planet with billions of other creatures, perhaps as significant as we are if we put aside our prejudices. We are increasingly realizing that it is artificial, self-centered, even unethical, to include within the zone of moral concern only members of our own species. This would make ethical outcastes of all nonhumans, including even higher animals (and, of course, we should not take for granted the metaphorics of "higher" and "lower," with ourselves at the top).

I will thus expand my focus to the conception and treatment of nonhuman animal bodies. We will see both what these have in common with and how they differ from our way of approaching human bodies. In previous sections, I have focused on ways we attempt to *relieve distress* through modern medicine, and might do a better job of it. Here, I will turn to the question of how we make ourselves *oblivious to the distress* of other living creatures and, consequently, *manufacture this distress* on an unprecedented scale through the institution of the factory farm.

Animals living under such conditions have been somewhat de-animalized by decades of selective breeding for passivity and food production, and then are held under conditions that prohibit expression of natural instincts and desires. Later on the book we will *meet* animals as other than just our *meat*. In chapter 12, we will learn of the companionate relations formed between animals and prisoners as these "discarded bodies" rescue one another. In the final chapter we will explore an even deeper bond, one in which humans are inspired to learn from and embody wild animal energies through practices of shape-shifting. We seek to channel the animal's perceptiveness and powers, not simply to eat its carcass.

But why start with factory farms? I choose this as a focus (animal experimentation would also have been apt) for many of the same reasons as I chose organ transplantation. This is a matter of great practical as well as ethical significance. It will also clarify what we imagine "bodies" in a generalized way to be and how such thinking leads to economic-technological applications. As in the last chapter, I will suggest the import of capitalism and Cartesianism in vectoring our ideas and practices—though I will press that analysis in some new directions. I will also thematize another hermeneutical context that until now has remained hidden: the pervasive anthropocentrism of much of the Western tradition. Of course, that which is most pervasive is often most hidden. It disappears through its very taken-for-grantedness.

The phenomenon of factory farming has, however, increasingly made an appearance in the public consciousness, as much as its handlers and we consumers conspire to look away. (The reader may be tempted to as well at this point in the book.) In slaughterhouses of the United States, some ten billion animals are killed each year. Even more disturbing are the unnatural conditions under which most of these animals live. They suffer extreme confinement and the frustration of their most ordinary instincts—for example, that of birds to spread their wings. Family and social systems are disrupted by overcrowded mass housing, leading to stress, aggression, and a variety of abnormal behaviors. Treated as "vices" that threaten production, these behaviors are often restrained by even more unnatural procedures—for example, cutting off with a hot knife the beaks of chickens living in high-density conditions to stop them from pecking each other. Bred and fed for rapid meat and egg production, animals develop severe anatomical problems and disease patterns that are only partially addressed—and often exacerbated—by a stream of hormones, food additives, and antibiotics.[1] These are indeed bodies that are *distressed* (etymologically, "pulled apart") and *stressed* ("pressed together").

Not only animals but humans suffer from factory farms, also known as concentrated animal feeding operations (CAFOs). Such operations are energy-intensive and largely petroleum-based, using up nonrenewable resources and releasing greenhouse gases. They produce large quantities of environmentally toxic waste that enters ground, air, and water, affecting the health of surrounding inhabitants. The fatty animal flesh produced by CAFO farming contributes to an epidemic of obesity among overfed Americans. Animal

diseases (e.g., mad cow disease) and the breeding of antibiotic-resistant bacteria also threaten human health.[2]

To effectively challenge the factory farm paradigm, it is important to understand it in depth. As we have seen, this means reflecting not only on the
technology, economics, and ethics of factory farming but also their historical
and metaphysical underpinnings. Again, we are interpreting a "text" through
disclosing or unconcealing (to use Heideggerian language) some of its most
significant contexts. How did factory farming become conceivable as an enterprise? What does its existence tell us about the nature of animal, human,
and machine, and their interrelationships as culturally constructed? Interpretation, of course, is always allied with praxis: From what we have learned,
how might the factory farm best be reformed or dismantled?

One way into such issues is to examine the term itself: "factory farm."
I will suggest that it contains within it a number of "hinges." A "hinge" (as
dictionary-defined) is a joint that holds two parts together while allowing
one to swing relative to the other. The word "factory farm" itself has parts
within parts. First, a "farm" is a kind of hinge between the human and the
natural/animal world. Farms are human constructions designed to meet human needs. Yet to access food, people must tend to nature, drawing on its intrinsic powers of fertility and growth. Historically, working farms used animals to assist in labor, manure the fields, and provide meat, milk, eggs, and
other products. In the words of the traditional American folksong popular
with children, "Old MacDonald had a farm . . . and on this farm he had some
chicks" and a cow, pigs, a geese, a horse, and so on. The cacophony of sung animal noises reminds us that this farm is a hinge, regulating the interactions of
MacDonald and his animal associates.

If a "farm" is a hinge, so too is a "factory." Often defined as buildings used for
the manufacturing of goods, factories also embody a complexity of beings
and relationships. They include not only the buildings but also the people—
factory workers, on-site supervisors, and more distant executives—who keep
it humming, along with the machinery that produces goods.

The term "factory farm" then constitutes a meta-hinge. It operates to join
and swing together farm and factory; agrarian and industrial; human, animal,
architectural, and mechanical. The open-aired farm, drawing energy from the
sun, is reconceived along the lines of closed-in manufacturing plants, most
often coal- and petroleum-based. Old MacDonald's cows and pigs are subsumed within a world of workers, corporate owners, machines, and commodity markets. This, of course, is precisely the kind of "farm" used by fast-
food corporations such as McDonald's. Unlike Old MacDonald's farm, a new

McDonald's farm is designed to maximize, on the factory system, large-scale, efficient, and highly profitable food production.

Admittedly, some such companies have made efforts to improve conditions. McDonald's itself, working with PETA (People for the Ethical Treatment of Animals) from 2000 to 2009, animal welfare expert Temple Grandin, and others, now contractually specifies animal-treatment standards to be employed by its suppliers, and has also announced a shift to using cage-free eggs[3] Though not the focus of this chapter, such on-the-ground reforms are important. Ultimately, however, they fail to challenge the fundamental paradigm of the factory farm and most of its intrinsic cruelties.

Again, we must ask, how did something as oxymoronic as a "factory farm," this hinge of all hinges, first become conceivable and constructable? This query will lead us to survey the respective roles and interlockings of three great "isms" in Western culture—capitalism, anthropocentrism, and mechanism. Here, too, the factory farm serves as a hinge for large-scale features of our culture.

Capitalism: Animals as Alienated Laborers

In the last chapter I discussed how the human body is subsumed within capitalism as producer, commodity, and consumer, a model into which organ transplantation is easily absorbed. Here I want to focus particularly on the "producer" dimension. In this section I will utilize the writings of Karl Marx, whose critique of capitalism is provocative and illuminating, even if his view of animals, as we will see, proves restrictive.

Famously, the early Marx discusses the fourfold "alienation" or "estrangement" (*Entfremdung*) that characterizes wage labor in a capitalist system.[4] The worker is alienated from the product of his labor, which does not belong to him or express his creative nature. Rather, it rules over him as something apart, something even hostile and oppressive, condemning him to toil and poverty. This alienation is realized not only in the object but also in the act of production. This is forced labor, dictated by another, and is often harsh, repetitive, and subhuman in a way that "mortifies his body and ruins his mind."[5]

Thus, humans are alienated from their species-being (*Gattungswesen*). This notion of Marx, drawn from Feuerbach, is complex, unclearly defined, and much debated, but it relates to a number of features that Marx took to be essentially human. Human beings, unlike animals, do not simply labor under the dominion of immediate physical need but produce freely and consciously, taking the whole of nature as a potential field of endeavor, working for goals beyond private self-interest, utilizing a full range of cognitive, aesthetic, and practical powers such that, ideally, one's work serves as a tool of creative self-expression. Not so for the wage laborer. "Estranged labor tears him from his species life,"[6] eradicating from work that which is truly human and humane.

As such, and finally, wage labor estranges "man from man."[7] Instead of forging genuinely human relationships, based on individual character and shared goals and affections, human interactions are governed by economic forces, rendering one an owner, another a worker, one coercive, another enslaved.

Marx's analysis of the nineteenth-century factory worker's plight applies as well to those within a contemporary factory farm. Many of the human workers in CAFOs suffer such modes of alienation. This can be low-paid work, often employing illegal and/or exploited immigrants, and under forcible control by the parent corporation. Alienated labor also extends to the fast-food establishments where these products are sold: in the last chapter, we saw the McDonald's worker who said, "You follow the beepers, you follow the buzzers and you turn your meat as fast as you can. . . . [Y]ou don't need a face, you don't need a brain."[8] Now, though, I will turn attention to the "animal workers" who are the chief producers of a factory farm. I'll but briefly sketch some ways in which they too constitute "alienated labor."

Alienation from the *product of one's labor* takes extreme form when the product is one's own flesh, built up through confinement and force-feeding followed by one's slaughter. Marx writes, "So much does labor's realization appear as loss of realization that the worker loses realization to the point of starving to death."[9] Such is curiously inverted when a meat animal is deliberately overfed, albeit in ways that induce nutritional deficiencies and incipient disease, before being killed. Other animal products, such as milk and eggs, are made in ways less lethal to the "worker." Nonetheless, these too are usually bound up with slaughter—for example, the killing of young calves and male chickens, while females are preserved for dairy and egg production.

It might be rightly said that since animals do not know their ultimate fate, they suffer less "alienation from the product" than would a human being in comparable circumstances. We can imagine a well-fed, oblivious chicken enjoying her brief life. But of course, this is unlikely on a factory farm. That the *product is alienated*—not one's own—is intertwined for Marx with *alienation from the productive activity*. Chickens, like most animals in factory farms, suffer conditions that are harsh and unnatural, designed to maximize production, not quality of life. For example, hens used for eggs may spend virtually their entire existence in artificially lit and environmentally manipulated barracks, confined some seven or eight birds to a small cage, feet perched awkwardly on wire mesh, unable to exercise natural drives, and tended to by perhaps one worker for every 150,000 chickens.[10]

As with Marx's wage laborer, this alienation from productive activity is also an *alienation from one's species nature*. Though Marx reserves the term "species being" to refer to humans' capacity for self-conscious, universalized free activity, he recognizes that animals have fixed species characteristics. Creatures have their natural habitats; their instincts for predation, aggression, seeking, playing, mating, and child rearing; their social rituals and pecking orders; and even their capabilities of high-level cognition, skill development, and emotional response that we are just beginning to appreciate. All these can be systematically frustrated in the unnatural world of the factory farm. Just as workers are "dehumanized" by alienated conditions, so, for example, is a pig, a highly intelligent creature, unable to express his or her pig nature in a crude confinement facility. Moreover, factory farms manipulate not only the environment but the genetic animal itself. Breeding for a single trait, as with large-breasted "white meat" chickens, can lead to animals who are deformed, neurologically or cardiologically damaged, and generally unhealthy, alienated from their original species character.[11] We thus see extreme manipulation of the animal body from the moment of its birth to its death, and even in its genetic preconstitution.

Finally, even Marx's notion of *"man's alienation from man"* is in a way applicable to factory-farm animals, taking both an inter- and intraspecies form. Traditional agriculture, as represented in "Old MacDonald's Farm," can permit a close and symbiotic relationship between humans and animals. Such relationships are severed by large agribusiness CAFOs. So, too, are the relationships between fellow animals. The instincts, rituals, hierarchies, and affective ties that organize animal families and societies are thoroughly disrupted.

In summary, as Benton writes, "the pathological distortions from the properly human mode of life which Marx attempts to capture in his concept of 'estrangement,' or 'alienation,' are in important respects paralleled in the modes of life imposed upon animals by precisely the same structures of social action."[12] Marx's analysis, thus extended, clarifies the "hinge" that links the fate of both humans and animals who are impressed into factory labor.

A hinge is always that which both connects and separates. This dialectic is seen in Marx's portrayal of humans and animals. On the one hand, Marx seeks to counter Hegelian idealism with a naturalistic conception of man. "Man is directly a natural being," a "*corporeal*, living, real, sensuous, objective being full of natural vigor."[13] Hence, man and animal are *connected*. On the other hand, he asserts that humans are importantly *separate* from the natural world insofar as they have freedom and self-consciousness.[14] He sees animals as tied to an instinctive fulfillment of pressing needs, whereas "conscious life activity distinguishes man immediately from animal life activity."[15]

This human/animal hinge, combining similarity and difference, is central to Marx's analysis. We can become alienated laborers only insofar as we are both *like* other creatures—caught up in a perilous struggle for corporeal survival—and *not like* other creatures, therefore bound to suffer when reduced to an animalistic existence. The horror of alienated labor, according to Marx, is that the worker "only feels himself freely active in his animal functions—eating, drinking, procreating, or at most in his dwelling and in dressing up, etc.; and in his human functions he no longer feels himself to be anything but an animal."[16]

In contrast to the natural hinge that connects/separates the human and animal, in Marx's view, capitalism creates an *unnatural hinge*. It swings together, even reverses, what should be separate: "What is animal becomes human and what is human becomes animal."[17] The worker is made brutish by labor's brutal conditions.

However, Marx's emphasis on the proper difference between humans and animals may limit his utility in any critique of factory farming. Marx envisions communism as taking over, even furthering, the productive powers established by capitalism. In his words, communism "will be the fully developed domination of man over natural forces, over nature in the strict sense, as well as over his own nature."[18] Marx's focus on human liberation did not extend to a concern with animal liberation.

More generally, there is a large scholarly debate about the relationship between Marx and environmentalism. Some view him as unfortunately Promethean, supportive of the development of productive powers that facilitate human control over nature, as exemplified in the last quote. Others read him as more ecologically sensitive and valuable. The latter authors, seeking a so-called greening of Marxism, point to Marx's naturalism and his quasi-environmentalist critique of the devastations wrought by capitalism.[19] Authors such as O'Connor[20] and Barry[21] seek to extend the Marxist paradigm to address contemporary ecological crises. For example, such crises clarify the impossibility of unlimited growth as forces of production outrun and exhaust natural conditions.

However, I will sidestep discussion of such scholarly debates. It does seem fair to assert, as Marx did, that his system remained fundamentally a kind of humanism. He is concerned with the quality of *human* life and society. He believes in appropriating the natural world as a setting for *human* expression. In Barry's words, "unlike radical green theory, eco-Marxism is firmly anthropocentric."[22] Although his critique of capitalism is useful for understanding the modern factory farm, we must then go beyond Marx to examine the role of this other "ism"—*anthropocentrism*.

Anthropocentrism: Animals as Subordinate

A predominant element of the Western tradition, broadly conceived, has been a focus on human beings as the pinnacle of nature and/or as having a unique supernatural significance. Nonhuman nature is often consigned to an instrumental role; it is important insofar as it serves human needs. There are always exceptions to be found to any generalization. Yet we find this anthropocentric orientation in much ancient, medieval, and modern philosophy and theology,[23] and in this regard, we have seen that Marx is no revolutionary.

Aristotle, for example, writes in book 1 of his *Politics*, "If nature makes nothing incomplete, and nothing in vain, the inference must be that she has made all animals for the sake of man."[24] St. Thomas Aquinas, in his grand synthesis of Aristotelianism and Christianity, reinterprets such notions theologically. Only rational creatures, insofar as they have dominion over their own actions and are made in the divine likeness, are cared for by God "for their own sake"—not so for animals, created to be "subordinated to others":[25]

> Through these considerations we refute the error of those who claim that it is a sin for man to kill brute animals. For animals are ordered to man's use in the natural course of things, according to divine providence. Consequently, man uses them without any injustice, either by killing them or by employing them in any way.[26]

Any biblical passages that seem to forbid cruelty to animals, Aquinas contends, are meant only to prevent the cultivation of mental states or actions that may lead us to harm other men.

Immanuel Kant famously concurs with such judgments in a modern idiom, defending them through appeal to reason and the categorical imperative: "So far as animals are concerned, we have no direct duties. Animals are not self-conscious and are there merely as a means to an end."[27] He suggests we should be kind to creatures only to assure we do not become hardened in our dealings with humans. Though Kant does not present his ideals theologically, he has been influenced by the long history of the Judeo-Christian tradition.

Just as there has been a "greening of Marxism," there are many contemporary thinkers who have sought to draw an environmental ethic from biblical sources.[28] The biblical notion of "dominion" need not imply domination, but can refer to the kind of loving oversight characteristic of God's care for the

world. While some biblical passages in this regard are clearly instrumentalist—
the human community will prosper better if it practices proper husbandry—
others point to the natural world, God's creation, as possessing intrinsic value
and interests independent of the human agenda.

We have seen this lately even from papal sources. Pope Benedict XVI,
then Cardinal Ratzinger, told a journalist:

> Certainly, a sort of industrial use of creatures, so that geese are fed in such a
> way as to produce as large a liver as possible, or hens live so packed together
> that they become just caricatures of birds, this degrading of living creatures to
> a commodity seems to me in fact to contradict the relationship of mutuality
> that comes across in the Bible.[29]

Pope Francis, in his encyclical on the environment, *Laudato Si'*, has an entire
section on "The Crisis and Effects of Modern Anthropcentrism," including
statements like the following:

> An inadequate presentation of Christian anthropology gave rise to a wrong
> understanding of the relationship between human beings and the world. Of-
> ten, what was handed on was a Promethean vision of mastery over the world,
> which gave the impression that the protection of nature was something that
> only the faint-hearted cared about. Instead, our "dominion" over the universe
> should be understood more properly in the sense of responsible stewardship.[30]

Still, as even the above quote acknowledges, this sort of reflection has often been subsidiary in the Western tradition. Religious doctrine and practice
has tended to be dominated by an assumption that the good for *human beings* is the focus of God's concern and so should be ours. The philosophical tradition has usually agreed, appealing to the uniqueness of human reason and
moral choice.

Though seemingly benign in intent, this anthropocentrism provides another conceptual and cultural underpinning for the cruelties of the factory
farm. It can posit animal bodies as resources for human exploitation. Though
Marx details the harshness of human factory work, we have also seen in the
West an evolution of moral concern and legal protection for workers. There
have been movements, albeit imperfect, to prohibit child labor, limit the work-
week, and protect the health and safety of laborers. Not so, not yet, or not
nearly to the same extent, has this happened for factory-farm animals. We
see a synergy of harshness when capitalism and anthropocentrism meet.

Embedded within this synergy is a paradox. Extending Marx's analysis
to the factory farm depends on making a connection between humans and
animals. Insofar as animals are treated *like* human workers, they fall prey to

similar modes of alienation. However, the role of anthropocentrism implies the opposite. It is precisely because animals are viewed as *unlike* human beings that we are seen to have no "direct duties" to their welfare; they can be abused without ethical restraint. When Jonathan Swift suggests in "A Modest Proposal" that we breed, fatten, and slaughter the children of the Irish poor for "a most delicious, nourishing, and wholesome food, whether stewed, roasted, baked, or boiled,"[31] we know this must be satire. What cannot be done to human beings, even the underclass, is, however, standard treatment for animals.

Again, we have arrived at something like a hinge, "a joint that holds two parts together." The factory farm depends on animals being treated *like* human beings (qua alienated laborers) and *unlike* human beings (insofar as they are not worthy of moral protection). What is the source of this hinge that can hold together both this similarity and opposition?

One answer: it lies in that which is neither human nor animal yet which, we will see, both links and contrasts them with each other—*the machine*.

Mechanism: Animals as Machines

As discussed in the previous chapter, early modern science, through the work of Galileo, Descartes, and others, ushered in a new world picture. Nature was no longer thought of as imbued with soul or purpose. Expunged were both the neo-Platonic ascription of occult sympathies and antipathies to matter and the Aristotelian notion of substantial forms with final causes they sought to actualize.[32] Instead, the world was reconceived according to the physics and mathematics of mechanics.[33] Matter was fundamentally passive, driven by forces in a machinelike fashion. Even living bodies were assimilated into a paradigm based on the inanimate: we have seen that Merchant terms this "the death of nature."[34] For example, Descartes makes a famous analogy in *The Passions of the Soul*,

> We may judge that the body of a living man differs from that of a dead man just as does a watch or other automaton (i.e., a machine that moves of itself), when it is wound up and contains in itself the corporeal principle of those movements for which it is designed along with all that is requisite for its action, from the same watch or other machine when it is broken and when the principle of its movement ceases to act.[35]

In the previous chapter, I focused on how Cartesian medicine approaches the human body through this machine paradigm. Organ transplantation is one corollary: if a piece of the watch breaks, replace it with another functioning part. However, for Descartes, humans remain unique in that our machine bodies are conjoined with an immaterial, immortal soul exercising thought, desire, and will. (The difficulties involved in his dualist position are legion— even Descartes recognized and wrestled with them.) His view of animals is more reductionist, a topic to which I will now turn.

In the *Discourse on Method*, Descartes argues that despite manifesting well-organized behavior and what can appear to be feelings and cognition, animals in fact possess no rational soul. Again, he refers to clocks and other automata to show how complex action can be accounted for mechanically.[36] That animals do not use language gives away the fact they do not think.

There is debate within the literature about whether Descartes really meant to argue that animals have no conscious awareness whatsoever, including that of pain. Certain scholars argue that Descartes did ascribe perceptual experience to animals, or was at least agnostic, not precluding that possibility.[37] On the other hand, the dominant tradition interprets Descartes in his original writings, subsequent correspondence, and replies to objections to be saying that animals are devoid of both sentient and rational consciousness.[38] However one views Descartes's stance, this modernist equation of the natural world in general—and animals in particular—with inanimate machines has profoundly influenced our practices.

We have largely focused on its influence within medicine. However, Descartes's medical studies were closely allied to animal bodies. During certain periods, he made almost daily trips to the butcher shop to obtain animal organs for dissection.[39] He also apparently engaged in vivisection, for example, describing in detail the pulsations one feels when slicing off the pointed end of a heart in a living dog and thrusting in a finger.[40] Descartes's paradigm and practices were taken up elsewhere. Nicholas Fontaine describes the Cartesians at Port Royal who, believing dogs to be unfeeling machines, beat and vivisected them with indifference, claiming their cries were simply like the noises made by a clock spring when touched.[41]

Earlier I wrote that the factory farm operates as a conceptual hinge. Its cruel practices arise because animals are treated both as *unlike* human beings (qua having no moral status) and *like* human beings (qua alienated factory laborers). I will suggest that the Cartesian worldview is the key to understanding how these opposites can be conjoined.

The farm can become a factory when the animal comes to be viewed as a machine, whether used for meat, milk, or egg production. *Unlike* human beings, these animal machines are seen as soulless, without intrinsic ends and desires or the capacity to experience pain and suffering. Hence, we are free to become their "masters and possessors," to use a Cartesian phrase, without ethical restraint. No limit is placed on our manipulation of their life and death. Moreover, we can effect this control using the knowledge gained by our analysis of these animal machines. This assists us to manipulate and accelerate their growth, alter their genetic stock to favor profitable traits, and maximize yields in artificial CAFOs while minimizing loss through antibiotics, dietary supplements, and mutilations. In an ironic twist on Descartes's dream of improving human health and longevity, the results for animals are often quite opposite.

Yet if the machine paradigm can *differentiate* animals from humans, it can also *link them together*. Historically, Descartes's religiously informed dualism often gave way to materialistic monism from which references to soul are expunged. The eighteenth-century treatise *L'Homme Machine* (Man-the-Machine) by La Mettrie,[42] French physician and philosopher, is one famous example. Mechanism becomes a guiding principle for our view and regulation not only of animals, but of human beings. Foucault comments,

> The great book of Man-the-Machine was written simultaneously in two registers: the anatomico-metaphysical register, of which Descartes wrote the first pages and which the physicians and philosophers continued, and the technico-political register, which was constituted by a whole set of regulations and by empirical and calculated methods relating to the army, the school and the hospital, for controlling or correcting the operations of the body.[43]

So, too, does the modern factory control the body machine via its manipulation of time, space, and motion to maximize productivity, and we have seen this is true as well of the factory farm. Human and animal bodies alike come to be subject to what Foucault calls disciplinary practices. (In later chapters I will look specifically at how prisoner's bodies are disciplined, as well as the relationships, both conceptual and practical, that develop between animals and prisoners.)

Many traditional cultures posit a close ontological relationship between humans and animals. We see this in mythology, the performing arts, sacred ceremony, and shamanistic practices. The human and animal worlds are porous and interconnected, allowing shape-shifting back and forth, the sharing of perspectives and powers.[44] (Such will be the focus of this book's last chapter.) Mechanism also posits a human–animal equation. However, this equation tends toward the monological and constrictive. The inanimate object, the machine, remakes both humans and animals in its own flattened image. The more creative possibilities of machines and human-machine cyborgs have been explored by authors such as Haraway and Mazis.[45] Nonetheless, historically, mechanism has lent itself to reductionist applications: living creatures are remodeled on the inanimate.

As evidenced by the factory farm, the paradigm of *"L'animal machine"* has proved even more powerful than that of *L'homme machine*. Whereas our sense of human intelligence, rights, dignity, and even divinity, has often played a powerful counter-role to "man-the-machine," animals have been less protected by any alternate metaphysics. There have been elements within the romantic, and subsequently the ecological, movements to recall us to the richness of animal being. In daily life, many enjoy the song of a bird or the personality of a cherished pet. But this sort of "love of animals" has failed to counteract the mindset that determines conditions for billions of factory farm animals.

The Big MAC

We have sought the origins not of "Old MacDonald's Farm" celebrated in children's song, but the new McDonald's farm of high-profit industrial agriculture. (Again, while using this company as an example, I do not mean to single it out for censure; it has adopted certain animal-welfare reforms.) In honor of the company's historic signature product, we might label what we have discovered as the Big MAC. In our historical/philosophical hermeneutic, the key structures underlying the factory farm have proven to be Materialism, Anthropocentrism, and Capitalism (hence, the Big *MAC*). Which, we might ask, is the true heart of the meal, the most important and foundational of these three forces? It depends on one's perspective.

In terms of cultural history, we might grant priority to anthropocentrism, which predates the advent of modern mechanism and capitalism. But we have seen, through a comparison of Marx's alienated laborers with animals used on factory farms, that anthropocentrism could be removed—animals and humans equated—yet key elements of the factory farm would be left intact.

Perhaps, then, capitalism is the central culprit, particularly if we view, á la Marx, economic structures and motivations as more significant than airy metaphysics. Yet in a transition to a communist state, again one can imagine factory farms left fully operative.

Philosophically, one might then view mechanistic metaphysics as the most powerful "engine" powering the factory farm. It helps us better understand how animals and humans can be treated both similarly (qua alienated labor) and differently (qua our lack of moral constraint in violating animal bodies). As such, it serves as a hinge holding together the disparate elements that form the factory farm. This institution seems inconceivable without the philosophy, science, and technologies associated with mechanism.

Ultimately, though, the three elements of this Big MAC might best be understood as a synergistic sandwich. The cultural tradition of anthropocentrism, the economics of capitalism, and the worldview and practices of mechanism interact in ways that are mutually enhancing—or from another point of view, maximally destructive for the animals subject to their rule.

Concluding Thoughts

Many, including myself, would hope not simply to understand but to significantly modify or dismantle the factory farm. Discussing just how to do this, and what would take its place, goes beyond the bounds of this chapter and my expertise. However, we have seen that praxis is ever informed by interpretation. A too-shallow reading of the "text" of the factory farm may lead to shallow reform efforts. In this hermeneutical analysis, I have tried to place the text back into three key contexts that have crucially shaped our praxis. The direction of one's attempts to transform this system may depend on which aspect of this Big MAC one takes to be most important. One can oppose, as many are now doing, the logic of the mass-production-and-consumption food industry; the theo-philosophical presumption of human superiority; and/or mechanist and behaviorist understandings of animal psychology.

If our Big MAC is synergistic, perhaps the best challenges will be as well, holding in view these different contexts and also what they have in common. In each case, the true species nature of animals (to use Marx's terminology) is obscured, rendered alien. Capitalism renders animals into producers, and commodities to be sold and consumed. Anthropocentrism tends to view animals as our inferiors, servants, and possessions. Mechanism reconceives the animal according to the model of an insensate automaton. What these logics thus all share is that *they do not allow the animal to be an animal.* The animal is not viewed as pursuing his or her own ends, inhabiting his or her own world, and exhibiting the unique powers and propensities characteristic of his or her species and individual personality. Any powerful challenge to factory farming would need to begin by reforming this limited view.

This has scientific ramifications. Much of animal psychology still remains veiled in mystery, our research limited by behaviorist assumptions, artificial laboratory conditions, and industrial agendas. There is a need for fuller study and appreciation of the richness of animal experience, including individual and communal thinking, creativity, emotions, and sociality.

This goes hand in hand with ethical ramifications. Whether animals are thought of as God's own creatures (as developed in ecotheology), ends in themselves (to use a Kantian logic), beings capable of suffering (as in utilitarianism), or embodied creatures coinhabiting the earth (as explored in phenomenology, ecofeminism, and deep ecology), animals have their own experience that demands our attention and concern. To *recognize* animals is to take seriously the moral and existential claims invoked by their subjectivity.

This is more than viewing animals as beings whose violation is prohibited. They are also *partners* with whom we share a world. For untold centuries, humans and animals have coevolved through symbiotic relationships. One of the ironies of factory farming is that in rendering animals totally subservient to humans, CAFOs also exclude most animals from the human community and vice versa. We never meet the cow until she arrives as our Big Mac.

Grandin and Johnson's recent book is titled *Animals Make Us Human*.[46] When animals are alienated from their species nature and our shared world, we, too, lose something essential. The counter to factory farming is not simply to negate a negative. Rather, it is to reintroduce elements of diversity, creativity, and "humanity" into our human-animal relations.

Factory farms do not create good landscapes, ecosystems, communities, health, or food for human beings. We have seen that the conditions for animals are abysmal. The loss of human-animal affiliation diminishes us all. (In chapters 12 and 13 we will explore such relations in a positive vein.) This chapter has asked how it is that factory farms became *conceivable*. As important is the question of how—remembering backward or thinking forward—they again can become *inconceivable*.

Rethinking Imprisonment:
The Life-World of the Incarcerated

In the last chapter, I looked at what becomes of animals incarcerated in factory farms. Yet we also cage a lot of people—who themselves may be viewed as "animalistic" by virtue of having engaged in criminal activity. (This connection between animals and prisoners will be explored in chapter 12.) I now turn my attention back to human beings, in this case those who have caused distress through their criminal activity and now suffer distress under conditions of incarceration. "Distress," we have seen in earlier chapters, comes from the Latin *dis*, meaning "apart," and *stringere*, to "press together" or to "stretch." Prisoners are both pressed together under overcrowded conditions and stretched apart—from their previous home, routines, and relationships.

We in the United States are said to be living in an "age of mass incarceration."[1] Contexts we've been examining in the last two chapters—such as the body taken up within capitalism—are clearly at play. The "prison-industrial complex" has proven an immensely profitable venture, if a kind of alienated labor for prisoners caught within it and often for the correctional staff overseeing them. Prisoners are used by states as a cheap workforce, and many companies, employees, and communities depend financially on aspects of the correctional industry. Incarcerating each prisoner can cost some $40,000 a year, generating vast revenues for a variety of receivers. Numerous prisons are now even operated as explicitly for-profit ventures run by private companies.[2] Again, the prisoner's body serves as producer, commodity, and consumer, all utilized within the logic of the marketplace.

Not only capitalism, but Cartesian metaphysics has done much to construct this vast machine of surveillance and punishment. The prison environment is often almost devoid of natural elements. Instead it is a highly planned, geometrical set of containers within containers (cells, cell blocks, inner and outer walls). Offenders are often warehoused like materials to be inventoried through daily "count-outs" or moved about because of security or space concerns. Thus is the human being treated like a Cartesian body-object.

However, in this chapter, I will not so much theorize about these contexts as turn instead to the words and experiences of the prisoners themselves. They are not merely objects, but subjects responding to the challenging world into which they have been inserted. Are they like the caged animals focused on in the previous chapter? In some ways yes, since they, too, are living beings whose natural desires are frustrated by confinement (see chapter 12). But in some ways the answer is no, humans are dissimilar. With their more, or at least differently, developed rationality and self-consciousness, human beings can reflect on their situation of long incarceration. They project into remembered pasts and imagined futures. They can devise mental strategies of self-liberation. Through interpreting their situation, they change it. In this chapter I am not so much engaged in my own hermeneutics of imprisonment as I am interested in the practical hermeneutics that prisoners themselves perform.

First, though, a little more in the way of social context and statistics. At the time of this writing, according to last report, in the United States we hold some 2.2 million people in prisons and jails.[3] In 1972, by way of contrast, the United States held a little over 300,000 inmates.[4] That this has increased sevenfold in the last three decades is a result of a myriad of factors, including the war on drugs with its focus on criminalization and punishment, an overall trend toward longer sentences, and the reduced use of parole. The incarceration binge has continued largely independent of criminal activity. Violent crime decreased for many years,[5] during which time the prison population continued to rise precipitously. All told, we now have 6.9 million people under the supervision of the adult correctional system, including those under probation or parole.[6]

Our incarceration rates are six to ten times greater than similar Western industrialized countries.[7] For example, we have held more prisoners in *one state* (California) than did the *nations* of France, Germany, Great Britain, Japan, Singapore, and the Netherlands *combined*.[8] The United States, though it has but 4.4 percent of the world's population, holds roughly 22 percent of the world's prison population.[9]

We might say the United States has embarked on a unique social experiment. In response to a complex variety of social ills, we respond with one solution: place a huge number of our citizens in cages. This strategy has impacted disproportionately minority populations whose social position is already disadvantaged. For example, some 49 percent of black men and 44 percent of

Latino men will be arrested by the time they are twenty-three years old.[10] About one in three black men will go to prison at some point in his lifetime, as opposed to one in seventeen white men.[11] Though composing less than 30 percent of the general population, more than 60 percent of prisoners are blacks or Latinos.[12] In Maryland, where I teach, the general population is about 30 percent black, but the prison and jail population is more than 70 percent black.[13]

A process has begun to reform the system, fueled by activists and op-ed writers, state officials facing budgetary overruns, and a realization among politicians across the ideological spectrum that mass incarceration has proven a humanitarian, financial, and practical disaster. Localities, states, and the federal government have put forth a variety of reformist recommendations, ballot measures, legislation, and policies. These are designed to reduce the use of mandatory minimum sentencing, find alternatives to incarceration for low-level property and drug-related crimes, and to address a few of the many flagrant racial inequities. However, this process has only begun and has many limitations and opponents. We can only hope for further and more dramatic changes in the future. At the same time, we cannot forget the huge numbers currently held within the prison system.

In this chapter, I will draw on work I did with inmates, mostly serving life sentences, in the maximum-security Maryland Penitentiary, then the oldest continually operating penitentiary in the Western world. It was a men's prison, as is the Jessup Correctional Institution where I currently volunteer and which is featured in later chapters. (Though I have done some teaching in a women's prison, I have met with administrative difficulties at that site. Consequentially, the material in the book will focus on men I have worked with— though the number of women locked up has been exploding over the last decades, raising its own set of issues about our incarceration binge and its radiating impacts.)

In the class here represented, I taught some ten to thirteen guys in a not-for-credit philosophy seminar that continued over eighteen months. We studied a broad range of texts, including several in continental philosophy by authors such as Nietzsche, Heidegger, and Foucault. The men used philosophical concepts to analyze their experiences ranging from life on the street to that on maximum-security lockup. The conversations were so powerful and illuminating that I began audiotaping them, somewhat surprisingly with the permission of prison authorities. From transcripts I produced edited dialogues that are published, with my own comments, in a previous book coauthored with the prisoners, *The Soul Knows No Bars: Inmates Reflect on Life, Death, and Hope.*[14]

This chapter relies on brief excerpts from these dialogues, but now newly and more systematically analyzed. My goal is to allow the inmates to speak for themselves but also, as a phenomenologist, to explore the essential structures of their experience. The voices we hear are mostly those of African American men from an inner-city environment, unusual for their level of educational achievement—largely secured through prison college extension programs that have subsequently closed down as a result of the 1994 Omnibus Crime Bill (more on this later).

I make no pretense that the men whose voices we hear are a representative cross-section of all inmates. If anything, categorical thinking about "all criminals" or "all prisoners" has tended to feed the incarceration binge. Yet I believe their words shed light on a range of human responses to imprisonment that manifest across personal, cultural, and institutional variants.

Aspects of the analysis are also applicable to other settings. Foucault argues that a modern regime of "discipline" operates similarly in the military, schools, workplaces, hospitals, and other institutions.[15] A careful division and manipulation of space, time, and movement creates "docile bodies" of its inhabitants, minimizing their resistance while maximizing their utility. We saw this at play with factory-farm animal bodies. Dyck et al. discusses how disciplinary structures can even infiltrate the home, as she explores interactions between low-income, older, chronically ill women and their (usually also low-income female) home caregivers.[16] "Nevertheless," Dyck writes, "this understanding of the body also opens space for resistance and the possibility that experiential knowledge is not determined by scientific discourse and disciplinary technologies on the body."[17] As Foucault recognizes, and we will see, dominant modes can and will be resisted by the individual, alone or banding with others.

This analysis is also continuous with earlier material in the book on medicine. When admitted to a hospital or nursing home, patients may find elements of their personal identity, clothing, history, home, and habits all stripped away, as they are installed within a medico-bureaucratic machine. In this they are not unlike inmates. Before that, illness and chronic pain themselves may have exerted a prison-like hold. Svenaeus uses the Heideggerian term "unhomelike" to capture such modes of existential displacement.[18] The sick individual feels trapped and alienated from her body, comrades, and customary contexts of meaning. Carel writes of the many struggles facing the seriously ill: "These issues can be summarized in one question: how should I face adverse circumstances over which I have no control?"[19] The same might be said of the prisoner. How to survive, perhaps to heal—even in the midst of limitation and deprivation? Using phenomenological tools, I will look at what imprisonment does to the experience of time, space, and body—and how these long-timers creatively respond.

Lived Time

Husserl,[20] Heidegger,[21] and other continental philosophers have distinguished between lived time and clock-and-calendar time. The latter is captured well by Newton's vision of a time that flowed forth equably, independent of observers. It is susceptible to mathematical measurement, divisible into standardized increments that can be plotted geometrically. By way of contrast, lived time, time-*as-experienced*, is a complex and variable phenomenon. Past, present, and future do not simply unfold consecutively as on a timeline. Heidegger suggests that, in a sense, the future comes first.[22] Our goals and anticipations organize our present activities, and even our interpretations of the past. Nor does experiential time unfold in standard increments. Time may slow down, as when we check the clock repeatedly during a tedious lecture, dismayed to find the minute hand all but paralyzed. At other times, we wonder "Where did the time fly?" A day of delightful play may seem gone almost before begun. Yet, after the fact, it might expand in pleasant memory, while the boring lecture contracts to insignificance.

Ultimately our experience of time has much to do with the rhythms of our daily lives and extended projects. Waking and sleeping, washing and eating, works begun and accomplished, friends and family encountered, special events, and the change of seasons, all combine to create a textured temporal field. Often, this field can be altered, even shredded, by "life on the street." The problems of the inner city—drug addiction, chronic poverty and unemployment, disrupted family life, community fragmentation, violence, loss of hope concerning the future—all have the power to distort lived temporality. Yet life on the street is nonetheless a life, with its own rhythms, goals, tasks, and interactions.

All this is radically disrupted by a prison sentence. Lived time is supplanted by an abstract Newtonian framework of mathematically measured calendar time. "Twenty years," says the judge. This is time turned into alien beast—or automaton, one might say, given its blind and abstract nature. Twenty years are to be removed from a person's life. They belong not to him or her but the state. Time itself has become something that *must be served*, an instrument of disempowerment. This is true not only on the macroscopic scale but in the intricate management of daily time to which an inmate is subjected. When you sleep, hours in and out of the cell, limited opportunities for action are largely predetermined by prison authorities rather than natural inclination. I have learned, for example, it is routine to do middle-of-the-night prisoner-counts, which can lead to chronic sleep fragmentation and deprivation.

In chapter 2, I discussed how chronic pain is a kind of dis-ease of *khronos*, of time itself. Similarly, long-term incarceration can trigger a massive disordering of temporality. The past may be brooded over as a scene for repetitive regret, if only at having gotten caught. The experienced present may be slowed almost to a halt by a lack of things to do, the boredom, the paucity of meaningful projects offered to inmates as they are warehoused for their duration. Experience of the future may be transformed, to use Minkowski's terms, from one of "activity" to one of "expectation." He writes, "Through its activity the living being carries itself forward, tends toward the future, creates it in front of itself."[23] However, "expectation" involves an inversion of lived time. While awaiting an event that we do not control, instead of moving toward the future, "we see the future come toward us and wait for that (expected) future to become present."[24] We are immobilized in anticipation. The expected future "absorbs, so to speak all becoming," allowing the present "only a shadowy existence,"[25] shriveled up and constricted. This is the predicament of many prisoners counting off the days and years on the way to an expected (or hoped for) release date. Instead of living richly and purposively, they are trapped in a diminished present, watching the future all so slowly march closer.[26]

We have also seen that rearrest is common postrelease. The passive prisoner may not emerge very different from when he arrived, or the inward alterations (such as bitterness and dependency) may be for the worse. So, too, is the position of someone excluded from a society that has moved on without him. For example, Maryland forbids prisoners access to Internet—but then they are released into a world and job market increasingly dominated by computers and smart phones. Many also find that, carrying the label of "ex-felon," their past gallops ahead to destroy their future prospects for employment and housing.

This constitutes but a brief description of the altered time that threatens those caught up in the prison system. But the individual remains capable of responding to and resisting such vectors. I now turn to a variety of strategies whereby inmates—in this case serving long or life sentences—rework temporality. Here they are discussing in class an excerpt from Eugene Minkowski's work on time, mentioned above:

DONALD THOMPSON: I think the problem is that guys in here spend most of the time just discussing the good ole days, the glory days, "When I had my car, these two jobs, or those five girls." Or "When prison was better" or "Instead of knives and machine guns we had forty-five magnums." If you try to talk about the future it's just not acceptable.

SELVYN TILLETT: I've seen guys with a couple life sentences plus some numbers behind it, saying "Yeah, my wife will be waiting for me like the old days." I be thinking, "Are you out of your mind?" I wouldn't say it cause they'd be ready to fight, but they're trapped in *that past*.

JOHN WOODLAND: Quite a few guys try to live in the past. I like living in the future, thinking about what my life is going to be. But I think one thing most of us try to avoid is the *present*. Because the present here is the most painful.[27]

Articulated here is a strategy of resistance I will call *escape*. Trapped in a painful present, the men seek ways to escape into the past or future. In its most deficient form, this can devolve into a sterile, even self-destructive escapism. The discussants are aware that dwelling in an idealized past can be a waste of time, perhaps even a setup for a repetition of bygone failures. Rather than actively advancing in life, one retreats to a static repository of memories.

But the strategy of escape need not always be escapist in the pejorative sense. Happy memories can be a source of strength and comfort. Or else, "thinking about what my life is going to be," as John does, introduces hope and ambition. We have seen that Heidegger writes of lived time as involving a series of *ecstases*, etymologically from the Greek for "standing outside."[28] To live in and for the future, like John, allows a door to swing open so one temporarily—and temporally—stands outside the prison cell. Freedom is not then something just to be "expected" at a future date, as in Minkowski's sense of debilitating expectation. Rather, imagining the future introduces an element of freedom into the prisoner's *current* life-world.

Resuming the discussion:

Q (AN ALIAS): I see it a little differently. To me, time is like a dragon I have to slay. If I can master the present, I will have used my time to *redeem* time. Then I can go back and offer something to people who never had to be in that situation. . . . I get up in the morning at 8:30 and I don't get back to my cell until about 10 p.m. Between those times I'm constantly involved in activities that are beneficial and what I want to do. I'm reading materials I intend to use in the future for political work, and philosophical literature, concentrating heavily. The time flies for me, you know? Sometimes I can't even find enough hours to complete what I wanted.

WAYNE: I call this *"doing time"*—when you use every available moment for your benefit. When you have time to sit back and mope and worry, is when *time begins to do you.*[29]

In contrast to the strategy of *escape*, I will call this the strategy of *reclamation*. The living present is reclaimed as a scene for fulfilling and purposive action. One is back to "doing time" instead of having time "do you." Q cites satisfying activities that give meaning and richness to his day, even one spent in prison. The temporal alienation introduced by the imposition of sentence is successfully overcome.

The strategy of *escape* emphasizes flight from an oppressive reality. The strategy of *reclamation* emphasizes redeeming that reality: the life-world is rehumanized. However, this polarity is far from absolute. Like the yin-yang symbol, such opposites bear within themselves seeds of one another, and can flow together and harmonize. This harmonizing of opposites, a Taoist ideal, also has its merits in a prison setting.

For example, we see this harmonizing in Q's description of being "constantly involved in activities that are beneficial . . . reading materials I intend to use in the future." Perhaps Q started by reclaiming the present, discovering the joys of reading possible even in prison. This reading may then have stimulated new visions of a life postrelease. *Reclamation leads to escape.* The progression can also be reversed. Perhaps Q liked to escape to an imagined future. Envisioning what he wants to do postrelease may have then helped Q find meaning in his prison days, including reading helpful materials. *Escape leads to reclamation.*

(For those interested, Q is the only class member who has subsequently been released, returning to his African homeland. Three of the original class members have died from disease at relatively young ages, and another from a possible suicide, though his mother thinks the guards killed him. Prison is hard to survive.)

Whichever movement came first, I will call this blending of escape and reclamation *integration*. From the Latin *integratus*, meaning "renewal" or "made whole," we see the power of integration in Q's ability to affirm his incarcerated present (and implicitly accept the past that brought him there) and to see this present as a route to a better future. The *ecstases* of time are effectively integrated, making whole again lived temporality. This can lead to an enhanced sense of the self's *integrity*, as it dwells in a reintegrated world.

Such strategies of *escape*, *reclamation*, and *blended integration* are equally applicable to an individual struggling, for example, with chronic pain. How to escape from the imprisoning present, retaining happy memories or hope for the future; yet also reclaim the richness available in each moment; and how to integrate these into a fulfilling existence that need not be dominated by disease; these are questions which the sick individual tries to answer through her manner of living. Though to my knowledge it has never been tried, it would be interesting to facilitate a conversation between the long-term incarcerated and the chronically ill. They might have much to share with and teach one another.

But the inmate also faces a series of daunting obstacles to integrative work embedded in our punitive prison system. Take the example of Q's copious reading. He is unusual in having been highly educated before being imprisoned for drug dealing. But some 70 percent of inmates have some degree of functional illiteracy, and prison schools and tutors are ill equipped for the massive remedial effort needed. Even for strong readers, prospects can be discouraging. Prison libraries are woefully underfunded and have restrictions on utilization. (Recently the head librarian of the Maryland correctional system told me—before quitting—that the state *had zeroed out* her budget for book buying.) Inmates and their families often have few financial resources to purchase books. Also, prisoners may be allowed only a small number of books in their cells because it is deemed a fire hazard. Those attempting to send texts in from the outside world (as I have done) may find this treated as a security threat; books are rejected because they do not come directly from the publisher. Certain types of literature—including, for example, religious materials—may have to be approved by a censoring authority. On and on it goes, as barriers within and without make it difficult to accomplish the integrative work discussed above.

Lived Space

Phenomenologists, Heidegger a prominent example, have also distinguished between geometric space and the lived spatiality of human experience.[30] The Newtonian conception of space, like that of time, is abstract and mathematizable. It can be plotted using Cartesian axes, as can any particular spatial point within it (the "point" itself being a theoretical concept, having no dimensionality). Space thus conceived is a contentless container, stretching uniformly and infinitely in all directions.

Spatiality-as-lived is something wholly other. It is oriented by our body, which vectors space into what lies ahead and behind, right and left, up and down, accessible or withdrawn from our sensorimotor powers. Moreover, our lived space is filled with meaningful places that orient our life.[31] There is the home in which we dwell, places of work and recreation, of social gathering and solitude. We experientially dwell not only in a house, but in nested environs—a neighborhood, landscape, city—that become a wider home shared by other "homies."

Yet all this is vulnerable to dis-place-ment. Just as the pronouncing of sentence rips the offender out of the temporal life-world, so, too, is she removed from a previous fabric of lived space. "Twenty years" means decades during which the sentenced cannot return to her home. She cannot wander the familiar neighborhood, nor see—except for dislocated visits—friends and family who dwelt there. As we will explore in chapter 12, even the world of nature is largely ripped away but for a patch of dirt or sky.

What does the prison put in place of these places? First, we might say it offers *constricted* space. The inmate's ability to roam freely has been forfeited. Hereafter, she will dwell in zones of severe restriction—the narrow cell, the tiered building, the hemmed-in yard, the prison compound.

This is also a *ruptured* space. Contrast the experience of walking across an open field toward a distant horizon with that available to an inmate. Everywhere bars, fences, barbed wire, tall walls, cut through space, separating limited *heres* from unreachable *theres*. The outside world, hitherto the place of all places, is severed from access.

We might also call this space as *disoriented*. The spatiality of home and neighborhood is organized by vectors of meaning, possibility, and preference. Far less so is the spatiality of prisons. They are often laid out in geometric grids, substituting that abstract Cartesian space for the more humane contours of ordinary habitations. Architecture here is dictated by issues of security and surveillance, not by the desires of the home dweller. Moreover, the prison usually stands in no meaningful relation to the natural landscape into which it is thrown or the rhythms of surrounding communities. A previous life-world of nested places gives way to space structured as an instrument of disciplinary control.

This can even give rise to a *reversed* spatiality. German phenomenologist Bollnow writes about the primacy of the "home," broadly understood, as centering one's life-world.[32] But prison tends to reverse all the meanings of home—security, privacy, comfort, freedom of choice. The guards are there to keep you in against your will, not protect you from intruders. Whereas the boundaries of home establish a zone of privacy, prison walls do the opposite; they compress you together, often in overcrowded conditions, with hundreds of others, some of whom may be dangerous. This is "maximum security" for the outside world, not for the prisoners. The "view" from your cell often faces more inward toward the tier, not outward like a window, and is there so you can *be viewed*. There is a door to your "home" cell, but you do not have the key. You are not free to go in and out as you please, but your adversaries, the guards, can, strip searching your cell without notice. You cannot even choose who lives with you since cellmates are assigned, and by definition your new companion will be a convicted criminal. And whereas "home" is a place where you can dwell in a settled way, here you can be transferred any time by administrative fiat.

This, then, is home in reversed caricature. Instead of establishing a positive center to lived spatiality, the prison "home" is like the epicenter of a flushing toilet, centripetally sucking away the world. Sveneaus's term for the state of those suffering from severe pain and illness—*unhomelike*—seems apt here as well. Yet again, inmate dialogues will reveal strategies that help rehumanize this world:

JOHN WOODLAND: We always had a concept around here about keeping yourself distant from prison activities and the prison mentality. Don't participate in a whole bunch of prison groups, don't get caught up in playing football, basketball, don't think about fixing no cell up to make it comfortable. Let it stay raggedy. You want to keep a mindset that this is not some place for me to get comfortable.

MICHAEL GREEN: I agree. I got a friend that every cell he moves in he paints to the max. I *refuse* to paint one of these cells or lay it out like it was home. To me it's just a place where you exist.

CHARLES BAXTER: [*laughing*] I understand what Mike's saying because I'm one of those dudes—I call my cell my *palace*. As a matter of fact I just got it painted last week and paid the dude four packs to do it. He painted the floors, my ceiling, the whole thing. I got my Oriental rugs laid down. I don't care where I'm at, I'm going to make it heaven while I'm there. Even in this hellhole, I'm going to find some heaven.

WAYNE BROWN: It's different being in a double cell. I could feel at home laying on my bunk. But when I got up and took one step to the wall, I felt like I'm in a danger zone 'cause I had somebody else on the top bunk. I was under their scrutiny. There's somebody watching. . . .

TRAY JONES: Yeah, when I used to sleep in a double cell, if I was in there with a person I didn't like, I felt like Wayne. But when I was in the cell with T—the only cell buddy that I really got along with—a bond developed, and in our closeness we were so brotherly. . . . It seemed like had *more* room in the cell with him than I do now when I'm alone. We'd play cards and talk, and it felt like there was a lot of room![33]

In this discussion, John and Michael emphasize a strategy of *escape*. That is, they cope with the disordered world of prison by refusing to become complicitous with it. Instead they imaginatively escape beyond its barriers, not allowing themselves to feel at home in a cell. Rather, they orient to the outside world, considering that their true home, albeit one from which they are temporarily exiled.

Charles adopts an opposite strategy, one that I earlier termed *reclamation*. He is determined to make himself as at home as possible in prison. If spatiality has become constricted, ruptured, disoriented, even reversed, Charles will do what he can to reverse the reversals. He will make of his cell a palace. With paint and oriental rugs, he will fight to humanize, even divinize, his surroundings into an earthly/heavenly home.

Wayne and Tray remind us that such strategies are never effected alone. A human being is always a social creature, inhabiting a world with others. As such, lived space is not constituted by the solipsistic individual but is a shared construction, deeply influenced by those around us. Wayne's life-world is constricted by the alienating gaze of a cellmate. However, Tray shows how the sympathetic *other* assists the process of reclamation. An experience of solidarity can radically expand and heal a lived space that was constricted and disrupted.

To further the analysis, I will add two more comments from our discussion:

CHARLES BAXTER: And the cell's where you actually get your schoolwork done, or work for organizations you're in, or work to get out of prison. Man is created from one cell, right, and as man grows he adapts into another cell, and that cell's also a place for growth and development. When you read the Koran and the Bible you'll see that different prophets went to the *cave* for comfort and isolation. And the cell's like that cave.[34]

TRAY JONES: My space ain't too restricted because I think of myself as on an *odyssey*. Even in here. I don't look at this as my home; it's just an experience that's necessary in order for me to get where I'm going. I believe I'm here because I lost my road. That's what I'm searching around for, the road to the larger society. In the meanwhile I'm supposed to be restricted in space. I take the stoic outlook—my space is supposed to be restricted but my ideas don't have to be, and that's where I find all my freedom. . . . When I was on the street, I had *less* space than I do in prison. I would only associate with the criminal elements. . . . Since I've been in prison, I've met people with sophistication, people from different races. . . . We meet here, and get a chance to rest and get out of our immediate world, and we can think about things we couldn't on the street.[35]

In these comments we hear eloquent statements of what I have termed the strategy of *integration*, combining elements of *reclamation* and *escape*. Both men positively affirm—and thereby reclaim—aspects of prison life that might otherwise seem alien. For Charles, who is a Muslim Imam, the limitations of the prison cell remind him of the prophet's cave, a place for growth and development. Tray, torn out of his driven world of drug dealing and murder, uses prison as a haven for thoughtful exploration. (While incarcerated Tray has written his own autobiographical memoir, *Eager Street*.[36]) Again, this process is assisted by others, whose diverse perspectives broaden his own.

Reclaiming the possibilities immanent within the prison world is the very tool that allows these men escape and transcendence. That Tray is pinned in place (serving a sentence of life-plus-twenty-years) has launched him on an odyssey. So, too, Charles, on a spiritual journey that progresses in his prophet's cave. This demonstrates the strengths of an *integrative* strategy. The very limits of prison space and time are used to trigger a life-world expansion.

Embodiment

I now turn to what has been implicit in my previous analysis; the place of the body in the inmate's life-world. As discussed in this book, the lived body is not just one object in the world but, as Merleau-Ponty's writes, "our general medium for having a world."[37] It is through our embodied perception, movement, symbolic expressions, and meaningful relations—not just through a purified rationality—that our life-world is constituted.

We have seen that prison tends to replace the richness of lived temporality and spatiality with a mathematized and dehumanized time and space. I will now suggest that this is correlative to a shift in embodiment. The lived body is naturally *ec-static*—that is, it stands outside itself through its ability to perceive across a distance, and desire and move toward its goals. It is ever engaged with a world beyond its own limits. But these projective capacities can also be blocked. A tall wall, for example, brings the body to a halt. We cannot see over or move through this barrier. The *imprisoned* body is not, then, an ordinary active subject but also a thing that is held, observed, and controlled. The prisoner, to a degree, is reduced to the status of an object.

Prison thus reminds us of the double-sided nature of the living body. It involves what Merleau-Ponty terms an *écart*—a fissure, or divergence.[38] The living body is always *both* perceiver and perceived, a constituting subject and a worldly object. But the restrictions of prison have the capacity to take this lived ambiguity and turn it into an experiential opposition.

We saw this happen previously in the context of pain and illness. The distressed body can seem "other" to the self, an alien thing. It is that which blocks one's will, undermines one's projects, causes suffering, may even threaten one's life.[39]

This is not quite the existential situation of the body incarcerated. Unlike illness, where an alien power arises *within* the body, the prisoner is more likely to experience hostile forces located *outside* in the system, guards, and bars. Social constraints, not one's own disabilities, immobilize the body. Nevertheless, the body can seem a coconspirator. If one did not have a body, one could not so be observed, disciplined, and punished.

As I suggested earlier, the points of equivalence can be pressed further once one considers the sick person as absorbed into medical institutions. When neurologist-author Oliver Sacks is hospitalized for a severe leg injury, he mishears the declaration that he will have an "operation tomorrow" as an "*execution* tomorrow" (emphasis added). On admission:

> One's own clothes are replaced by an anonymous white nightgown, one's wrist is clasped by an identification bracelet with a number. One becomes subject to institutional rules and regulations. One is no longer a free agent; one no longer has rights; one is no longer in the world at large. It [is] strictly analogous to becoming a prisoner. . . . One is no longer a person—one is now an inmate.[40]

As with incarceration, this powerless state results from both internal and external forces: one's own body has rendered one vulnerable to coercion.

Another imperfect analogy to the situation of the prisoner would be that of women in a patriarchal culture. As de Beauvoir discusses, women are often identified particularly with the body and taken up as an object for the male gaze and use.[41] Insofar as women internalize this gaze, they come to regard their own bodies as those things in the mirror that must be rendered properly attractive, fit, and constrained to be socially acceptable. Whether one "fails" or "succeeds" in this task, it is binding—in fact, *double-binding*.[42] For example, if sexually cautious, a woman may be labeled "frigid," if sexually active, a "slut." Whereas Merleau-Ponty writes about the body's "I can" structures of ability,[43] Young writes that women often internalize an "I cannot." They learn an objectified style of embodiment that limits their capacities—for example, how to "throw like a girl" rather than using their full powers.[44]

Certain similarities are evident in the prisoner's situation. He or she is also made into an *other*, an object under the omnipresent gaze of watchers. Furthermore, the inmate's body is everywhere constrained. The institution reinforces the experience of the "I cannot"—I cannot move freely, leave the prison, secure privacy, pursue my goals. The prisoner's bodily location, dress, and actions are largely dictated by the state. A woman in a patriarchal society may be reined in even by subtle reinforcers—e.g., "You look pretty in that dress." In a prison situation, the forces of confinement can be much more blunt, fashioned of bars and barbed wire, the legal and illegal restriction of rights, officers with rifles watching from guard towers, threats of longer sentences and solitary confinement. (Of course, women can also be objectified and subjugated in brutal ways, as through rape and domestic violence.) Both sorts of cases provoke alienation from one's body. In Zeiler's words, a "disruptive movement that breaks the lived body apart . . . means that she or he cannot but attend continuously to her or his body as an object," rather than focusing on the world *through* the lived body.[45] The prisoner, like women in a sexist society, watches his or her body being watched.

An alienated embodiment can also result from living as a "minority" member in a racist society. (We have seen that the majority of inmates in the United States are African American or Hispanic.) In *Black Skin, White Masks*, Frantz Fanon writes about a formative encounter with a young boy who becomes frightened at seeing a "Negro." Confronted with his own blackness, culturally associated with primitiveness and defect, Fanon feels "imprisoned." "My body was given back to me sprawled out, distorted, clad in mourning."[46] The imprisoned body, like the black body in Fanon's description, is associated with violence and deficit, objectified by a fearful social gaze, appropriated by hostile others. Thus, the experience of *both* being a member of a minority group in a racist society *and* imprisoned may lead to synergistically intensified distortions.

A Platonic dialogue speaks of *soma* as *sema*—the "body" as a "tomb" (*Gorgias* 493a). Prisoners may in fact feel the deathly weight of an embodiment that renders them vulnerable to harsh discrimination and incarceration. It is not unusual to consider suicide as a way out of this living death. I mentioned that one of our class members—O'Donald—just seventeen when he joined us with a life sentence, may have killed himself.

Yet there are other ways out. I will now explore how embodiment can be reclaimed or escaped in vitalizing modes. I begin with an inmate's remark, continuing on the theme of whether the prison could be a "home":

TRAY JONES: But you can never really have a home in here. Because the officers could come with the key anytime they want and uproot you. Like right now, everything that I own I brought out with me (my toothbrush and all) because *I'm the cell*, my own body, rather than some hole cut out of space.[47]

This comment reminds us that as much as prison renders one's body the possession of the state, it can also reaffirm the body as the *self's* true possession and identity. We saw similar paradoxes operative in cases of illness and pain. The sick person may feel both alienated from the body and yet more closely tied to it, hyperaware of its functions and solicitous of its well-being in a way that was unnecessary in health. So, too, may the inmate become identified with and solicitous of the body. With so much else of the world ripped away, one's embodied power can be *reclaimed*—guarded and cultivated with care.

This strategy of *reclamation* takes many forms. Tray Jones affirms the body as a zone of privacy and security. Often the inmate's first task is to bolster the lived body against possible assaults from guards or other inmates. Many prisoners also develop the body's capacity and skills through weightlifting, sports, yoga, and various forms of manual labor, insofar as these are available. Inmates also employ their bodies as a locus of self-expression. A tattoo or a certain style of walk, dress, or mode of speech can help assert power and individuality or participation in a collective (all too often, a gang). Prisoners have also produced amazing artistic creations with the most limited resources. Then, too, the body can be a source of pleasure. Even within a depriving environment, gratifications of music, movement, sexuality, and drug use often remain obtainable as much as the authorities try to restrict them (or, alternatively, make a profit on them).

The presence of others can assist in bodily reclamation. As discussed in chapter 8 on organ transplants, the body is not just one's own possession: we inhabit "intercorporeal being"[48] as our life ever intertwines with that of those around us. Tray mentions the threat posed by invasive guards. Yet earlier he spoke of a brotherly cellmate whose presence expanded lived space when "we'd play cards and talk." The communion of prisoners with one another, sympathetic employees, and outside visitors can help the inmate reclaim embodied wholeness.

This is a challenge in the face of the disciplinary gaze. Foucault discusses how the structure of the "panopticon"—an architectural form that keeps its inmates always potentially visible to the authorities—serves to maintain control over potentially rebellious bodies.[49] The inmates have read this material and respond:

MARK MEDLEY: When you're virtually under twenty-four hour surveillance— like the new prison in Jessup—there's also a way you can *resist* or *escape*. Autistic thinking. Total absorption in fantasy. "I'm building an island and this is what my water source will be, and the kind of plants I'll have . . ."

You can absorb yourself in this for hours and hours and resist being conditioned by the discipline.

CHARLES BAXTER: I was in Supermax, and a lot of the brothers in there, they
escape by a lot of reading and studying—African history, the Bible, the
Koran. They realize they're being watched, but they escape to something
that gives them, you know, hope and inspiration.

DONALD THOMPSON: But there's another side. Before I came here I was
very violent. It didn't take much for me to strike out at another person—
different ways—a baseball bat, a brick, a gun. But since I came in here I've
had one fight. Knowing that I'm being watched has made me control this
violence. And as time went on it helped me discipline myself, 'cause my intellect eventually kicked in.[50]

Donald's comment is an example of the strategy of *reclamation*. He has found
a way to turn even the disciplinary gaze—potentially alienating and disempowering—into a source of personal power. He cannot escape being watched,
yet he uses this to help him overcome his own violent impulsivity. From Foucault's point of view, this is the triumph of discipline: it has been internalized to
the point where individuals police themselves. Yet Donald experiences it as his
own triumph. He is glad that he has attained more self-mastery.

Comments by Mark and Charles remind us that the imprisoned body cannot only be *reclaimed* but strategically *escaped*. Mark, rather than affirming
discipline, as does Donald, chooses to escape it via fantasy. Through "autistic
thinking" he all but vacates the body, giving it over to the authorities, but
as a lifeless thing. Charles makes reference to the escapist power of reading
available even when confined in Supermax—a place where the "worst" inmates are isolated in their cells twenty-three hours a day. Our very study of
philosophy in prison might have served as such a strategy of escape: we fly
free together over all the bars and barbed wire through the elevating powers
of the intellect.

Is the body genuinely escaped through such activities? Not exactly. The
very means by which the inmates "transcend" the body are rooted in the
body's own capacities. Mark distracts himself with visual imagery, constructing a quasi-perceptual scene that calls on body memories. Charles holds a
book in his hands and scans it with his eyes, using his brain to process symbols
and formulate thoughts. We gather in class to have our philosophical discussions. The words there spoken are now recorded here in this book. The body
is as involved in activities of the higher intellect as it is in weightlifting or sex.

Yet, as I discuss in *The Absent Body*, certain activities, because they put
out of play or background large regions of the body, and involve modes of

projection and self-transcendence, *can seem as if disembodied*.[51] As you read this, for example, you may be sitting still. The body's movements are then reduced to subtle eye scans and subvocalizations. The physical words on the page or screen become as if transparent to the meanings they signify, which are processed by brain activity unavailable to our senses. When reading we may feel transported out of our immediate locale to other times and places or a world of nonphysical ideas. Such factors combine to create an experiential sense of escaping the body, of being "pure mind."

Strategies of *integration* combine elements of body escape and reclamation. We see this implicit, for example, in Charles's comments. Even in the extremes of Supermax bodily confinement, he and his "brothers" can reclaim their situation at the same time they use it as a launching pad for transcendent escape into matters of intellect and spirit.

The Penitentiary

Let us step back for a moment and reflect on the setting where all this unfolds. The notion of the "penitentiary" was first formulated in the late eighteenth and early nineteenth centuries. (I mentioned that the Maryland Penitentiary, where these classes took place, was the oldest continuously operating penitentiary in the Western world, having first opened—or closed?—its doors in 1811.) The penitentiary movement was designed to improve the treatment of criminals by doing away with the evils of corporal and public punishment. Instead it employed what it took to be a scientific, utilitarian, and spiritual approach to reforming the inmate's soul. Quakers and other religious men were leaders of this movement to humanize and spiritualize the treatment of criminals. The prison cell was modeled, to a degree, on the monastic cell. Prisoners were to be kept in isolation from each other, given time to reflect on their sins and repent, emerging cleansed by the experience.

We have seen that certain prisoners do accomplish something like this in prison. They use the very conditions of confinement to enlarge the self and its life-world. They experience a genuine and positive existential reformation. In doing this work described above, inmates, often unknowingly, thus operate in harmony with the penitentiary's stated intent.

However, as Guenther documents, from the start the humanistic goals of the penitentiary were combined with the intent to inflict severe punishment.[52] At the prototypical Eastern State Penitentiary, inmates were kept in almost absolute isolation, disoriented spatially, deprived sensorially and socially, even masked or hooded when leaving their cells. Critics of such a system quickly emerged, including famous men like Alexis De Toqueville, Hans

Christian Andersen, and Charles Dickens, charging it with a level of inhumanity that perhaps exceeded previous modes of punishment. In Guenther's words, Dickens recognized that "in practice this withdrawal from concrete social relations did not establish in prisoners the habits of reflective, penitent souls; rather it brought about a general demolition of their personhood, not an infliction of this or that *part* of the person, but a generalized incapacitation of their Being-in-the-World."[53] The modern penitentiary still poses this threat; we have seen the men struggle, in the face of assault, to rebuild a shattered life-world. In the next chapter, we will see their collective criticism of the penitentiary in its current form, and their suggestions for how it could be re-formed into a genuine place for growth and learning.

The typical modern-day US penitentiary does little to further such ends, and much to undermine them. Conditions are harsh and overcrowded. Solitary confinement, while no longer the norm as in the original penitentiary, is vastly overused, constituting a form of psychophysical torture built into the system.[54] Treatment by prison authorities can be dehumanizing, demeaning, and radically disempowering. Opportunities for educational, therapeutic, and occupational advancement are sadly deficient. The prisoner seeking positive transformation battles hostile forces at every turn.

I will give a few examples. Due to a change in the status of the prison to medium security, most of the men whose voices we have heard were abruptly transferred en masse to other prisons. The sense of community we had painstakingly built was shattered. This is not unusual in a prison culture where close relationships and inmate communities are often seen as security threats to be countered by transfers. Around this time, I was also excluded from teaching for a year for a protocol infraction. The governor of Maryland (a moderate Democrat) announced he would not approve the parole of any inmate serving a life sentence, even when receiving positive recommendations from the parole board. Lifers' self-transformative work, this says, will neither be recognized nor rewarded. This serves to undercut just the sorts of motivated prisoners featured in this piece.

Soon thereafter, the "Violent Crime Control and Law Enforcement Act" made Pell Grants, which fund higher education for low-income Americans, unavailable to all prisoners. This has continued to be the operative law in the intervening decades. The immediate result was a whole-scale closing down of prison college extension programs. For example, before 1994, seventy publicly funded postsecondary prison programs existed in New York State alone—now there are none.[55]

This seems to me a tragedy for incarcerated men and women, for those in the larger society who have an investment in their well-being, and even for all simply concerned with public safety. While more than three-quarters of offenders are rearrested within five years of release, a meta-analysis by the Rand Corporation, funded by the US Justice Department, found on average a 43 percent reduction in recidivism for those who participated in educational programs while in prison. An estimated $5 were saved for every $1 spent on correctional education.[56] As I write this, the Obama administration has just announced a pilot program, at limited sites, to again make Pell Grant funding available to prisoners for college education—we at Jessup, where I now work, have applied to be one of those first sites.

Yet, whereas Charles envisions the cell as a prophet's cave for learning and growth, all too often it is more like Plato's cave in the *Republic* (bk. 7, 514a–521d). To illustrate the state of the unenlightened, he uses the metaphor of prisoners chained within a cave. Their necks are fastened so they cannot turn to see the light at the cave mouth. All that is visible to them are dark shadows cast on the wall by puppets. These they take to be reality, having no object of comparison.

Though metaphorical, it seems an apt image of many a prison. Educators, counselors, and others who might bring "light" from the outside world are often woefully absent. The inmates are left primarily amongst "shadows"—the society of often contemptuous authorities, other criminals, and personal memories of a previous misspent life. For most, there are few activities of a positive nature to pursue. The entire environment reinforces their identity as a "criminal," taking an act from their life, perhaps the worst thing they have ever done, and saying "*this is who you are.*" Not surprisingly, on release from the cave, the inmate is often poorly equipped to reenter the broader society. Incarceration has torn prisoners from the fabric of their previous life-world. It has punished and disempowered them. The prisoner who emerges is often angrier as a result, and more dysfunctional. He or she is out of touch with new cultural developments and technologies that others take for granted. Then there is the permanent label of ex-con, making it harder to find a job, housing, and benefits, and to forge a new identity. Is it any wonder that the rate of recidivism is so high for released inmates? Of course, this then reinforces a stereotype that rehabilitation does not work, justifying harsher sentences and prison conditions.

I have heard it said that if a mad scientist wished to create a system designed to *increase* criminality, he or she would come up with something like our modern prison system, now caging more than two million Americans and peripherally effecting tens of millions more of their dependents, family members, neighbors, and friends. Happily, we are in the midst of a social reconsideration of the practices that undergird mass incarceration. But this may come too late or in too limited a fashion to help many now in prison, at least the sort of men I work with.

To focus only on the grimness of it all is an ever-present temptation, whether for inmates or academics. However, a prisoner cannot long afford this mentality if he or she is to survive, even flourish, over the many years of incarceration. And for scholars to focus solely on the horrors of the prison system—real as they are—can risk overlooking the power of the individual to escape, reclaim, integrate even the harshest of conditions. The prisoner is not only the passive object of punishment. He or she is also an active constitutor of a life-world, capable of creating freedoms.

Rethinking Prisons:
The Enlightened (and Endarkened) Prison

This chapter turns from a focus on personal strategies to a concern with transforming institutional conditions. There is a limit to the freedoms that can be obtained by individuals when they remain embedded within structures that are static or actively destructive. In chapter 5 we tried to rethink the hospital and the nursing home in humanizing ways. Here we turn to an institution even more in need of reforming. Perhaps it is time to be penitential about our modern-day penitentiary: that is, admit what it does wrong, how our criminal justice system can at times be criminal, how our departments of correction are themselves in need of correction, and then make needed changes. What might the process and result look like? How could a prison better support the healing work of *escape, reclamation, integration* that we have just been describing?

We asked these kinds of questions in another class I held not long ago at the Jessup Correctional Institution (JCI). This serves as both a medium- and maximum-security men's prison midway between Washington and Baltimore. JCI's clientele range from lifers, some thirty or forty years into their "bits," to new-timer youth caught up in gang violence. Of the roughly 1700 JCI inmates, the majority are African American, many hailing from the tough and drug-ridden streets of East and West Baltimore, as all too often featured on TV shows like *The Wire* and in the news, as with the 2015 civil unrest in Baltimore surrounding the death of Freddy Gray while in police custody. Still, any surface impressions fail to do justice to the complexity and diversity of the men and their respective backgrounds.

My JCI class included some of the prison's "elite," long-timers unusually committed to reflection and self-transformation. Though we primarily read original texts of a philosophical and psychospiritual nature, that semester we happened to use *The Soul Knows No Bars*, the same book from which I quoted in the last chapter.[1] In dizzying meta-fashion, we had dialogues about the book's dialogues, including men who had been involved in the original project (like Tray Jones and John Woodland) commenting on their words from many years earlier. But our focus was also on the future. We were working together on this question of what prison could and should be. What if prisons were not like Plato's cave where chained men watch the play of puppet shadows? What if, instead, they were places for genuine change and enlightenment?

This could lend itself to utopianism, but our conversations remained rooted in concrete experience. This, not professional training as criminologists, was the source of the men's expertise. Prison was not something they had studied but lived. They had witnessed the power for soul destruction or life enhancement in a warden, caseworker, family member, a ticket for an infraction, a glimpse of the sky, an overcrowded cell, an educational class, a contemptuous look, an unguarded shower.

The challenge was to speak honestly of such experiences but also to translate this specificity into general principles. If we could articulate the fundamental attitudes that characterized the "enlightened prison," these could be used to suggest, validate, and measure the success of all features of an institution: programs for inmates, employee training, architectural elements, and many more.

The enlightened prison, we concluded, would embody the following five core attitudes: *hope, growth, recognition of merit, individuality,* and *community*. These would stimulate and support the positive efforts of individuals described in the previous chapter. In the absence of these attitudes, you have the "endarkened" prison—a category into which, as we have seen, all too many penitentiaries would fall. Such a place tends to inculcate opposite characteristics, which we termed respectively *despair, stasis, recognition of demerits, classification,* and *isolation*.

I will describe these ideas as they emerged in discussion and written submissions, without myself providing much of a scholarly apparatus. There are phenomenological and hermeneutical elements to the analysis: the inmates are describing their lived experiences and how they interpret them. However, I will not use the theoretical terminology found elsewhere in the book, including the last chapter. Here, I will stick more to terms and concepts used by the men.

There can be a problem to such claims to "bear witness" to the voices and suffering of others, for one's own voice can never be eradicated. As James Hatley, a friend and colleague, remarked when reading through a draft of this material,

One issue in particular [you] ought to confront squarely would be the charge from practitioners of a hermeneutics of suspicion that the very gestures of claiming one has refrained from interpreting the words of others is perhaps the most dangerous mode of interpretation there is. Can one really speak for others without the very assumptions at the core of one's own sense of things not having intervened? History is replete with those who have attempted to do so only to re-inscribe the violence they were hoping to undo.

It is true that I did intervene at multiple points, asking certain questions, guiding discussion, even suggesting categories I thought would best capture the men's insights. I did, though, check with them to see whether the terms I was using were valid and showed them a draft of this material to provide a chance for correction or supplementation. I also suggested they submit their own words in writing, and I have quoted from these documents below— though again, it was I who made the selection. This issue is also at play in the previous chapter where I worked with audiotaped comments, but ones that I chose and edited.

Perhaps it is best to refer back to a concept earlier introduced, that of the *dia-logue* (etymologically, the "speech between"). What is presented here are the truths that emerged in the speech between the men and myself, a conversation in which I was an active participant and commentator, but hopefully also a good listener and faithful recorder. I sought to stay true to both the spirit and, in many cases, the letter of what the men had to say.

Other challenges can be made to this material. One may find the prisoner recommendations naïve and idealized. Perhaps they call for too radical a change in the existing system. Conversely, these ideas may seem to some readers insufficiently radical because the inmates do not speak here of dramatic sociopolitical change or the abolishing of all prisons. (This material was originally drafted for a journal issue focused on prison reform, not prison abolition, so the latter topic was not our focus.) These may be worthy goals, and other authors and activists give them full voice. At the same time, these prisoners are *realists* in their own way. They know what has *really* made their lives miserable or, on occasion, better. In this conversation, that remains their focus and their source of authority.

Hope versus Despair

"Abandon all hope ye who enter here." So reads the sign over the gates of hell in Dante's *Inferno* (Canto 3, l.9), and it would work well for many a modern prison. Far from assisting a "penitential" process of self-examination and positive change, we have seen how penitentiaries often foster *despair* (etymologically, to "lose hope"). The men described how hope can be extinguished at several stages of their criminal justice process. This begins with the contempt and callous mistreatment of the defendant demonstrated during trial proceedings, when attorneys on both sides joke with each other like members of an old boys' club; the shock of a long or life sentence (with strange extensions such as "double-life-plus-twenty"); a harsh introduction to the "slammer" that slams you mentally and physically; loss of access to friends, family, resources, and kind words; a gathering sense of regret, bitterness, confusion, and depression, all of which endarken the spirit. This is reinforced by the many indignities of prison life. "Can you imagine," wrote one man, "having your cell searched and torn apart by a person whom you graduated high school with? . . . having money missing from your inmate account and being unable to do anything? . . . your release date comes and your case manager hasn't filed the appropriate paper work? . . . your family tells you they've sent pictures of the family reunion [but] the mail room lost them? . . . etc." The men speak of imprisonment as a descent to the underworld, a confrontation with death from which some, though not all, return.

The enlightened prison assists resurrection. It would be a citadel not just of punishment and deprivation, but of *hope*, as in a dictionary definition: "the feeling that what is wanted can be had or that events will turn out for the best." Some men said hope in prison is an imperiled, almost irrational feeling, and men sunken so low are in need of encouragement lest it die off. The enlightened prison is one that supports, philosophically and practically, opportunities for positive change. The criminal past need not rule all. The future does not yet lie in ruins. It remains a realm of possibility that can stimulate and organize present action—allowing for that work of *escape, reclamation,* and *integration* described in the last chapter.

Several men told stories of better prisons they have been incarcerated in, or their own ability to rise above dismal surroundings and pursue education, reach out to family, do legal research and filings on cases, make progress toward parole, or simply grow in meditation, prayer, and wisdom. With hope, they felt, a man can maintain a healthy relation to time even when "serving time" of unimaginably long duration.

Of course, it mattered greatly, several said, to have someone who cares. This could be a mentor: an older prisoner, spiritual teacher, caseworker, or volunteer; a family member who stands by through thick and thin. Positive programs within the prison, recognition of accomplishment, possible paths to release—these also give hope (and will be discussed later in more depth). Hope is both the *product* of positive institutional and personal reforms and, in a curious way, their *precondition*. One or two men spoke of how, ideally, everyone—legislators, judges, wardens, correctional officers, parole boards, family, society at large, and inmates themselves—have to hold onto hope or prison is just a gate to hell.

Growth versus Stasis

Hope is associated with possibilities for change and growth. Yet many prisons, according to these men, are monuments to *stasis*. Stasis is present in the architecture—imposing, constraining, inescapable—and the bureaucracy, unmovable in its exercise of power. The main "job" of the inmate at such institutions is simply to *stay put*. He or she has been *put away*, in this cell, tier, prison, for a prescribed number of years or even the entirety of a life. As explored in chapter 10, an inordinately lengthy *time* is thus to be spent in a severely restricted *space*, rendering both time and space confining and disoriented. This is compounded in a prison where there is little to do (except watch TV, eat, or walk around a bit) and little to see (the patch of sky out a cell window, the dining hall, the dirt yard).

By contrast, the men described the enlightened prison as a place for *growth*. This is valued, supported, expected. After all, a human being is a living thing, and living thing, as one man said, must grow or die. They described the many forms this had taken in their lives, all of which and more would be available in the "enlightened" prison: GED tutoring for those developing high school–level competencies; higher education programs for those simply in love with learning or seeking skill enhancement, employability, and special expertise; Twelve Step groups to help break addictive patterns; therapeutic groups and environments like the Quaker-initiated "Alternatives to Violence Program," which a number of my students participated in with great enthusiasm; a well-stocked library (individuals spoke of books that had changed their lives); prisoner-run service groups that help others inside prison or through outreach (e.g., to gang members and youth-at-risk), enhancing one's own self-esteem and leadership skills; classes in yoga and meditation; resources for the creative arts; access to computers; job training; work-release programs; the list can go on and on.

Like a university, the enlightened prison would embrace growth and change as central to its mission. As one man writes, even "architectural elements are very necessary for light to shine in. The design would be more like a college campus, plenty of windows, skylights, and flowers."

Realists that they are, many men in my class expressed skepticism about whether the prison system, and society at large, really wants to empower inmate growth. I wondered, do we have not only the vision but also the money for such things? However, given the more than $40,000 a year tab for housing a Maryland inmate, such programs and features, which reduce recidivism, could well prove cheap by comparison. A couple of men characterized our prison system—holding more than two million Americans who, as we have seen, are mostly black or Latino—as a contemporary form of enslavement. The true goal, then, is to keep the "slaves" under control, limited in intellect and ability, dead in spirit. More than a note of cynicism filtered into such conversations. The men had witnessed too much to believe that the "American dream" of self-improvement well rewarded was operative inside penal institutions. Here, instead, they saw a shadow side of America, infected by racism, classism, and a focus on capitalist profit.

Nevertheless, these men refused to acquiesce to either passivity or bitterness. Many were living proof of the possibilities for multidimensional growth even while incarcerated. They have secured advanced degrees; written books, newspaper articles, and publicly performed plays; developed artistic skills; pursued religious study and meditation practice; won statewide and even national awards; received fellowships and political support for large-scale community programs, and so on. Yet these men also know themselves to be "exceptions to the rule." They described a system that tends to favor stasis, and thereby retrograde movement, as many inmates are made worse, not better—less employable, less self-sufficient, less able to negotiate the legitimate world—by their extended prison time. We have seen that, with high rates of recidivism, return to prison is prevalent postrelease.

Many inmates become complicit in their institutionalization. My students expressed frustration with some at JCI: immature youth, distracted short-timers, or long-timers who have given up on their cases or are narcotized by TV. One wrote to me of those who "affected by this inhuman and psychologically degrading environment" become "addicted to the dependency of institutionalization, selfishness and lack of responsibility. . . . They know it's wrong and no good for them but they lack the psychological and emotional discipline and will to free themselves from its grasp." The enlightened prison would do what it could to prevent or treat this paralysis.

A parenthetical comment: though some inmate recommendations may seem hopelessly idealistic in an American context, one can look to other prison systems, for example, those characteristic of Scandinavian countries, to see such principles put into practice.[2] A criminal-services fact sheet from Norway states: "During the serving of a sentence, life inside will resemble life outside as much as possible. You need a reason to deny a sentenced offender his rights, not to grant them. Progression through a sentence should be aimed as much as possible at returning to the community." Larson describes a Finnish prison scene: "Your cell phone lies on a shelf, next to a TV and CD player, inside a prison that lets you go to paid work or study. There is no perimeter wall. Prison staff will help you with free-world social services to cover a missed month's rent on your family's apartment. Another will help you look for work, or for the next stage of education."[3] This is not just about "coddling" criminals, but assisting them to put their criminal identity in the rear-view mirror.

Recognition of Merit versus Demerit

When an inmate makes positive changes, these need to be recognized and rewarded. Several men spoke with great frustration about how this is not currently the case in our "endarkened prisons." You may have crafted a new understanding of self and world or a building desire and ability to help others—but find yourself with no realistic way to act on these. Or you pursue education, develop skills, achieve credentials, even take on leadership roles, but realize the prison administration, parole board, and governor couldn't care less. There is *no recognition of merit.*

Such recognition typifies progress in the outside world: you accumulate accomplishments that build your college application, job resume, and the like. However, in the criminal justice system, I was told, assessment is largely reversed. You are defined not by your demonstrated merits, but by *demerits.* The "convict" first became one by virtue of demerits, a conviction for alleged criminal activities. The criminal justice system then continues this focus on demerits. Infractions—having an altercation with a guard, failing to show up for a count-out, being caught with contraband—are meticulously ticketed and punished. Such records can lead to loss of privileges for the men, lockup, administrative segregation (solitary confinement), transfer to another institution, or extension of sentence.

But what, conversely, does it mean to "do well"? Primarily, to have a *lack of demerits.* Far from offering positive recognition, "good behavior" is defined as the negative of a negative—one has *not* done something one is *not* supposed to do. According to the men, while personal accomplishments are noted, they count for relatively little in the mathematized calculation of their record. I pondered this: it's as if the best a student in my Loyola class could hope for, even at the end of a semester of excellent papers and presentations, was a note in my grade book to the effect that she had not been observed disrupting class. I can imagine how demoralizing this would be to my Loyola high achievers.

My prison class likewise included a number of high achievers. One of them, a lifer, handed me a sixty-page single-spaced curriculum vita filled with

significant accomplishments (including the publication of well over one hundred articles and letters) largely done while in prison. In an enlightened institution, such work would not only be supported by the correctional infra-
structure, but rewarded through the granting of commendations, privileges,
promotions through the system, and accelerated release. Another man, one of
the organizers of our class, showed me a "Merit-Based Movement" program he
and others had helped develop, which involved a detailed calculation of merit
points earned through participation in educational, vocational, and addiction
programming, and other noteworthy accomplishments. Not surprisingly, it
was never implemented. The enlightened prison, however, would emphasize
the development and honoring of strengths and achievements.

Individuality versus Classification

The recognition of merit is an aspect of a broader issue: the struggle in prison
to realize yourself as an *individual*. "Who am I, really, and who do I want to
become?" seemed a central life issue for the men (as perhaps for all of us). I
heard people searching to articulate their unique identity, value, and destiny.
A number of them talked about how their criminal behavior was rooted in not
being true to themselves. "I was trying to fit in." "I lost myself for a while." "I
was just a stupid kid." Without a sense of positive identity, you can end up acting out in "powerful" but pathological ways, and/or submerging yourself in
a gang affiliation.

How to find yourself, but in a healthy fashion? The men talked about the
importance—and in today's overcrowded and noisy prisons, the rarity—of
solitude and privacy. "I find my peace," one writes, "early in the morning,
when mostly everyone is asleep. There is no loud noise, the quietness in the air
is so beautiful, calming and peaceful." Time to think, remember, dream, and
rediscover your authentic self. Yet we also define who we are by what others
reflect back. The enlightened prison would be a place that recognizes and
supports the positive individuality of those it houses.

But in today's prison, the individual is viewed primarily as a member of
an unsavory class. You have been convicted of an act classified as a criminal offense, which then comes to constitute your identity. You have not just
been found guilty of a crime; *you are a drug dealer, murderer, thief,* or *rap-
ist*—a representative of a class of people (or, as we will see in the next chapter,
of "subhuman predators"). All the unique and positive aspects of your history
and character are submerged in this *class-ification*.

Prison is a place that ceaselessly reinforces a class identity. Your right to
dress as an individual is taken away: in Maryland, you are issued a uniform

that both labels you as different from those in the outer world and makes you the same, *uniform*, with other convicts. For administrative purposes, your name is largely replaced with a number.

In class, the men also brought up a different and, for them, especially hurtful and counterproductive form of classification: the punishment of entire groups for the infraction committed by a single person. One inmate stabs another and the whole prison is placed on lockdown. Someone violates a work-release program and commits a widely publicized crime—end of the program. A large number of men who were making good use of work-release in Maryland, laboring hard at their jobs and integrating well with the outside world, were all suddenly remanded to prison. Even the *possibility* of a single high-profile crime plagues politicians worried about reelection. They decide that no lifers will be paroled on their watch, no matter what the individual's accomplishments or the positive recommendation of the parole board. This is the position taken since the early 1990s by a number of Maryland governors, one of the very few states in the country where the governor had to personally approve every such parole. Governor Glendening, referred to in the last chapter, has now admitted that his actions "made the parole process much more political than it should be and that he would 'not have a problem' with a change in state law to remove the governor from that process."[4] (New legislation has somewhat, though not entirely, mitigated the governor's role.) Again, such one-size-fits-all policies treat the individual simply as a member of a class. He or she can be punished in advance for the actions, or *possible actions*, of any other class member.

The enlightened prison would treat each person as an individual. He or she is not simply categorized according to crime, sentence, addiction, race, or socioeconomic status. The more I got to know the people in my class, the more their individuality came to the fore: this one a painter, that one a student of contemporary physics, another an avid meditator, or a Washington Redskins rooter, or a fan of Epictetus and Nietzsche. I heard some of their complex family histories, involving a mother who had held the family together in tough times or the traumatic death of a brother in a young man's arms. One person had previously been a criminal lawyer, another an ob-gyn, a third had run a business selling jet skis. The enlightened prison is an institution that illuminates, even celebrates, the complex humanity and individuality of its residents.

Often the men spoke of the key role of personal relationships in preserving a sense of self. One wrote of a case manager who was clear and respectful in her communications: "I made sure that I was able to see and converse with Ms. Mowan weekly, and the more I spoke with her, the less burdensome my sentence became." Another recommended having correctional officers assigned to a single tier, rather than constantly transferred from one to another; now they never get to know the inmates as people and do not treat them as such. The value of personal recognition was clearly expressed by a man writing of his graduation from a college extension program in the days before Pell Grant tuition funding was withdrawn from inmates:

> It was not a great moment because I graduated with honors. It was not a great moment because I gave a speech. It was a great moment because my son, Rashaun, was there. He was 11 years old, and it was his first opportunity to see me in a positive way. It was the first time that I didn't feel like a prisoner who only had a few minutes left on his visit to talk to his son, or the drug dealer convicted of murder. I was his father the valedictorian who was preparing to give a speech. I could see in his eyes that he was proud of me. And that was a great feeling that I will never forget.

Over years of teaching inside this prison, I have witnessed men honoring one another's individuality through appreciative comments, gestures of friendship, mutual applause and fist-bumps at the graduation ceremony with which we end each semester. A prison must have hierarchy and security, but in an enlightened prison this recognition of the individual would also pervade the organizational structure and be demonstrated by the warden, administrative chiefs, correctional officers, case managers, volunteers, parole board, and the family and friends whom the prison would make welcome. The emphasis in such an institution is not only on *taking away*—your freedom, possessions, clothes, name—but on helping *to give back* a sense of positive identity, as in the previously mentioned Scandinavian model.

For some, this is the recovery of an earlier lost self to the throes, for example, of addiction. For others, it may be an entirely new experience. "I hate the term 'rehabilitation,'" said one of the men. "It implies I'm recovering something I used to have. But I never had it to begin with." The development of healthy individuality is a maturational challenge. Not everyone is ready for it. The men in my class were quick to acknowledge that many in JCI were mired in violence or ignorance and uninterested in change. But the enlightened prison would invite a process of individual growth and self-expansion, with the person held responsible for follow-through.

Community versus Isolation

As the above discussion suggests, healthy individuals are formed and recognized within healthy *community*. Obviously, such is often lacking or actively discouraged in prisons. Convicts are removed from family, friends, and the community in which they reside, but which they have "offended." They are thrown together, often in overcrowded and insecure conditions, with hundreds or thousands of other men who themselves have committed antisocial acts. Prison administrators discourage close ties between guards and inmates, for such can compromise command and security. So, too, close ties among inmates may be deterred. They can lead, in the eyes of authorities, to the forming of power blocs and conspiracies. Men have told me that a prisoner with too many friends or too much power may simply be transferred to another penitentiary. "Diesel therapy," one prisoner called it. Then, too, the whole spirit of penal institutions and their members can undermine attempts at community. Anger, fear, aggression, distrust are pervasive elements among inmates and staff given their personal histories, current experiences, and the institutional mission. Several men voiced contempt for the correctional officers for treating them with contempt. Thus the circle turns.

"Hell is other people," says a character in Jean-Paul Sartre's *No Exit.*[5] To spend long years in an overcrowded prison, with two men crammed into a cell barely adequate for one, constant noise echoing down the tier, no hope of escape, a lack of trust for those around you; this would be hell indeed. Paradoxically, such overcrowding can also lead to a spirit of *isolation.* Forgotten by the larger world, looked down on by prison authorities, and having to fight for survival with other inmates, each person stands alone. "The jungle's creed reads; the strong must feed off any prey at hand," one man wrote. "Prison is a jungle. It's a matter of do or die." This stark aloneness is not to be confused with restorative "solitude." Quite the converse: when you can rarely get away from others, never feel safe and quiet, it is unlikely that one will find internal solace and solitude.

What encouraged me, though, was the extent of positive community among the men despite all these impediments. This was not the false community of clinging to a violent gang or to a powerful exploiter/protector for security. This was a community of mutual respect and affection: men in the class had known each other in some cases for decades, struggled and worked side-by-side in harsh conditions, taken advantage together of positive opportunities, and bonded through their many experiences. This was not always true. There were the antagonisms one might expect from rough-edged men who had too long been forced to live at close quarters. But at least in our classroom, these were restrained by an etiquette of politeness and mutual respect. Everyone's voice was welcomed.

The enlightened prison would seek to support such community. Opportunities for solitude would be complemented by activities with and for others. Again, we return to the importance of providing classes, groups, and programs.

There are also curricula that directly enhance community building and defuse threats to its existence. One of my inmate class members writes of the
Alternatives to Violence Program used in JCI and nationwide:

> Some inmates here are like a time bomb, which can explode at any time and
> without any warning, resulting in a violent or deadly situation in a fraction of
> a second. A good, alert, open minded and wise inmate who utilizes the AVP
> tools is like an experienced member of a bomb squad who dismantles a bomb
> before it explodes, preventing death and destruction. I believe we must be vi-
> sionaries, open-minded and proactive.

He contends that, due in part to such programs, violence in JCI has declined.
The enlightened prison need not compromise security: it can and should be a
safer prison for inmates and correctional officers alike.

This is especially true insofar as the latter are included in the sense of
community. This may seem naïve or even dangerous—the guards are there
to *guard*, not to fraternize and thereby "let down their guard." But they, too,
have to live within this tightly wound world. They, too, need to feel and be
more than just "the enemy." One inmate spoke of an enlightened warden who
created an annual charity run in which correctional officers and inmates had
to participate together. This began to break down the barriers of hostility that
had pervaded the institution. (Again, Scandinavian systems may provide a
model: in Norway's Halden Prison, "the guards socialize with the inmates
every day, in casual conversation, often over tea or coffee or meals."[6])

However high the barriers of walls and razor wire, several men also spoke of
the crucial nature of contact with those outside. A friend or family member who
kept in touch, sent a package, came to visit, could make all the difference. So,
too, volunteers who enter to share their skills; or having access to the Internet
so you can learn what is happening in the world and ready yourself to participate in it; work-release programs that allow you to temporarily leave prison,
reclaiming a public identity—the enlightened prison supports such visits and
ventures. It is not solely about creating barriers—locked cells, segregated tiers,
towering walls—but about assisting people to surmount the barriers that keep
them in isolation. To me, and I think *us*, that is what our class, and this chapter
are all about: men speaking to each other, but also to those in the wider world.

The Simurg

The *Conference of the Birds* is a twelfth-century Sufi allegorical poem by the
Persian author Farid ud-Din Attar. The plot is nicely summarized by the Ar-
gentinian writer Jorge Luis-Borges:

The faraway king of the birds, the Simurg, drops an exquisite feather in the middle of China; weary of their ancient anarchy, the birds determine to find it. They know that their king's name means "Thirty Birds." They know that his royal palace stands on the Kaf, the circular mountain, which surrounds the earth. They undertake the almost infinite adventure. They fly over seven valleys, over seven seas; the next-to-the-last one is called Vertigo; the last, Annihilation. Many of the pilgrims desert; others perish. Thirty of them, purified by their labors, set foot upon the mountain of the Simurg. At last they contemplate it: they perceive that *they* are the Simurg, and that the Simurg is each one of them and all of them.[7]

The "enlightened prison" is like the Simurg—an ideal that is sought for, but seems far away, almost impossible to reach. Why even discuss and write about it in our class? Many inmates have "deserted," others "perished," caught in the "vertigo" and "annihilation" of inner-city streets and nihilistic prisons; yet there are those who labor on in their quest. "They undertake the almost infinite adventure" of life still available even to a lifer. Seeking the enlightened prison, they catch a glimmer of it as a reality, here and now.

In our class discussion, I experienced among the men the very things of which they spoke: *hope* for a future still alive and beckoning; a dedication to *growth* in mind and spirit; the *recognition of merit*—their own and that of others as we listened respectfully, argued, laughed, and on the last day of class, shared cake and applause, celebrating both our *individuality* and *community*.

We were exactly thirty in our class (in the acknowledgments I list the names of each of the men), looking in a sense for the Simurg, the "thirty birds." We discovered that for now we *are* the Simurg. Wherever people search within, and with others, for the "enlightened prison," right then it begins to manifest.

Rethinking Prisoners and Animals: "They're Animals" and Their Animals

As discussed, we now cage more than two million men and women in our U.S. prisons and jails. Billions of animals likewise live in prisonlike conditions the world over, raised for eggs, meat, and milk production before their slaughter. Previous chapters have addressed the situation of, and the institutions within which we house, prisoners and animals. In this chapter, however, I turn to the *relationship between them.*

In the first section, "They're Animals," I will discuss the way criminals are viewed in the social imagination. They are often typified as animalistic in a way that justified modes of harsh treatment *otherwise reserved for nonhuman beings.* The second section is entitled "Their Animals." Here focus shifts toward the rich relationships between prisoners and the animals with whom they interact. I will draw again on comments from prisoners at Jessup Correctional Institution (JCI), this time participants in a philosophy class that raised these topics. (The membership of this class overlapped but was not identical with that represented in the previous chapter.) More specifically, I worked closely on this material with one incarcerated individual, Vincent Greco, whose contribution to this chapter is invaluable. He helped administer the JCI Scholars Program (our prison education program), among his many other efforts, and is a prison-reform activist and educator on the inside and out. He was recently released from JCI after serving thirty-three years.

They're Animals

We have seen in previous chapters how prisoners are often categorized and condemned as fundamentally flawed persons. An examination of public discourse suggests something further: that criminals are metaphorically portrayed as *subhuman*. They and their crimes are called "savage" and "bestial." They are "predators" or, in a term fashionable in the 1990s to describe young gang members, "superpredators" thought to be radically impulsive and brutally remorseless.[1] The "criminal" is thus related in the social imagination to the "animal"—not actual animals, who are diverse in their species nature and often complex and highly social beings, but the *animal-as-imagined*, savagery unconstrained by reason or morality. In Mason's words,

> We call someone an "animal" when we want to insult and debase him or her. . . . We describe horrible human beings as "animals," "beasts," or "brutes" (an old word for "animal") when we want to describe their egoism, insatiable greed, insatiable sexuality, cruelty, senseless slaughter of nonhuman beings, and the mass slaughter of human beings.[2]

This imagery is used in prosecutorial appeals to judge and jury; in media descriptions of crimes and their suspected perpetrators; in everyday conversations where fear and anger are expressed, mingled with incomprehension: "What kind of animal would do such a thing?"

In the United States, this metaphoric dehumanization goes hand in hand with long-lived racial stereotypes. People of color, such as African Americans and Latinos, have historically often been viewed by European Americans as less than fully human, justifying enslavement and other modes of oppression and mistreatment.[3] It is no accident that such groups are those focused on by the criminal justice system and, as we have seen, vastly overrepresented in the prison population.[4] This discriminatory treatment—with, for example, blacks incarcerated at six times the rate of whites—has been related to what criminologists call "black threat" or "minority threat"—the notion that such *others*, being savage and predatory, are peculiarly dangerous and in need of control.[5]

Within the mass media and other public depictions of the criminal, Sloop finds a racialized bifurcation that began in the 1960s and has carried forward:

> The first of these represents the male prisoner in a fashion similar to that of the 1950's, a prisoner who is primarily "human" and generally Caucasian, needing only help and understanding in order to escape the mental fetters that place him in prison. The second male prisoner of the 1960's, one increasingly depicted as African-American, is constructed as violent, tending toward rape, and generally irredeemable; he needs and deserves punishment.[6]

The equation of *criminal—person-of-color—violent animal* leads to disproportionate and inhumane uses of caging and solitary confinement, which then seem to confirm the existing stereotypes of the human-beast.

Of course, sometimes people do engage in brutal actions. In our JCI class, Michael writes, "The prisoners that stalk their victims, rape, molest, rob, murder—certainly act as animals in the wild." Arlando Jones III (Tray) talks about how conditions may make it necessary to act savagely—for example, when living in a violent neighborhood, protecting territory in the drug game, or stuck in a maximum security (yet insecure) prison. It is a "jungle," and human beings can be reduced to a Darwinian struggle for survival.

At the same time, our interactions over the years have made clear to me that people in prison are first and foremost *people*—reflective, emotional, and subject to the same fears, pressures, and social and economic influences as are "upstanding citizens." In fact, any attempt to reify the criminal/citizen boundary is doomed to fail—ordinary people are likely to commit criminal acts in the course of a day, and "criminals" have done many worthy things in their lives. In the words of classmate Zaeed Zakaria, "We are humans just like anyone else. . . . But in an instant these same people have made a poor decision or got caught up in something . . . in the blink of an eye this person's past is forgot and [they are] viewed as an animal—they become less than human—this person is treated if they were born in prison and had no life prior to this one."

This then seems to justify inhumane practices. Shaylor gives a striking example from the solitary confinement unit in a California women's prison:

> Guards speak to and about the women as though they are sub-human. A pamphlet. produced by the Warden's office . . . lists times for daily "feedings." Guards constantly use racial epithets, many of which are gendered, to refer to the women. They call the prisoners "dogs," "niggers," "bitches," "whores" and "black bitches": women refer to their cells as "cages." When women are denied privileges, they are put on what guards refer to as "dog status." . . . The fostering of a perception of prisoners as less than human allows state employees to deny the women any semblance of dignity and to abuse them without compunction.[7]

It would be unfair to simply demonize the correctional officers—they too are under fierce institutional pressures, and dehumanizing the prisoners may be an emotional and professional coping strategy. Yet paradoxically, it is the cruel behavior exhibited by guards, institutions, and by extension, the larger society, that could be said to be *inhuman*, or at least *inhumane*. It is not just those imprisoned, but all of us, who are diminished by such patterns of mistreatment.

ZOOS, CIRCUSES, AND FACTORY FARMS

If prisoners are viewed as animals, what does that make prisons? JCI's Zaeed Zakaria compares them to zoos. "Zoos in essence are prisons designed to cage the wild animals in, to confine and restrict and to manipulate for one's purpose. It is a way to show . . . how one group has power over another." A story was told in class about an inmate who—when groups, including college classes, legislators, and judges, would be taken on tour of the prison—would jump about, scratching his body while making monkey noises. This was his ironic commentary on being exhibited like a caged animal, as he simultaneously adopted and refused this role.

Jeremi Lewis of our class was reminded more of the circus. "The guards frown down on us and speak to us as if we lack an understanding or compassion. . . . We are prodded, humiliated and subjected to strip searches which are dehumanizing, as is being encaged. We are to them amusement like circus tigers jumping through hoops of flame as the sound of the whip echoes in the ear."

In zoos and circuses, animals are displayed for the entertainment of the general public. We see this to some extent in the plethora of TV shows and movies that feature criminals being captured by police or confined in prison, all for a salacious thrill, the satisfaction of seeing good triumph, and/or the curiosity that leads us to peer into dark places. Now and then our collective gaze thus penetrates through the bars and barbed wire. However, for the most part, prisoners are shielded from public view. This deprives them not only of freedom, but of rights and protections, even the fundamental right to be seen, heard, and remembered. Hidden away, so too are the abuses to which they are subject. The brutalities described by Shaylor above might not survive a thorough airing in the press.

Foucault writes about how the public spectacle of punishment—torture and execution exhibited for the entertainment, edification, and intimidation of the general public—gave way after the eighteenth century to a system of punishments largely hidden away. Instead of publicly inflicting pain on the body of the condemned, that body is confined within institutions of discipline that meticulously order and document its movements through space and time. Prisoners are kept under a system of constant surveillance and microregulation. "Thus discipline produces subjected and practiced bodies, 'docile bodies.' Discipline increases the forces of the body (in economic terms of utility) and decreases these same forces (in political terms of obedience)."[8] As mentioned in chapter 10, Foucault traces out disciplinary mechanisms within the modern penitentiary, but also sees them at play in the school, army, hospital, asylum, and factory.

Though he, himself, says little about disciplinary institutions for animals, Foucault's analysis can be extended to the modern factory farm examined in chapter 9. As Cole writes,

Many intensive "farming" practices are similarly suggestive of the production of docile bodies through spatial distribution, surveillance and "correction." Technologies of confinement such as battery cages, "broiler" sheds or "veal crates" all share the motif of "correcting" nonhumans for their "wasteful" use of energy (read: feed, for which read: economic cost) to sustain their own biological processes. Mutilations are designed to ameliorate the economic costs of "aggression" that result from confinement technologies (that is, result from the actions of the human captors who design, build and maintain them), such as the amputation of horns, tails or beaks or the "clipping" of teeth.[9]

CAFOs (concentrated animal feeding operations) thus operate as extreme disciplinary institutions. Animal bodies are caged, fattened, impregnated, medicated, and in various ways forced and tracked along a production line that leads to slaughter.[10] As described in chapter 9, along the way they suffer the frustrations of their most ordinary instincts, such as that of a chicken to walk about and spread its wings. They are nutritionally deprived and/or overfed, often developing severe anatomical problems and diseases as a result. Families are separated, social systems disrupted. Unable to establish a normal social order, animals struggle to survive in stressful and overcrowded conditions. Their consequent aggression is treated by the "mutilations" Cole mentions above, such as slicing off chickens' beaks using a hot knife.

Comparisons to human incarceration are not difficult to make. Doing so will allow us to relate more explicitly the material presented in the last chapters respectively on factory farms and penitentiaries. In the United States, prisoners often live in overcrowded conditions, packed together in barracks or with two inmates inhabiting a small cell built for one. Stress, aggression, and disease are the result. In one telling example, the Supreme Court recently ruled that conditions in the California system, holding nearly double the amount of prisoners it was designed for, violated the inmates' constitutional rights. In his majority opinion, Justice Kennedy notes, among many other such details, "a correctional officer testified that, in one prison, up to fifty sick inmates may be held together in a twelve-by twenty-foot cage for up to five hours awaiting treatment."[11] A lower court had called it an "uncontested fact" that "an inmate in one of California's prisons needlessly dies every six or seven days due to constitutional deficiencies."[12] Extreme overcrowding, insufficient facilities, and the lack of adequate care for physical and mental illnesses result in high suicide and death rates.

All this is reminiscent of factory-farm conditions—for example, that of egg-laying hens confined six-to-eight in a small wire-mesh cage, with a single worker monitoring as many as 150,000 chickens.[13] Some bird "wastage" through disease and death is deemed an acceptable cost given the economic efficiency of large-scale egg production. Similarly, human wastage is too often deemed acceptable in our prisons, given the aim of disciplining those disruptive to the social order. The yield in behavioral docility is also complemented by economic utility. Not only do inmates constitute a population of cheap labor producing goods for state governments but, as earlier discussed, their very warehousing generates significant wages and profits for construction companies, food servicers, telephone companies, correctional officers, municipalities, and, increasingly, private corporations who are contracted by the state to build and run for-profit prisons.[14] Incarcerating one inmate can cost/generate some $40,000 a year—that's a lot of eggs.

Along the way, the inmate experiences caging and a disordered sociality comparable to the CAFO-confined animal. Rather than seeking a "restorative justice" that might reintegrate offenders, we remove them from family and community and place them in overcrowded conditions among hundreds or thousands of other criminals, producing what can be a chaotic and dangerous environment. The struggle to survive in such conditions and establish a "pecking order" can lead to gang affiliations and individual violence. All this calls forth more intrusive disciplinary measures such as prolonged solitary confinement, essentially a form of torture that can cause or exacerbate mental and physical illnesses.[15]

One might ask whether it is worse to cage animals or humans. Peter Singer has argued that under some conditions animals suffer more than humans because of their cognitive limits—for example, when being taken to a veterinarian an animal may panic, not understanding that treatment will be brief and salutary. In other conditions—for example, having cancer—an animal may suffer less, unafflicted by anticipatory dread.[16] Which applies here? Recently, Arlando Jones III (Tray) has told me, unsolicited, that human suffering from incarceration is clearly worse. "Humans just need more space than other animals. It's fundamental to the human spirit." Yet at another time he also said (as previously quoted), "My space ain't too restricted because I think of myself as on an odyssey. I take the stoic outlook—my space is supposed to be restricted but my ideas don't have to be, and that's where I find all my freedom."[17] Perhaps both sides of this paradox are true—that the more abstract, projective modes of understanding available to humans can be a source of great suffering—when imprisoned one reflects on the stupid mistakes of the past and all the rich possibilities of life slipping away—and yet this same intellect can expand lived time and space, establishing a sense of mental and spiritual freedom unavailable to the caged animal. Chapter 10 surveys some of the emancipatory strategies incarcerated persons employ.

To ask, though, who is worse off may disguise the fact that both situations cause great suffering and often in similar ways. Up until now, this chapter has referred to "humans" and "animals" as if separate categories, but of course humans *are* animals. Guenther writes that without acknowledging this, we cannot fully understand the destructive effects of solitary confinement:

> What the opposition between humane and inhumane treatment fails to grasp is the degree to which it is not primarily as *human beings*, with a presumably inherent sense of dignity and freedom, that we are affected by solitary confinement and sensory deprivation, but as *living beings*, sensible flesh, with corporeal relations to other embodied beings and to an open field of overlapping experience in a shared world. It is as *animals* that we are damaged or even destroyed by the supermax or SHU, just as our fellow animals are damaged or destroyed by confinement in cages at zoos, factory farms, and scientific laboratories.[18]

We have come full circle. This section is entitled "They're Animals." This turns out to be true, but not in the sense with which we began—that criminals are *different from us, subhuman*—savage, bestial, brutish—but the opposite— that criminals are animals insofar as *they are human like ourselves*. As Guenther writes, people are also animals, living beings, sensible flesh, in corporeal relations with other embodied beings and a shared world. That world is radically truncated for the factory-farm animal and the prisoner alike. Not only isolated from family and community and subjected to harsh treatment, the incarcerated person is permitted little contact with the natural world of trees and rivers, flowers and fields, and other nonhuman animals. However, and happily, this is not the whole story.

Their Animals

Though living in a largely denaturalized environment, often one in which (nonhuman) animals are forbidden for sanitary and security reasons, nonetheless prisoners have trans-species encounters with other animals. We might think of these animals as themselves bandits. They sneak across fences, steal food, break the rules. In a sense, they share in the inmates' own incarceration. In another sense, they are wild and free in a way that may lead to prisoner envy. They may also be feared, loathed, or respected—and sometimes loved. We will briefly survey a series of such relationships, using written accounts I solicited from JCI class participants, particularly those of coauthor Vincent Greco, which range across tame creatures to wild; state-sponsored programs to illicit encounters; the scampering rat to the soaring bird.

PESTS AND PETS

There were five or ten groundhogs running around the institution. When I was exercising, there was a groundhog who crawled under the fence and sat right next to me. Another time I saved a cricket—put it on the grass. If you're in tune with yourself you become in tune with how special life is, no matter how small. The same Creator gave both humans and animals life.[19]

The prisoners describe such relations with a varied range of wildlife (and "low-life"): skunks, foxes, bugs, cats, fish, rabbits, mice, rats, among others. The rodents in particular can be viewed by inmates and staff alike as pests. To keep them out and himself protected, Greco himself had to build a smallscale version of his own prison:

> I found that I had to have a three-foot-high door board and use steel wool as barbed wire across the top to block the mice and rats from entering the cell and eating all our food. At night I would hear the mice or rats climbing the door board only to run into the barbed wire—some tried their paws—but never succeeded.

Such highlights the unsanitary, even disease-ridden, conditions that can be found in many penitentiaries, conditions from which, of course, the prisoners have difficulty escaping.

At the same time, even these pests can become pets. "Prisoners were breeding rats. They made elaborate cages and plastic running tubes in their cells. I suppose we could call these animals prison hamsters and guinea pigs" (Greco). Michael writes,

> [I] discovered a mouse eating my commissary. Stayed up one night and captured it with a trap—I let it go on the tier but it came back to my cell the next night. After about thirty days of chasing the mouse I was able to wash it and feed it *every* night. After about sixty days the mouse actually came on my bed and rested. . . . I went on lock-up and to my surprise I did not miss the sunshine, the yard, recreation, TV, population—what I did miss was my pet mouse.

This from Vincent Greco:

> Where there are rats there are cats. One day we found a litter of cats, about a day or two old, in the bottom of the elevator shaft; the mother had died. I climbed down and got them out and I took one back to my cell. She had to be fed with an eye-dropper but she grew up just fine eating tuna from the kitchen. I had the cat—Spud—for several years . . . I built her shelves so she could jump around the cell and left the T.V. on for her when I went to work.

After several years I decided to free her. l sent her home to my mother after a big fanfare and party. I still have the picture with her and me in the visiting room with a sign saying "Spud makes parole."

As Guenther was quoted above, person and animal meet "as *living beings*, sensible flesh, with corporeal relations to other embodied beings and to an open field of overlapping experience in a shared world."[20] Prisoner and pet are incarcerated together, sharing the same food and conditions. At the same time, they liberate each other—*Spud makes parole*—but also, in a sense, Vincent Greco "made parole" through Spud, even while imprisoned—because they formed a relationship that transcends the prison context. The prisoner, often thought of as an "animal," shines forth his humanity by acts of caring. The animal, in this case Spud, is free of the judgments that a human might make. He does not see Greco as a prisoner—simply as a friend and caregiver. Prisoners dwell in institutions that reinforce their criminal identities, ceaselessly reminding them that they are defective and malicious. The uncritical gaze of an animal helps one to experience and express a better self.

Another aspect of the close relationship between prisoners and their animals is their shared vulnerability to arbitrary modes of power. Greco recounts how one prison ordered mounds of kitty litter to help bolster the cat population to keep down the number of rats. But at another time,

> the prison administration decided they wanted to get rid of the cats. They told us at 9:00 in the morning that we had until 2:00 to have someone pick up our pets or the SPCA would get them. My mother could not make it until after work. The Assistant Warden said I had to tell my mother to pick him up at the SPCA. What was unknown was that the SPCA's policy is to immediately euthanize feral cats. My mother went only to find that my cat had been killed.

In his article, "Killing Time on the Prairie," Mobley writes about a Colorado prison inhabited around the edges by a colony of prairie dogs to which he and many others had become devoted. When it was learned the animals were under threat from the authorities, the prisoners contemplated a food strike or work stoppage. Provisions were stockpiled in case of lockdown or riot. Nevertheless, in the name of safety and security, the entire prairie dog colony was exterminated. Mobley, understanding the parallel relationship between the prisoners and animals, and their co-vulnerability to carceral cruelties, by then had become a vegetarian. "After a time it didn't feel right for me to support any 'system' that treated living beings in impersonal, mass-produced ways."[21]

JCI SERVICE DOG PROGRAM

On the positive side, one of the ways in which prisons have helped both "humanize" and "animalize" their environments is through prison-based animal programs (PAPs).[22] These programs accomplish a variety of goals, including rehabilitating animals for community adoption, training service dogs for those with various physical and mental disabilities, supplying companion animals as inmate pets, caring for injured wildlife that are then released, farming, taming wild horses, and even breeding and protecting endangered species.[23] Survey results suggest that a majority of states have some such program in their prison system, with dogs the most popular animal in use.[24] This recently appeared at JCI in the form of a program run by Canine Partners for Life, founded in 1989 to train service and home companion dogs for people with cognitive and physical disabilities. (Most PAP programs are facilitated by outside organizations, with the prison's cooperation.) As Greco writes,

> Bud, Jakster, Smidget, and Riblet came into the institution as eight-week-old puppies. Needless to say JCI was immediately transformed. Some prisoners, including myself, have not interacted with dogs [pets] for over thirty years. We did not realize just how much we missed it. While it must be acknowledged that there are people who just don't like dogs, and in addition who believe that prison is not a place for dogs, I can see the upbeat effect that the dogs have on our community.
>
> The Warden's decision to place the dogs in D-building was calculated. Historically it has had a reputation for violence and placing dogs in that environment has contributed to the reduction of violence. In fact the program seems to enhance consciousness toward humanity awareness. Animals have a real calming effect on a community and that seems to be even truer for a closed prison community.

JCI Warden John Wolfe (an appropriate name) is a big supporter: "I know the dog program has had an overall positive impact on both the inmate population and the staff because it brings a sense of normalcy to the situation. . . . Pets bring comfort, joy and companionship to peoples' lives."[25]

This positive take is echoed by prison administrators across the country. Of sixty-one respondents to a national survey, sixty said that they would recommend such programs to fellow administrators, reflecting a remarkable unanimity (the only dissenter expressed concerns that the program had not proved revenue-generating). When asked to identify any negative aspects associated with the program—for the inmates, staff, or facility—60 percent reported *none*.[26]

The many benefits of these PAPs noted by administrators and/or prisoners include a calmed environment, which can reduce the incidence of aggression,[27] and the development of inmate vocational skills that contributes to experience with goal setting and practical problem solving, and an enhanced sense of responsibility and discipline. At the same time, these human-animal interactions grant more freedom for the expression of feelings, including those involving love and tenderness not easy to access in a harsh prison setting. Toxic anger and self-hate can build up over the years. These can be released and diffused when caring for, and being cared for by, an animal.[28] The result is an embodied relational therapy that could not be duplicated just through talk and self-help programs. Greco suggests how deep things can go:

> Trust and loyalty, or the lack thereof, is a component of the darwinistic social milieu of prison. I suppose everyone has been betrayed by a thought-to-be friend or lover. However, how many pets have actually turned on us? The loyalty of a dog is next to none. . . . I've also seen one person who became a caretaker of a dog and it seems to help resolve the guilt he [many of us] feel over not being with our loved ones during their time of need. . . . Being a caregiver to an animal in such an enclosed environment parallels to some degree the experience of care-giving to a sick loved one.

There are many "stakeholders" brought together and benefited by this transspecies relationship. The prisoner, caring for a pet, is reminded of his or her younger self and of loved ones, able to care for them vicariously. The affection directed from and toward an animal can transcend racial and gang divisions, and the division between prisoners and correctional officers. The common project is endorsed by warden and inmates alike. The animals themselves, while confined in an unnatural setting, can also benefit from sustained care and attention (and sometimes PAPs use animals that would otherwise be euthanized). According to one account, "inmates produced exceptionally well-trained dogs, a result that may be linked to the amount of time that inmates can devote to the dogs."[29] And this, of course, will also benefit the animals' future owner, perhaps struggling with a disability.

> I guess waiting for a year while your canine partner is being trained in the prison is like being in prison and waiting for a year-long delayed release. Try placing yourself in the shoes of someone confined to a wheelchair or bed, who will be receiving a significant amount of freedom because prisoners are training their canine partners. . . . Programs like this reflect the humanity of prisoners. Sometimes we are portrayed as selfish people who have no regard for the law. However, these present a different image, for [prisoners] have given

up a considerable amount of time and effort to train dogs in order to give some unknown people a sense of independence and freedom. (Greco)

We have seen how chronic illness can lead to a kind of "solitary confinement," like that of Philoctetes' exile discussed in chapter 1. The sick or disabled person can feel cut off from others and the world at large. Greco recognizes that dog training not only helps to liberate the inmate but also the disabled person for whom the animal will represent a world-expanding companion.

As Greco notes, the dog trainer not only changes internally (one man said, "as the puppies improve, you improve yourself as well"),[30] but also changes others' views, helping to reconnect inmates with the larger society. It is harder to say of prisoners that "they're animals" when seeing them care for their animals.

THE GEESE

Drive to JCI and one is surprised to see the otherwise grim environs livened by the unexpected presence of geese flocking on the grass by the outer parking lots, squatting or waddling about the prison yards, as if transforming them into the picnic grounds of a public park. Donald Gross explains:

> I've defended the geese in prison against abusive prisoners and guards by thoroughly explaining to them that this Jessup area is the geese's sanctuary. This area, behind these prisons, has been designated as one of the geese's migratory stops on their way down south as they left Canada. There's a reservoir out back which was made for them, and food is placed out daily. They're protected in this area which is why they remain and breed here. So for real, we're violating *their* space.
>
> I've gotten into arguments with inmates and officers in regards to me feeding the geese. Their arguments consists of I shouldn't feed them because they shit everywhere and it's like walking through a minefield. My reasoning is that the administration/police shits down on us on a daily basis metaphorically by denying us what we're supposed to be getting, so don't mis-direct your anger at the geese for being what they are.

The geese thus inhabit the boundary between the wild and the tame, the rejected and the welcomed. The JCI area serves as a designated sanctuary. However, unlike the service dogs, these creatures are not particularly condoned by the administration or always by the prisoners. But when Donald Gross says "don't mis-direct your anger at the geese for being what they are," he seems also to be speaking of himself—"the administration/police shits down on us on a daily basis." The geese shit, but not on him. In fact, they reframe his dwelling place not only as prison, but as a protected wildlife sanctuary.

Greco has taken up a similar battle and absorbed his own lessons:

> Many people hated the geese because they defecate all over the compound. Nevertheless, most people enjoy the goslings (born in late April or May—a sign of Spring) and the parents' dedication to them, beginning with sitting on the eggs for a month or two, regardless of how people try to shoo them off. Then after they are born the parents' dedication to the goslings is truly intriguing. Also I believe that some people have mixed feelings of this amazing act of nature because of their own relationships with their parents. One thing I can say for sure is that I never saw a parent goose physically abusing or just plain ignoring one of their goslings. They are extremely attentive and dedicated parents.
>
> I, of course, love to feed the babies. They will come and eat right out of your hand. . . . I had to be careful because many people still disliked them. One day the Warden was walking with some staff and I was coming out of the building and my goslings saw me and they ran right up to me and stopped bobbing their heads for the food. I tried to play it off but they snitched me out.

Through the geese, Greco gets to *see* the caring and nurturing parent— one that many inmates have missed out on or themselves have failed to be. He now gets to *be* that parent, feeding the babies. In this shit-filled environment, such nurturing shines forth as a gift given to—and from—the goslings.

Zaeed Zakaria comments:

> When I first seen a goose my eyes widened and my heart began to feel joy because I was looking at a creature Allah created. I felt sincere peace, but more so I was inclined to feel humble and to feel compassion. Why? I don't know why, but I also felt envious of this creature. Not in a bad way but more so as one admires a plane as it flies overhead with a destination. These geese, these living, breathing creatures of God, know from where they came, they know where they are going, they have an aim, a goal. We know from where we came but then life stops. No direction, no goal. The geese have chosen this destination—a destination in which I find no liberty.

The paradoxes are dizzying. The geese, migratory creatures capable of flying thousands of miles, have chosen to settle for much of the year at JCI— the very place to which the prisoners are unwillingly bound. In an urbanized world (JCI lies in the Washington, DC-Baltimore corridor), the prison offers a sliver of green space. This maximum-security penitentiary actually does provide security for the birds, even if not always for the inmates—Jessup prisons have been the site of many stabbings. This place that tears men away from their parents and children is for the geese a family breeding ground.

While such ironies may seem cruel, they also have a redemptive aspect, as the above prisoner-comments attest. We will explore in the next chapter how, for indigenous peoples, totem animals associated with the tribe and channeled by the shaman provide a spirit of help and guidance. Animals, after all, possess special skills, sensitivities, and powers that humans do well to access.[31] The geese can similarly be seen as nature's or Allah's gift to an otherwise grim JCI. They teach about sanctuary, nurture, family, freedom, and purpose.

This also alters some of the restrictive patterns of prison spatiality and temporality discussed in chapter 10. The geese provide an avenue for what we called "escape"—flying free, at least imaginatively—but also a "reclamation" of an enriched, expanded sense of space and time. The spaces of wild nature and the temporality of the seasons are reintroduced; the prison yard becomes the site (sight) of new birth.

In ancient India, the *hamsa*—often translated as "swan," but more accurately a species of wild goose—is associated with the transcendent spirituality of the renunciate.[32] The *hamsa* is reputed to be able to separate milk from water, representing the power of spiritual discrimination. Its soaring flight, as the world melts away far beneath, exemplifies the freedom attained by the enlightened being. (I have meditated with the mantra *"hamsa"* which dates back to the *Upanishads*, and will say more about this in the next chapter.) In my study with the prisoners of inspiring works of philosophy and spirituality, I have sensed the essence of the *hamsa*, as our discussions soar and dip, fly over and beyond all the bars and barbed wire, before coming again to settle right where we are. In the last chapter, I equated the men with the Simurg, the "thirty birds" of the Sufi allegory. They search for their king, only to find out he is none other than themselves, purified by the quest. Perhaps the spirit of these "thirty birds" is truly that of the JCI geese, merging with the spirit of the men.

Conclusion

"They're animals." This is the place where we began—the social caricature of prisoners as savage, bestial, subhuman. Ironically, the result of being so viewed is to remove prisoners from relations with actual animals and with their own animality. That is, they are captured in a geometrized, technological place of cold buildings and barbed wire—one that offers little contact with beauty, sensual pleasure, or wild nature. One is lucky if there is a single straggly tree in an otherwise barren yard—after all, that tree represents a security hazard, a place where people might hide or weapons be forged. This is a "dehumanized" world, yes, but largely insofar as it is *denaturalized*. In a sense, the prison environment is *all too human*.

Thankfully, this can be somewhat relieved by the presence of animals. Possibilities of cross-species communication—care, affection, protection, growth, and learning—breathe life back into the institution. (In chapter 5 we saw something similar happen when the introduction of animals and other natural elements help transform nursing homes into "Eden Alternatives.") Prisoners and animals find and rescue one another, an unlikely conjunct.

Or is it? With billions of animals caged in factory farms and millions of people caught up in our cancerous carceral growth, perhaps these are natural partners. They provide each other mutual aid, one by one.

Yet one by one is not sufficient. It is important to shift the character of coercive institutions by seeing through and beyond the dominant ideologies that subserve them. As Nocella writes, "Simultaneously working to end both racism and speciesism is difficult, but it is essential. . . . Just as speciesism underlies the agricultural-industrial complex, racism underlies the U.S. criminal justice system and prison-industrial complex."[33]

All such "isms" are variations on a fundamental *reductionism*. Prisoners and/or people of color are reduced metaphorically to "animals." But actual animals are reduced in turn to mere meat-production machines, as if devoid of feeling, cognition, and social bonds—that is, they are *de-animalized*. Seeing prisoners and animals in loving relationships helps shatter all this falsity.

Rethinking Humans and/as Animals: The Art of Shape-Shifting

In the previous chapter I focused on the relationship between prisoners and animals. This was interpreted in two ways—the metaphoric equation of the groups in the public mind and the actual relationships that can develop between them, often loving and mutually beneficial. The latter even suggest the possibility of cross-species mergings—man and dog, man and geese—enacted through imaginative identification and embodied practices of care.

What if we press even further on this idea of animal-human connections? What if we universalize the notion in two ways—we extend the focus from prisoners to people in general, and from animals to other natural entities as well? After all, humans and animals are not isolated creatures, but always in relationship with the environing earth.

I will end this book on a positive note, examining how a reclaiming of a close *corporeal* bond with the natural world can help us revitalize the human world. Along the way, we rediscover that these are not two different worlds. The conceptual dichotomy so prevalent in the West that separates humans and animals, or humans and nature, is a false one. But we need to do more than simply think beyond it. We need embodied practices that are relational and liberating.

It may seem that we have traveled far from the focus on illness and pain with which the book began. Philoctetes, moored on a desolate island, is a distant memory (though we will return to him in the end). Nor will this final chapter further address factory farms and penitentiaries, our dehumanizing and de-animalizing institutions.

While these concerns remain implicitly present, I want to end by broadening this discussion. Many of us in the contemporary world have some form of a distressed body. We cannot help but live in relationship to distressed, and distressing, institutions and environments. In addition to the vulnerabilities to which the flesh is prey, our contemporary lifestyle can breed insulation, isolation, and therefore alienation—from our bodies, one another, and the earth. I have discussed capitalist imperatives of maximized production and consumption, as well as the Cartesian mechanistic view of matter. Such developments have facilitated great command over nature, but also helped cause global climate change, toxic pollution, habitat disruption, reduction of biodiversity, and species extinction. Then, too, we humans have become so entangled with our electronic devices that we have difficulty looking into each other's eyes, let alone noticing what we do to other creatures and habitats. We are in need of both personal and communal healing.

Earlier, for example in the chapters on touch and organ transplantation, we saw the importance of human-to-human bodily communion. This chapter seeks to extend that focus now to the more-than-human world.[1] As embodied, we are denizens of the wide earth. Real-izing this (that is, making it real) allows us to mend and expand. We can be more in touch—and not just with people, but other natural beings, and thereby with ourselves. *Distress*, we may remember, comes from Latin roots meaning "stretched apart." Paradoxically, in stretching apart from our human identity—in reaching out to other, different life forms—we may come back to ourselves made more whole by the encounter.

This may sound like hollow idealism. I want to introduce more phenomenological and sociological specificity by turning to practices of "shape-shifting." At the same time, this last chapter will remain more suggestive than definitive. I will rethink some cultural patterns that already surround us, but remain largely unseen as part of the taken-for-granted. To use Heideggerian language, this is a hermeneutics of *dis-closure*. The goal is to open up a range of phenomena, and their essential connections, in ways that invite new modes of investigation and praxis.

Let's start small. A child, pretending to be a cat, makes claw-fingers and lets loose a threatening hiss. A yogi, arching his back, lifting and opening his chest, assumes the cobra pose (*bhjangasana*). Donning a deer head, a young man readies to participate in the deer dance, a reenactment of the hunt traditional to the Yaqui tribe of northern Mexico and Arizona. An American football player pulls on his helmet emblazoned with a Bronco, symbolizing quickness and power. A dancer assumes the role of a graceful swan. An audience is enthralled by the latest Spiderman mega-hit. A meditator sits in full lotus posture (*padmasana*), letting consciousness ground and open.

What do these diverse performances have in common? They involve a kind of shape-shifting in which the human body incorporates elements of the natural world. This may be accomplished through imitation, implication, and imagination, but it is never purely conceptual. Shape-shifting is a carnal gesture and transformation. The human body longs to open beyond itself—to explore, play with, learn from, and internalize the many nonhuman bodies it encounters. We witness an eagle soaring overhead, or the fierceness of a wolf, a floating cloud, or steadfast boulder. Such entities seem to embody different forms of skill and awareness. We are mystified, companioned, intrigued by their presence. We long to experience such styles of being from within.

As befits this topic, we will see that shape-shifting as a phenomenon can disguise itself such that it becomes easy to overlook or devalue. Yet we do so at our peril. Our human body longs to be protean, open to inspiration from the more-than-human world.

Beginnings

I will not theorize about the "origins" of such human-nature shape-shifting. Notions of an originary moment or structure tend to be conjectural and univocal in a troubling way. However, we can begin by inquiring into some of the ways in which shape-shifting itself can be said to begin.

For the individual, we see it leap forth first in childhood play and exploration. In the swaying of trees in the breeze, the opening of a flower, the child encounters styles of movement that seem to echo and call forth her own mood and gestures. Looking into the eyes of a pet cat, the child receives back a gaze no less piercing than that of her younger brother. Yet the cat body is alluringly strange, even in its familiarity. What is it like to arch one's back, scamper across a room, hiss and purr? Only one way to know: turning arms into forelegs, dropping to the earth, swishing her bottom, she becomes a child/cat, transformed through performance. Possibilities are explored, lessons learned, joys heightened. (For example, as a young boy I discovered it would enhance the pleasure of a morsel of cheese if I nibbled it like a mouse, clutching it in my hand-paws.)

The boundary between human and nonhuman, even animal and plant, living and nonliving, inner and outer, is porous in the child's world, allowing for an ease of shape-shifting. Philosopher Arne Naess calls the "deep ecology" movement that he helped found,

> largely an articulation of the implicit philosophy of five year old children who have access to at least a minimum of animals, plants, and natural places. These children experience animals as beings like themselves in basic respects. They have joys and sorrows, interests, needs, loves and hates. Even flowers and places are alive to them, thriving or having a bad time.[2]

We see this not only in imitative play but in children's toys and entertainment. A cuddled teddy bear, as its name suggests, is toy, bear, and person, all. Books and movies overflow with animal protagonists—talking bunnies, mice, dogs, pigs, bears—who have anthropomorphic features (over time, Mickey Mouse was made to look less like a rodent and more like a baby with a rounded head). The child vicariously delights in these interspecies transgressions. *Animation*, particularly congenial to such conjurings, keeps alive in our mechanized culture the ancient spirit of *animism*—a worldview in which everything is alive, aware, and intertwined.[3] Hence, the popularity of such "performers" as Bugs Bunny, the Lion King, and Winnie the Pooh, to name but a few from my culture.

Going back to life's beginnings, it may be not only the child but the mother who is gifted with a primordial sense of shape-shifting. Returning to an account of breastfeeding mentioned earlier, Simms writes:

> Nursing a baby is such a primal event. It is the miracle of becoming food for another being, of sustaining life out of oneself. We share this with all other mammals: wolves, dolphins, cats, but, above all, I felt connected to cows. The stillness and earthiness of the cow spoke to me most during those early days on the bed with my new baby. Milk, milk, everything was milk. And I felt heavy and complacent, bovine and earthy, content to empty myself out in an infinite stream.[4]

In the chapters on touch and organ transplantation, I mentioned breastfeeding as a prototype for the intimacy of human bodily exchange. Here we see how it also connects us to a wider circuit of more-than-human embodiment.

"Beginnings"—the theme of this section—can be understood not just in terms of personal development, but anthropologically. We become lost in the mists of prehistory, but it may be telling that much of the first artwork we have, such as the Paleolithic cave paintings of Lascaux, France, or the even-older paintings of the recently discovered Chauvet cave,[5] are of large animals—stags, rhinoceroses, horses, bear, cattle, bison. The exact use and meanings of such paintings is unknown, but Schechner surmises they may have been embedded in a context of ritual performance—dancing, singing—perhaps related to hunting or fertility.[6] The portrayal and performance of animals seem to have been central to the arising of the human arts.

Regarding "beginnings," we also see animal/human blendings reflected in the creation stories of indigenous peoples. These, the world over, often refer to some variation of "First Beings" who make or repair the world. As Mason writes:

Whatever the origins of the land and seas, the First Beings in them are invari-
ably animals. Typically they are animals with human abilities . . . and in many
cultures they are the ancestors of human beings. Generally, this first being is
the most wily and intelligent animal in the tribal area. Among North American peoples, it is the mink, raven, or bluejay in the Northwest; in the Plains,
it is the coyote or grandmother spider; in the Northeast, it is the white arctic
hare.[7]

When humans come into the world, they are taught to make fire, tools, clothing, and to perform the proper rituals, by these animal ancestors.

This sense of close cross-species kinships remains central in many indigenous cultures, invoked by story, dance, and ritual. Tribes may have an affiliation with a totem animal establishing group identity and exemplifying certain
modes of power and protection. Animals often have keen senses, as well as
instincts, strength, and skills, that surpass those of the ordinary person; character traits, such as courage (as in our expression, "brave as a lion"), indus-
triousness ("busy as a bee"), or wisdom ("wise as an owl") that we do well to
emulate; and powers both natural and spiritual—like the soaring of a bird in
flight—that far transcend yet can inspire our paltry earthbound self. The bea-
ver shows us how to dam; the wolf, how to live in families and track in packs;
the fox, which fruits are edible, which poisonous; and so on. For the vast majority of our existence, humans have been hunter-gatherers coinhabiting the
land with other species that have taught us so much.

As important, we have learned about hunting not only by imitating the
skills of predators but through studying the ways of prey. To track an animal
one needs to *embody* it from within, coming to know when it will emerge from
hiding, where its hunger would lead it, what it will see and smell from its van-
tage point. This takes sensitivity cultivated through training and performance.
Lawlor writes about Australian aboriginal culture:

> The most powerful hunters are also spectacular dancers and singers who can
> imitate the movements and sounds of animals and birds. . . . [These are] em-
> ployed as lures and decoys during the hunt. The intelligence and sensibilities
> of the animal become alive within the consciousness of the hunter and his kin.
> *In this way, the quarry first becomes part of the hunter in spirit before becoming
> part of him in flesh.*[8]

Though hunting, of course, involves meat eating, it is hard to overemphasize
the difference between this and food production on the factory farm. In the
latter, we do not need to study and emulate the intelligence of our prey animals.
Instead, we have bred them into docility, destroyed family bonds, restricted

natural impulses—that is, remade them into products ready for industrial pro-cessing. This is not simply their cause of death, like the hunt, but a reductive transformation of the animal's entire life. The human has not shape-shifted with the wild animal so much as disciplined its wildness almost out of existence.

In indigenous cultures, sensitivity to animal life is still alive, and there will always be performers who excel in this art. Shape-shifting underlies not only the hunter's skill but also the powers of the shaman, who dwells on the border between human culture and wild nature.[9] Abram, a phenomenologist who is also a sleight-of-hand magician, used his talents to gain the confidence of tra-ditional shamans in Sri Lanka, Indonesia, and Nepal. He discovered that in their healing work they were not so much traveling to a *"supernatural"* realm, as has often been the account given by Westerners, but were communing with the *natural* powers that everywhere surround us. One Nepalese magician, So-nam, trained Abram to become fiercely attentive to ravens. "But Sonam was after something specific: he wanted me to feel the experience of meeting up *with myself* inside the bird. To feel the two sides of myself joining up with each other over there, in the torso of the raven."[10] Sonam was himself so expert at merging with ravens that one day he startled Abram by appearing to him *as a raven*—then seeming to reassume his human form. (Abram uses phenom-enological tools to try to make sense of this mystifying experience.) I quote at length Abram's valuable summary statement:

> Learning to dance another animal is central to the craft of shamanic traditions throughout the world. To move as another is simply the most visceral approach to feel one's way into the body of that creature, and so to taste the flavor of its experience, entering into the felt intelligence of the other. I have witnessed a young medicine person in the American Southwest summon the spirit of a deer by dancing that animal, have watched a Kwakiutl magician shuffle and dip his way into the power of a black bear, have seen a native healer dream her body into the riverdance of a spawning salmon, and a Mayan shaman contort himself into the rapid, vibratory flight of a dragonfly. In every case, a subtle change came upon the dancer as she gave herself over to the animal and so let herself be possessed, raising goose bumps along my skin as I watched. The care-fully articulated movements, and the stylized but eerily precise renderings of the other's behavior, were clearly the fruit of long, patient observation of the animal other, steadily inviting its alien gestures into one's muscles. The dancer feels her way into the subjective experience of the other by mimicking its pat-terned movements, and so invoking it, coaxing it close, drawing it into her flesh with subtlest motion of a shoulder, or a hip, or a blinking eye. . . . Merely call-ing to the creature in one's imagination will never suffice; one must summon it bodily, entering mimetically into the shape and rhythm of the other being if the animal spirit is to feel the call.[11]

This art of shape-shifting undermines and outruns Western dualisms of body and spirit, earthly and divine, nature and culture, animal and human.

Sacred Performance

Blendings of human-natural forms are central not only within shamanistic practice but many sacred traditions of Western and Eastern "high culture." Ancient Greek deities such as Zeus, god of sky and thunder, and Poseidon, god of the sea, embody natural powers. Some can assume animal form, as when Zeus takes on the body of a bull or swan to effect his seductions. This mythological world is also filled with river and forest nymphs, chimera and griffins, and half-human, half-animal centaurs and satyrs. The last were particularly associated with the god Dionysus, whose Bacchanalian rites formed one of the sources of Greek theatre. It led most directly to the satyr play, a tragicomic genre featuring a chorus of these bawdy figures, half-men, half goat or horse, played by actors in animalistic masks. This interspecies shape-shifting allowed performers and audience alike to sympathetically explore themes of "bestial" drunkenness, sexuality, and humor.[12]

Turning toward Asia, we see the blending of god/human/animal forms within Hinduism. Its divinities are accompanied and empowered by an animal consort. For example, Saraswati, goddess of wisdom, language, learning, the arts, and philosophy (and thus my personal favorite) is portrayed as a beautiful many-armed woman riding atop a white swan (*hamsa).* The swan or goose, we have seen, represents purity and spiritual discernment, the renunciates's ability to soar free of worldly temptation.[13] Saraswati and swan *together* embody the divine energies that lift us to spiritual heights.

Other Hindu deities themselves have animal forms, like the elephant-headed Ganesh, powerful enough to remove all obstacles, and Hanuman, the monkey-god who plays a central role in the *Ramayana.* Hanuman, a fierce warrior, healer, and devotee of Ram—yet with a simian spirit of mischief—is worshipped in temples, the subject of many stories, and honored through monumental statues.[14] He is also a popular character in the masked and shadow puppet versions of the *Ramayana* performed in India and Southeast Asia.

Sacred performance, in the broad sense, is not confined to temple or stage; it is also enacted in the bodily practices of devotees. Well-known in the West is the Hindu *hatha yoga* tradition of working with *asanas* (poses), many named for and adapted from animals, including the fish, cobra, frog, lion, eagle, and dog poses. According to legend, ancient yogis living in the forests were able to observe how animals stretched and invigorated themselves, rested and healed.

Humans thus designed yoga postures in imitation. Some *asanas* reflect other natural, though nonanimal, inspirations. When assuming the tree pose (*vriksasana*), I feel a bit of the solidity and flexibility that keeps a tree rooted even in a blustery wind. Mountain pose (*tadasana*) allows me the experience of being firmly grounded even while stretching toward the heavens.

This human-natural shape-shifting finds expression not only in outward postures but in "inner" alignments of breath and awareness.[15] A Hindu teaching, dating back to *Upanishads* including the *Mundaka*,[16] is that you can realize Brahman (the unlimited Divine) by entering the "cave of the heart."[17] Traditionally, seers (*rishis*) meditated in caves at the foothills of the Himalayas. One can conjecture that over time they learned to interiorize the mountain stillness, the womblike depth of the cave, until these *outer* forms became embodied as an *inward* place of meditative focus.

To take another personal example, I frequently use the mantra *hamsa*— mentioned in the last chapter—breathed in and out through the *hridyam* or "heart center."[18] This sacred sound embodies many significances.[19] It is said to be a contraction of *"aham sa"* ("I am that"), referring to the unity of Self and All. *"Ham-sa"* is also said to be the natural sound of the breath's inhalation and exhalation, such that we unknowingly repeat this mantra thousands of times a day from birth. *Hamsa* also means "swan," or more accurately the "wild goose" that migrates high in Indian skies, symbolizing the *samnyasin* (renunciate) who flies free of the entangling world. In chapter 11, I compared our thirty prison-class members to the *Simurg*, the thirty intrepid birds of the Sufi allegorical poem. In the last chapter, I mentioned the close relationship, maybe even the identification, that some prisoners find with the geese who live at JCI. When meditating on *hamsa*, I sometimes visualize an inner goose flying toward the sun, each breath a flap of its graceful wings as it soars toward enlightenment.

Switching traditions, and exchanging movement for seated meditation, I also perform in a low-level way Crane-style *qigong* (*chi kung*) that I learned in a class. (Prisoners at JCI now have an opportunity to study this with a teacher.) Flowering from an ancient Taoist and Buddhist tradition, and practiced extensively to this day in China, *qigong* involves gentle movement and breathing exercises designed to preserve health, energy, flexibility, and tranquility through circulating *qi* (*ch'i*), vital energy.[20] In a flow of five movement sequences, I enact my crane body by stretching upward to the sky, spreading my wings, flexing my long neck.

Qigong is closely related to *taiji* (*tai chi* or *t'ai chi ch'uan*), a movement practice that can be considered as martial art, dance form, exercise, and meditation. According to legend, *taiji* was invented by a fifteenth-century monk,

Chang San-feng, who witnessed a fight between a bird and a snake. He saw how the soft and yielding can overcome the hard and inflexible: wherever the bird attacked, the snake was able to yield and thereby avoid being killed. Creaturely inspirations are present in many *taiji* forms. These include, to name a few, Snake Creeps Down; Winds Sweeps the Plum Blossoms; White Crane Spreads Wings; Lion Shakes its Head; Embrace Tiger, Return to Mountain; Wild Horse Leaps the Ravine; Golden Cock Stands on One Leg; and Swallow Skims the Water. One classic text describes the *taiji* martial artist's moves as such:

> The ward-off arm is extended at an angle like the crescent moon. . . .
> The hand is like a deer looking backward. . . .
> Push is employed like a tiger pouncing on a sheep;
> Waist, legs, arms and hands perfectly coordinated. . . .
> Pull-down is like a monkey plucking peaches;
> After sinking, grasp obliquely, enticing the opponent to steal.[21]

The master's body is thus in-formed by natural inspirations.

Such shape-shifting is also central to East Asian art. For example, in Chinese brush painting, when seeking to portray flower, mountain, or river properly, it is recommended that you contemplate them for so long, and with such depth of attention, that they penetrate your heart/mind, allowing you to express them from within. To paint a bird properly involves becoming one with the bird without losing your human artistry. The painting then invites the viewer to share in this contemplative experience.

Once we look for it, we discover sacred shape-shifting even in unexpected places. For example, the Buddha is often seen as having withdrawn in solitary meditation from the world of suffering. Yet he remained connected to the natural world, achieving enlightenment after sitting all night beneath the Bodhi tree (a *Pipal*, or banyan fig) and touching the earth to proclaim his awakening. Then, in Narada Mahathera's words:

> As a mark of profound gratitude to the inanimate Bodhi tree that sheltered Him during His struggle for enlightenment, He stood at a certain distance gazing at the tree with motionless eyes for one whole week. Following His example, His followers in memory of His enlightenment still venerate not only the original Bodhi tree but also its descendants.[22]

According to folklore, since the Buddha has the power to produce rain, the Bodhi tree is now endowed with similar magical abilities.

We might think of this as a symbolic way of saying that the body/mind of the Buddha and tree have interfused. The once restless prince Siddhartha has learned to sit with still body and mind, finally resolving all the insufficiencies and cravings of human-animal life. (In a recent meditation weekend, when my mind was pulling me hither and yon, I imagined myself holding on to Buddha's tree for dear life.) Buddha's consciousness, we might say, has absorbed the qualities of tree-being: it has become rooted yet receptive, stationary yet flexible, connected to the nurturing energies of the universe. The tree is earth-bound, yet reaching upward toward sun and sky. As Marder writes, "Despite their undeniable embeddedness in the environment, plants embody the kind of detachment human beings dream of in their own transcendent aspiration to the other, Beauty, or divinity."[23]

In his groundbreaking work (pun intended) on "plant-thinking," Marder more generally draws attention to the richness of plant life often overlooked or denigrated in the Western philosophical tradition. Our shape-shifting is not constricted to human-animal blends, but is seen also in our deep resonances with the vegetal world. We find an echo of this not just in Buddhism but in Christian spirituality. When a priest offers bread, intoning the words from the Last Supper, "This is my body which will be given up for you," and offering wine as Jesus's blood, the ritual invokes a mysterious transformation. While supernatural in significance, it is rooted in natural relations. Our body is sustained by, and akin to, bread; our red blood looks and flows like grape-distilled wine. The vegetal world mysteriously passes into us, and gifts us with life. In the Eucharist, this "ordinary" shape-shifting serves as that which recalls us to God's extraordinary love.

Secular Performances

We have briefly surveyed the role of human-nature shape-shifting in many "sacred" performances: shamanic healings, Dionysian theatre, yoga, *taiji*, meditation, and worship. Yet we can say that shape-shifting is no less present in the "secular" world—while acknowledging this very division of sacred and secular is itself provisional and porous.

To start with a superficial example (from the Latin *superficialis*—"of or pertaining to the surface"), shape-shifting presences in the world of fashion. Through clothing, which alters the outward face of the body, we can transform our appearance and identity in ways that may be inspired by the natural world. A young woman dons a leopard-print dress, a motorcycle gang member rides in leathers, the aging matron wraps herself in a fur: how alluring to put on a real or imitative animal skin, embodying qualities—sexuality, toughness, elegance—associated with these creatures. Warranted criticism of the cruel factory-farm system that produces some of these skins (as discussed in chapter 9) should not blind us to the primal, quasi-shamanistic urge that lies beneath.

One cannot only wear animal skins, but carve animal art right onto our own. Snakes, eagles, dragons, lions, and other creatures are popular choices for tattoos in many cultures, shape-shifting human flesh into an animal image. Honoring my special feeling for *hamsa*, I am just about to get a tattoo on my shoulder of two geese in flight. (This came from a deal with my twenty-year-old daughter—if I get a tattoo, she will not get a motorcycle license.) Symbolically my flesh will take on animal form.

We see shape-shifting also at play in the sports world. Various animals embody qualities, somewhat superhuman, that athletes strain to achieve as they operate at the very limits of human performance. For example, in American football, an aggressively violent but sometimes strangely beautiful game, some fifteen of the thirty-two teams have animal identities. These are represented in the team names and mascots, the color and design of their jerseys, and the images emblazoned on their helmets, such that the players take the field as interspecies hybrids. The National Football League boasts five birds— the Falcons, Cardinals, Seahawks, Ravens, and Eagles—honoring, perhaps, the prominence of the aerial pass in football. Representing the ferocity of the hunt are Lions, Panthers, Bengals, and Jaguars. Three teams are named after horses, swift and powerful, like football halfbacks and receivers: the Colts, Chargers, and Broncos. Then there are the Rams and Bears (try to tackle one of these creatures on the open field!) and, as a gesture to bioregionalism, one sea-dwelling creature, the Miami Dolphins. (My own city's representative, the Baltimore Ravens, has the distinction of being the only football team named from a poem—hometown boy Edgar Allan Poe's "The Raven.") These athletes are like modern hunter/shamans incorporating the powers of wild creatures.

Shape-shifting also shines forth in the performing arts. Earlier we referred to the intertwining of theatre with religion and ritual, as in the Dionysian satyr play or the shadow puppetry of the *Ramayana*. One of the inspirations behind this chapter is a Yale Repertory production of Ovid's *Metamorphoses* that I saw as a teenager, directed by Paul Sills. I still remember the enchantment produced when Philemon and Baucis, an elderly couple who have been hospitable to the gods, are rewarded by being transformed into two trees, oak and linden, their trunks and branches forever intertwined. As the actors embraced, merging into one another and the earth, the effect on stage was magical. Again, we see that not only human-animal but human-vegetal shape-shifting is a rich topic for exploration. There is a way in which trees proliferate beyond themselves, giving and receiving, in exchange with earth, sky, and other plant life, that embodies ideals of selfless merger.[24]

Western theatre, however, has often tilted toward an anthropocentric focus. A number of reasons for this can be adduced. Performance stages increasingly became human constructions, set off from the natural world. On stage, humans usually interacted primarily with one another. While elements of nature remain key framing devices—in Shakespeare, for example, think of *King Lear's* stormy heath, the woods of Elsinore in *Macbeth*, or the wild settings and creatures of *The Tempest* and *A Midsummer Night's Dream*—drama largely focuses on human character development and interactions. (Chaudhuri discusses the rare counterexample wherein animals play a central dramatic role.[25]) Even "higher animals," while trainable for performance, cannot deliver dialogue as humans do, nor "act" in the full-fledged sense—that is, understand they are portraying a fictional character and conjure a seeming world independent of reality.

However human-animal shape-shifting remains alive and well, particularly within certain genres. In a ballet like *Swan Lake*, the choreographer and performers take up the shamanic role of dancing to life the body and spirit of the creature. Costuming, the graceful and sinuous use of limbs, torso, head and neck, all combine to create the woman-swans who populate the ballet.

We also find this art alive and well in musicals, with their elaborate and fanciful costuming, sets, and special effects. Referring to the theatre of the moment, I think of *Cats*, a strange transmogrification of T.S. Eliot poems featuring dozens of human-felines; Disney's *Lion King*, with its African-inspired animal costumes and puppets; *Beauty and the Beast*, exploring magical shape-shiftings between the human and bestial, animate and inanimate; *Shrek*, with its talking donkey and human-ogre shape-shifting; *Spiderman*, featuring a flying superhero infected with arachnoid powers. As "family musicals," these are designed to appeal to children who, as we discussed, are closer to the animistic worldview of human-animals blends.

"Movies," based on a perceptual illusion of movement, can also create a modern-day shamanism, using lighting, costume, music, acting, cinematography, editing, and special effects. To take a few recent (hugely popular) examples at this time of writing, the *Batman* films showcase a hero whose noble attributes merge with the sinister-nocturnal aspects of his totem creature; the *Twilight* movies feature "werewolves" (or, more precisely, descendants of shape-shifting Spirit Warriors of the Quileute tribe); *Avatar* portrays the indigenous "Na'vi" people, both humanoid and animal-like, and their ways of merging with other life-energies on the planet Pandora. This film also explores shape-shifting as technologically mediated: its hero, Jake Sully, via a computerized linkage, is able to move and sense remotely through a Na'vi body, or "avatar." We see here a futuristic version of the ancient art of embodied merger. This can also serve as a meta-commentary on the art of film itself: after all, through advanced technology, a master showman-shaman like director James Cameron vicariously transports the movie viewer into another body and world. The primordial art of shape-shifting is renewed through twenty-first-century computer graphics.

While easy to dismiss as popular entertainment, the global impact of these films should not be overlooked. When last I checked, of the top twenty gross-ing movies of all time, *nineteen* of them (the sole exception being *Titanic*) take viewers into worlds redolent with shape-shifting, including *Avatar, Toy Story III, Alice in Wonderland, The Avengers,* the *Lord of the Rings* films, the *Pirates of the Caribbean* series, and the *Harry Potter* movies. (This list may be revised by the time you as reader encounter this book, but I invite you to check whether the fundamental point does not still hold.)

The political messages of such films obviously vary. While *Avatar* valo-rizes environmentalism and the wisdom of indigenous peoples, other super-hero films can seem aggressively pro-military or be used to promote obscene levels of consumerism. In any case, the box office results of these global enter-tainments remind us that human-nature shape-shifting remains a powerful presence in the contemporary, as the archaic, world.

"Performance," Schechner writes,

> must be construed as a "broad spectrum" or "continuum" of human action ranging from ritual, play, sports, popular entertainments, the performing arts (theatre, dance, music), and everyday life performances to the enactment of social, professional, gender, race, and class roles, and to healing (from shaman-ism to surgery), the media, and the internet.[26]

I have but briefly suggested ways in which shape-shifting manifests across this broad array of performances, including, on Schechner's list, ritual, play, sports, entertainments, the performing arts, social roles, and healing.

Kinship and Alterity

This leads to a series of more foundational questions. From what sources does this call to shape-shift arise? What, if anything, is its telos? Why is shape-shifting such a persistent urge, and how is it significant to our humanity and sociality? I will begin by discussing various modes of *kinship* that link us to other natural entities, later turning to modes of alluring *alterity*.

First, we share and are nourished by a *material kinship* with the earth and all that inhabits it. In the chapter on organ transplantation, I wrote about how our bodies are never simply "ours" but emerge from and merge with other bod-ies. Yet it is not simply other human bodies that birthed us. We are made of fundamental stuff, ancient elements often created and cast off by supernovae, now ingredient in our solar system and planet. Our bodies thus resonate with the universe around us. Our bones are stony, stiffened by calcium. Our blood is like sea water, with many of the same electrolytes flowing through our veins. Our life is dependent on ceaseless exchanges with the environment as we breathe, eat, and drink. We inhale the oxygen that trees exhale as waste, chew a carrot, or piece of chicken, and through the magic of the visceral body shape-shift it into human flesh.[27] I earlier quoted Wang Yang-ming, sixteenth-century neo-Confucian philosopher:

> Wind, rain, dew, thunder, sun and moon, stars, animals and plants, mountains and rivers, earth and stones are essentially of one body with man. It is for this reason that such things as the grains and animals can nourish man and that such things as medicine and minerals can heal diseases. Since they share the same material force, they enter into one another.[28]

Switching to the framework of contemporary evolutionary theory, the famous biologist Edward O. Wilson hypothesizes that, through our millions of years of living in natural settings, particularly the savannahs of Africa, humans have evolved an adaptive "biophilia." Etymologically meaning "love of life," Wilson defines "biophilia" as "the innate tendency to focus on life and lifelike processes," or "the innately emotional affiliation of human beings to other living organisms."[29] It is not, he suggests, a single instinct, but a complex of learning rules that are mediated by cultural training and includes within it instinctive biophobias, as humans often have for snakes. (After all, other life forms can threaten as well as nourish us.) While his notion is controversial, research studies have suggested a human affinity for certain natural features and landscapes that trigger positive emotional states, lessen stress, promote wellness, and perhaps assist creative and higher-order cognition.[30] Our urge to shape-shift with the natural world may be one expression of this biophilia.

Our kinship with the natural world, material and evolutionary, extends to our relationship with plants. As Aristotle said in *De Anima*, plants share with us the quest for nourishment and the capacity for reproduction.[31] Like plants, we are rooted in particular places, yet grow upward and outward in search of fulfillment, participate in diurnal and seasonal rhythms, and are nurtured by symbioses and threatened by competitors.

Yet our relationship is particularly close with animals. In Aristotle's language, we share with these creatures an "animal soul" in that we perceive, desire, and move to fulfill our ends. We also share similarities on the level of visceral, musculoskeletal, and sensory organs. We are kin even to lizard and fly, in that they too have eyes, seek food, and are vulnerable to danger. We cannot follow the bird in flight, but can flap our arms like wings or seek a higher "bird's-eye-view" on the world.

We have special homologies with other mammals. Like a lion or wolf, we are warm-blooded, have four limbs, know what it is to climb to a height, survey a landscape, feel the wind in our face, and birth and nurse our young. Earlier we saw Simms express her particular feeling of connection to cows as she breastfed her infant with mother's milk, and "felt heavy and complacent, bovine and earthy."[32]

Our kinship is thus not only material and evolutionary, but *experiential*. This, of course, is a controversial claim. Philosophers, such as Nagel in his famous article, "What Is it Like to Be a Bat?," have at times disputed that we can know anything of the subjective experience of other species.[33] But other philosophers have asserted, rightly I believe, that profound commonalities of experience do allow us to commune with other creatures.[34]

Kinship is not identity. There is also difference and alterity in these cross-species encounters. Of course, this is true with other humans as well. I cannot truly know what it is like to be quadriplegic or to be an aboriginal tribesman with a cultural training incommensurate with my own. Yet even here, we would have things in common, for example, a capacity to feel pain or to use language.

Our resonance with other animal bodies also ranges across a continuum of kinship and alterity. I know little about what it is like to be a clam. Its bodily constitution and life-world are extremely different from mine. On the other end of the spectrum, I share much with my dog, like me a four-limbed mammal, and one of a species that has been bred over thousands of years for compatibility with humans.[35] That is, the canine, too, has been literally shape-shifted to assimilate humanlike modes of behavior. Dogs, it is said, are the best "anthropologists," carefully studying and responding to human expressions and gestures. We, too, may have been reshaped by this coevolution. Grandin refers to new theories and evidence that human family and pack behavior, atypical of other primates, may have been learned from our wolf companions. It has also been discovered that our midbrain olfactory bulb has shrunk over time; perhaps, in our symbiotic relationship, we let our dog/wolves handle the smelling while we focused on planning and organizing.[36]

Experientially, I have delighted in this human-dog kinship. (Having my first pet when in my 50s perhaps made me even more appreciative to this new presence.) We throw open the door, and Maggie and I together enjoy the rush of activity and sudden expansion of space as our walk commences; we race each other across a favorite field; then, growing hot and tired from this scampering, we drag our tails home to flop down in an air-conditioned house.

There is still alterity even in the midst of this kinship. I will never understand the world of intricate smells that Maggie tracks with her more than 200 million olfactory receptors (I have but a paltry 5 million), and she will never fully grasp the speech and thought I produce with my hypertrophied forebrain. Still, as Acampora writes, "though there are deep phenomenological differences between distinct kinds of animals, these do not constitute an absolute existential divide—for instance, they do not hermeneutically preclude communicative interrelationships."[37] Maggie understands my facial expressions and inflections, my simple words, like go! and wait!—and I understand she is telling me walk-time! when she gets frenetic, wags her tail, and jumps against the door repeatedly.[38] She, as I, participates in a carnal intentionality directed toward the world, and a gestural language of sound and movement through which we connect. At the same time, alterity adds alluring mystery to our relation. What does she mean when she looks deeply into my eyes? Why did she choose just that bush to pee on? What would she do if she actually caught a squirrel? The fact that she cannot answer in human speech makes her style of being-in-the-world more, not less, fascinating.

The framework provided by twentieth-century phenomenologists such as Straus[39] and Merleau-Ponty[40] helps us to explore and explain interspecies relations. As we have discussed, renouncing the "logocentric" dualism that has been prevalent in the West—the assumption that a human being is foremost a rational mind or soul tethered to a material body—they investigate how our perception, movement, experience of space and time, even our language and thought, are profoundly *embodied*. We are not solitary minds, as per Descartes, having to infer the existence of an external world and other consciousnesses. Rather, our lived body always prereflectively finds itself embedded in a life-world that we inhabit with other embodied subjects. In Merleau-Ponty's words:

> It is precisely my body which perceives the body of another person, and discovers in that other body a miraculous prolongation of my own intentions, a familiar way of dealing with the world. Henceforth, as the parts of my body together comprise a system, so my body and the other person's are one whole, two sides of one and the same phenomenon.[41]

The laughter or tears of another elicits my own by empathic resonance. I follow the gaze of a companion to discover what she is looking at. That which my friends desire or scorn I usually learn to as well, absorbing their stance on the world. I am part of an embodied circuit of co-subjectivity.

Most continental philosophers, Merleau-Ponty included, have focused on human-to-human sociality. Derrida, in *The Animal that Therefore I Am*, particularly critiques Descartes, Kant, Heidegger, Lacan, and Levinas, for this resolute anthropocentrism: "The experience of the seeing animal, of the animal that looks at them, has not been taken into account in the philosophical or theoretical architecture of their discourse. In sum they have denied it as much as misunderstood it."[42]

Yet there are hints in Merleau-Ponty of how one might expand his phenomenology of the lived body to include cross-species relations. "There is a kinship between the being of the earth and that of my body (*Leib*)" he writes, and "this kinship extends to others, who appear to me as other bodies, to animals whom I understand as variants of my embodiment, and finally even to terrestrial bodies since I introduce them into the society of living bodies when saying, for example, that a stone flies."[43]

We might call animals in particular the *other others* that, no less than human *others*, call out for existential and moral recognition. Not only we have faces, but so do dogs, cats, birds, wild animals, all of whom gaze on us, and gaze *with us* on the world. We dwell with them in an embodied relation that Acampora variously terms "transpecific intersomaticity," "symphysis," and "humanimal conviviality."[44] Other animals offer us not only companionship, but an embodied style that, both through its kinship and alterity, suggests to us new possibilities, pleasures, and powers. Hence, me as a child nibbling cheese like a mouse; the shaman studying, and embodying, the ways of the raven; the hunter dancing the deer; the ballerina dancing the swan; the yogi assuming the cobra pose; and on and on, in our intersomaticity.

Nor is this restricted only to our encounters with animals. In the quotation above, Merleau-Ponty notes that even terrestrial bodies can be experienced as alive. We have seen that "in the beginning" historically, developmentally, and phenomenologically, boundaries between the living and inanimate, the subject and object, body and world, are porous. We are inspired by the rush of the wind, and the tree that clings to earth despite it, and the majestic immobility of the mountain that remains long after the wind has swirled and departed. We bring these forms into our visceral and sensorimotor organs, our meditation and play, our consciousness and speech. We embody these powers, these styles of being, be they defined by later thought as "animal," "vegetable," or "mineral." In Abram's words, "Each being that we perceive enacts a subtle integration within us, even as it alters our prior organization. The sensing body is like an open circuit that completes itself only in things, in others, in the surrounding earth."[45] One inhabits the world not just as an *I* but part of a *we*, enriched and expanded by more-than-human being.

Shape-Shifting Imperiled

In some cultures, terms like "art" or "religion" have no meaning because they are so ingredient in all aspects of life that they cannot be objectified as a special domain. So it may be in an indigenous culture concerning the kinds of shape-shifting we have been describing. It is simply the condition of dwelling in the world of forest and sky, cliff and river, amidst our many animal cousins. However, a reason we now can and should thematize shape-shifting is that its performance has become imperiled. My previous discussions might suggest the opposite—for example, the pervasiveness of shape-shifting in blockbuster film. Yet this may also speak to a yearning for a magic that has receded from our everyday life. Yes, it is there in child's play, but then is trained out of us as we reach adulthood and stop pretending to be cats. Yes, it is there in the yoga pose or the *taiji* form, but for most these are specialized practices meant to lift us, for a particular time, out of our norm in which we work away at our computers.

What is it, operative in our culture, that has significantly diminished the power and presence of shape-shifting? I will briefly survey a few factors. First, as mentioned, Western culture is significantly tilted toward anthropocentrism and logocentrism. Theologians have taught us that humans alone are made in the divine image, possessed of an immortal soul, granted dominion over the natural world. Philosophers have pointed to our unique powers of reason, language, and moral choice; our capacity for self-determination; and our understanding of mortality.

Accompanying this focus on what "sets us apart" is a fear of reverting to, or being overwhelmed by, our animality. We scold a wayward child: "Don't wolf down your food" or "You eat like a pig." As previously quoted, Mason writes:

> We call someone an "animal" when we want to insult and debase him or her. It is an epithet applied to the cruelest, most heinous criminals. . . . We describe horrible human beings as "animals," "beasts," or "brutes" (an old word for "animal") when we want to describe their egoism, insatiable greed, insatiable sexuality, cruelty, senseless slaughter of nonhuman beings, and the mass slaughter of human beings.[46]

These are actually behaviors far more characteristic of humans than other creatures, but they are ascribed to animals in the social imagination. Rather than feeling inspired to shape-shift with other animals, we thus seek to *eradicate the animal within*, thought of as containing libidinal and violent energies that lie below the surface.

In the last chapter, we saw how criminals are metaphorically equated with animals, as in the Mason quotation. They are viewed in the media and popular imagination as bestial, savage, and predatory. This then justifies their mass caging and the deprivation of human rights. By locking away "the animals," segregating them from "human society," we thus literalize our denial and fear of the animal within. "*We are not animals, they are,*" we say, as we point a finger at prisoners—who, we have seen, are all too often people of color. Biophobia and racism thus synergize.

Another particularly modern version of nature alienation arises with the mechanistic worldview of early modern science discussed in previous chapters. Natural entities in general, and animals in particular, come to be viewed as machinelike. The same physical forces and chains of cause and effect that determine the motions of inanimate things are seen to underlay biological processes.[47] The tree is a machine for turning sunlight into bark and leaf; the chicken, a factory for producing eggs and breast meat, and its behaviors understood as genetically encoded instinct and patterns of stimulus response. After studying with indigenous shamans and developing the embodied sensitivity to animal consciousness discussed earlier, Abram describes what happens when he returns to this Westernized context:

> I began to lose my sense of the animals' own awareness. The gulls' technique for breaking open the clams began to appear as a largely automatic behavior, and I could not easily feel the attention they must bring to each new shell. . . .
> I found myself now observing the heron from outside its world, noting with interest its careful high-stepping walk and the sudden dart of its beak into the water, but no longer feeling its tensed yet poised alertness with my own muscles. And, strangely, the suburban squirrels no longer responded to my chittering calls.[48]

Our attitude toward and dominion over nature has not only deadened our response, but brought about very real deaths. We have discussed the cruel factory farms to which animals destined for our table are consigned. At the same time, patches of wilderness shrink, and so too the numbers of wild creatures deprived of their habitat. Animals, once so central in human culture, increasingly become fewer and marginalized in our communities, reduced to something like a zoo-spectacle we visit.[49] We earlier quoted Naess who called the deep ecology movement "largely an articulation of the implicit philosophy of five year old children who have access to at least a minimum of animals, plants, and natural places." But can we now assume even that minimal access? Many of us are firmly embedded in urban "mindscapes" more than natural landscapes. We thus lose the allure and opportunity of shape-shifting.

Accompanying this psychic and practical shrinking of nature and animal is an expansion of *the reign of the machine*, as discussed in earlier chapters on organ transplants and factory farms. Our mechanistic view of the world has led us to remake it accordingly. We dwell amidst our technologies. We speed to work in a car that enhances our motility through engine and wheels. We ride the elevator up, obviating the need for a step-by-step climb. We stare at the computer screen or the smartphone, connecting to an information grid. Even our thinking shifts in accord with computers; we "Google" information and "word-process" language, as I have done in composing this book. Our corporeal capacity to shape-shift into new forms is thus directed primarily toward machine linkages. Powers that might previously have been sought through human-animal shape-shifting—speed, flight, connection, inspiration—instead are realized through human-technology blends. We become cyborgs.[50]

In some ways, this can enrich our lives. The book you are now reading would not have been produced without the benefit of multiple technologies. It allows our minds to meld. To take another more medical example, Mazis explores how cochlear implants expand the world of someone with profound hearing loss.[51] Nor is there a clear boundary between culture and nature, the technological and organic. My dog is a product of culture—centuries of breeding and domestication—as much as of nature, and together we like to hop in a car and drive to a favorite trail. Still, my dog is not the same as my car. Something is lost if machines, rather than natural beings, become my primary interlocutor. I do not experience the same play of kinship and alterity.

In one sense, compared to the animal, the car and I have far less kinship. With its fiberglass body and internal combustion engine, my car cannot participate in the organismic world of sense and desire. It may be that I perceive it as having something like a face (a deliberate construct of car designers) or that it is styled after an animal—there are "Jaguars," "Mustangs," and "Stingrays" on the road. I may give it a personalized name and feel affection for it as if it were alive. Wilson writes, "Mechanophilia, the love of machines, is but a special case of biophilia."[52] But ultimately the machine is not a true companion. Etymologically, a "com-panion" is one with whom I *share bread*, something I cannot do with a car but can with my dog. She, like me, knows a hungry stomach and the pleasures of eating. My body-car linkage gets me where I'm going, maybe even directs me there with a GPS synthetic voice, but ultimately I ride alone. The car and I do not share a life-world.

We can see this as a *deficit of kinship*. The car is *too other*, devoid of animal consciousness. Yet this can also be understood as the reverse, *a deficit of alterity*. In a sense, the car is *not other enough*. Putting aside futuristic developments of artificial intelligence, our machines do not manifest true independence of origin and awareness. The car, elevator, computer, smartphone are things that humans have made to advance human purposes. They are anthropocentric in construction and intent. This cannot be said of the zebra, the wolf, or even the "domesticated" dog, who still maintains a fierce will of her own. Nor can it be said of mountain and ocean. These natural entities are not simply our creations, but confront us as *genuine others*, autonomous powers.

"Diversity" is a value much lauded, at least on college campuses. It is expanding and enriching to interact with others different in race, nationality, religion, gender, or socioeconomic background. Yet in a machine-dominated world, we lose another form of diversity, equally important—not simply *biodiversity*, as other species and ecosystems are destroyed, but also what might be called *bio-experiential diversity*. Humans have the ability to experience with and through a diversity of natural bodies. We can dance *Swan Lake*; meditate like a mountain; complete a *taiji* sequence like "Swallow Skims the Water"; sit on the beach, becoming fluid like sand, vast as the sky, slow and rhythmic like the sea; cavort with our dog; watch *The Lion King* with a thrill of vicarious pleasure; or stretch into cobra pose in a yoga class. These provide us with rich bio-experiential diversity.

Of course, not all shape-shifting is "created equal" in terms of its redemptive power. One might question any attempt to equate watching the latest blockbuster Spiderman movie or a football game, even if it is the Tigers versus the Rams, with doing *taiji* or yoga, or building a direct relationship with a real animal. Earlier expressed concerns about the alienating synergy of capitalism and Cartesianism are still operative for the film and football game. They are used to generate big money, often employ or refer to advanced technologies, and celebrate bone-crushing violence. There are reasons to believe that doing the lion and eagle poses as a yogic practice would be more healing to our distressed bodies then watching the Detroit Lions demolish the Philadelphia Eagles while we lie on the couch eating potato chips.

Still, teasing apart the uses and abuses of different modes of shape-shifting is a task for future exploration. I have but tried to suggest the many forms these trans-species mergers can take, sacred and secular, that are often hidden in plain sight.

We do well to keep this theme in mind during academic work lest we slip into an unconscious anthropocentrism; so, too, in our individual and communal lives, lest we become recklessly inattentive and destructive toward the natural world and toward our own lived bodies.

Wind and sky, mountain and river, dog and cat, bug and bird; we can incorporate their embodied styles. Thus we explore our animality and the protean richness of being human.

★

Philoctetes, as we saw in chapter 1, was bitten by a snake when he transgressed the sacred precinct of Chryse. He is exiled to a wild island, which I used as a metaphor for the exile that accompanies serious pain and illness. In the course of this book we have also spent time with other exiles—animals in factory farms, prisoners in cages. These are all distressed bodies.

But distressed bodies can become de-stressed. Ruptures can be healed. Though a snake poisoned Philoctetes, it was not satanic. It was guarding a sanctified region, serving as the instrument of a goddess. We have seen that animality and wild nature are themselves godly. From where the poison emanates, there, too, the healing. Our own bodies, which make us vulnerable to pain and death, also open us to life. To heal, we do better to embrace animality, wildness, embodiment, than to flee from these. Shape-shifting is an example of how to go deeper into the human body through journeying beyond it.

Of course, this is no easy task when one has a distressed body. The body can both anchor and exile us, as Philoctetes knows. Our culture pursues a fantasy of escape from this fate through a kind of *deus ex machine*—not simply the "god *from* the machine" used in ancient Greek plays (including *Philoctetes*) where a deity was lowered onto the stage—but the modern god *of* the machine. That is, we now make gods of mechanical devices and institutions that promise mechanistic control. We pursue the fantasy of the pill that cures all or the transplant to replace our organs when they wear down. We plug into our electronic information and entertainment feeds. We more literally feed ourselves through "factory farms," processing animals as if they were meat machines. We even house those humans deemed dangerous in a "prison-industrial complex." We worship so many *gods of the machine*.

We would do better to honor our living bodies and the more-than-human world in which we dwell. It is thereby that we enact the sacred. We are not simply exiles, but intertwined with one another. We can yet come home—or discover that we never left to begin with.

Acknowledgments

This book would not be what it is, and might not be at all, but for the many ideas, voices, and modes of support generously provided by others.

The topic of chapter 1, Philoctetes' wound, was gifted to me by Dr. Richard Selzer. Working under him as a medical student, I received an exquisite teaching on compassion in the healing arts, as well as life-changing encouragement to follow my philosophical interests. Chapter 3 on touch was inspired by the work of four accomplished healers, Suzanne Crater, Leyan Darlington, Heather Dorst, and Nancy Romita. They have left their healing touch on me, this chapter, and many others with distressed bodies. In another vein (and nerve), I want to thank the skillful and caring surgeon, Dr. Eric Williams, who has done so much to relieve the chronic pain that forms a focus of chapter 2.

Chapters 3, 4, and 5, rethinking medical therapeutics, were coauthored in their original forms with Dr. Mitchell Krucoff, Department of Medicine/Cardiology, Duke University Medical Center. I want to thank him for sharing his experience, inspiration, and lifelong friendship. I am grateful for his permission to use this material here.

Regarding the "hermeneutical" chapters in this book, I would like to thank Dr. Edward Gogel and Fr. Robert Smith, whose recognition of the important link between medicine and hermeneutics was the initial inspiration for my own forays into this field. Kaitlyn Smith provided valuable research assistance for chapter 8 concerning the latest advances in organ transplants.

Chapter 11 on the enlightened prison was written with the help of a class of the "Jessup Correctional Institution Scholars." These spirited class members included the following, all of whom I thank: Douglas Scott Arey, Kenneth Bond-El, Dalphonso Brooks, Craig Cobb-Bey, Anthony Davenport, Jeffrey Ebb Sr., Vincent Greco, Eric Grimes, Donald Gross, Tyrone Herrell, Edward

Hershman, Warren "Ren" Hynson, Michael Jeffrey-Bey, Marvin Jenkins, Arlando "Tray" Jones, Kevin Jones-Bey, Fortunato Mendes, Wesley Moore, Shaka F. Muhammed, Shakkir Talib Mujahid, Christopher Murray, Lakhem Ra-sebek, Michael Razzio Simmons, Clarence Somerville, Michael Thomas, Gregg Dallas Wakefield, Mike Whittlesey, Jacobi Williams, John Woodland, and Zaeed Zakaria. A couple of the men, Arlando "Tray" Jones and John Woodland, have been respected friends since the 1990s—their voices are also present in chapter 10.

Chapter 12 on prisoners and animals was coauthored in its original form with Vincent Greco. I am thankful for the valuable material he provided and his permission to use it here—he is a generous spirit. I am also grateful for the administrative work he did in building our JCI Scholars Program, which now involves many professors from area institutions offering a wide variety of free college-level classes to more than one hundred participating inmates. (Thanks as well to Joshua Miller for his spirit and expertise in building this program; the same goes for Daniel Levine, other giving faculty members, and our JCI students, so appreciative of access to a liberal arts education.)

There are many others whose help I wish to recognize. Frederik Svenaeus provided invaluable comments and suggestions on a draft of this manuscript, which have notably improved the book. So, too, Kirsten Jacobson, whose friendship and comments on the book I have so valued. James Hatley is another trusted colleague and reader who particularly helped with suggestions for the book's third section.

Then there are others whose fingerprints (electronically speaking) are on the finished manuscript. Marion Wielgosz did invaluable and painstaking work on endnotes and formatting, always with positive energy and expertise. I can't begin to repay the number of hours she put in whipping things into shape. Gina Brandon helped with important word processing tasks. Lisa Flaherty, in her unique and spirited way, provided administrative assistance. Lisa Wehrle did meticulous and excellent copyediting on the manuscript.

It was a joy to work again with T. David Brent, also my editor at the University of Chicago Press for *The Absent Body*, my first book from twenty-five years ago, to which this is something of a sequel. Since then we have both had some trying experiences with "distressed bodies," but are happy to be alive, kicking, and collaborating on this new project. I have also had the pleasure of working with Ellen Kladky, Editorial Associate at the press.

Other colleagues who have encouraged, inspired, and supported me along the way to this book include David Abram, Mavis Biss, Rick Boothby, Ed Casey, Bret Davis, Tris Engelhardt, Catriona Hanley, Mary Rawlinson, Tim

Stapleton, and many others I can't begin to name. Money and institutional support are important too. I want to thank Loyola University Maryland, as well as the Philosophy Department, for a generous series of Summer Research Grants and a funded sabbatical to help bring this book to fruition. Loyola's Center for the Humanities provided ancillary assistance.

And then there is my family, or families really. My father, Harold Leder, a New York City internist, exemplified for me a style of humanistic medicine that I still advocate for in this book. I remember as a child when he would take me around Manhattan on Saturday house calls to visit sick patients (that was indeed another era). His kind spirit pervades this book. So, too, my mother's, who got her M.A. at Columbia in English literature when in her fifties, so valuing the world of books and scholarship.

Of my present family, I cannot say enough. My daughters Sarah and Anna-Rose have been patient with their father upstairs typing away on the computer, and brought great joy to my life when I came downstairs. Sarah Leder also provided valuable research associate work on a couple of the chapters. Our dog (my first ever), Maggie, is a primary inspiration for chapter 13 on shapeshifting. She has helped teach me about the pleasures of animal-human blending. Finally I come to Janice McLane, my wife and fellow philosopher. Her assistance with my "distressed body," and in helping me find the time, energy, and mental health to write this manuscript, has made all the difference. She is a kind and giving soul. That is why this book is dedicated to her in gratitude.

I am also thankful to the following publishers for permitting me to present material that was revised from the following original sources in which they appeared:

Chapter 1: "Illness and Exile: Sophocles' *Philoctetes*," *Literature and Medicine* 9 (1990): 1–11. Copyright © 1990 The Johns Hopkins University Press. Reprinted with permission by Johns Hopkins University Press.

Chapter 2: "The Experiential Paradoxes of Pain," *Journal of Medicine and Philosophy*, forthcoming.

Chapter 3: "The Touch That Heals: The Uses and Meanings of Touch in the Clinical Encounter," with Mitchell W. Krucoff, *Journal of Alternative and Complementary Medicine* 14, no. 3 (2008): 321–27.

Chapter 4: "'Take Your Pill': The Role and Fantasy of Pills in Modern Medicine," with Mitchell W. Krucoff, *Journal of Alternative and Complementary Medicine* 20, no. 6 (2014): 421–27.

Chapter 5: "Toward a More Materialistic Medicine: The Value of Authentic Materialism within Current and Future Medical Practice," with Mitchell W. Krucoff, *Journal of Alternative and Complementary Medicine* 17, no. 9 (2011): 859–65.

Chapter 6: "Clinical Interpretation: The Hermeneutics of Medicine," *Theoretical Medicine* 11 (1990): 9–24. With kind permission from Springer Science+Business Media.

Chapter 7: "Toward a Hermeneutical Bioethics," in *A Matter of Principles? Ferment in U.S. Bioethics*, ed. Edwin R. Dubose, Ronald P. Hamel, and Laurence J. O'Connell (Valley Forge, PA: Trinity Press International, 1994), 240–59.

Chapter 8: "Whose Body? What Body? The Metaphysics of Organ Transplantation," in *Persons and Their Bodies: Rights, Responsibilities, Relationships*, ed. Mark H. Cherry (Dordrecht: Kluwer Academic, 1999), 233–64. With kind permission from Springer Science+Business Media.

Chapter 9: "Old McDonald's Had a Farm: The Metaphysics of Factory Farming," *Journal of Animal Ethics* 2, no. 1 (2012): 73–86.

Chapter 10: "Imprisoned Bodies: The Life-World of the Incarcerated," *Social Justice* 31, no. 1–2 (2004): 51–66.

Chapter 11: "The Enlightened Prison," with the Jessup Correctional Institution Scholars, *Special Issue: The Beautiful Prison: Studies in Law, Politics and Society* 64 (April/May 2014): 19–32.

Chapter 12: "Prisoners: 'They're Animals' and Their Animals," with Vincent Greco, in *Philosophy Imprisoned* (Lanham, MD: Lexington, 2014), 219–34.

Chapter 13: "Embodying Otherness: Shape-Shifting and the Natural World," *Environmental Philosophy* 9, no. 2 (2012): 123–41.

Notes

Chapter One

1. All quotations, cited parenthetically by line number in the text, are from David Grene's translation of Sophocles' *Philoctetes*, in *The Complete Greek Tragedies*, ed. David Grene and Richmond Lattimore (Chicago: University of Chicago Press, 1959–1960), 2:401–60. Copyright © 1957 by The University of Chicago. Reprinted by permission of The University of Chicago Press.

2. Eric J. Cassell, *The Healer's Art: A New Approach to the Doctor-Patient Relationship* (Cambridge, MA: MIT Press, 1985); also see his *The Nature of Suffering and the Goals of Medicine* (New York: Oxford University Press, 1991). Also see H. Tristram Engelhardt Jr., "Illnesses, Diseases, and Sicknesses," in *The Humanity of the Ill: Phenomenological Perspectives*, ed. Victor Kestenbaum (Knoxville: University of Tennessee Press, 1982), 142–56; also see Engelhardt's *The Foundations of Bioethics* (New York: Oxford University Press, 1986).

3. Michel Foucault, *The Birth of the Clinic*, trans. Alan M. Sheridan Smith (New York: Vintage, 1973).

4. S. Kay Toombs, *The Meaning of Illness: A Phenomenological Account of the Different Perspectives of Physician and Patient* (Dordrecht: Kluwer Academic, 1993). Also see Havi Carel, *Illness: The Cry of the Flesh* (Stocksfield, UK: Acumen Press, 2008), and Isabel Dyck, "Hidden Geographies: The Changing Lifeworlds of Women with Multiple Sclerosis," *Social Science and Medicine* 40, no. 3 (1995): 307–20.

5. Loretta Kopelman, "The Punishment Concept of Disease," in *AIDS: Ethics and Public Policy*, ed. Christine Pierce and Donald VanDeVeer (Belmont, CA: Wadsworth, 1988), 49–55.

6. Richard M. Zaner, *The Context of Self: A Phenomenological Inquiry Using Medicine as a Clue* (Athens: Ohio University Press, 1981). Also see Drew Leder, *The Absent Body* (Chicago: University of Chicago Press, 1990).

7. Carel, *Illness*, 25–29, 61–88.

8. Lisa Diedrich, "Breaking Down: A Phenomenology of Disability," *Literature and Medicine* 20, no. 2 (2001): 209–30.

9. J. H. van den Berg, *The Psychology of the Sickbed* (Pittsburgh: Duquesne University Press, 1966).

10. Elaine Scarry, *The Body in Pain: The Making and Unmaking of the World* (New York: Oxford University Press, 1985), 3–6.

11. Peter Conrad, "The Social Meaning of AIDS," *Social Policy* 17 (Summer 1986): 51–56.

12. Jean Seligmann and Nikki Finke Greenberg, "Only Months to Live and No Place to Die," *Newsweek*, August 12, 1985, 26. As cited in Conrad, "Social Meaning of AIDS," 55.

13. Carel, *Illness*, 37.

14. Fredrik Svenaeus, *The Hermeneutics of Medicine and the Phenomenology of Health: Steps Towards a Philosophy of Medical Practice*, 2nd rev. ed. (Dordrecht: Kluwer Academic, 2001). Also see his "What is Phenomenology of Medicine? Embodiment, Illness and Being-in-the-World," in *Health, Illness and Disease*, ed. Havi Carel and Rachel Cooper (Durham, UK: Acumen Press, 2013).

15. Tony Perry, "Greek Classic Resonates at Camp Pendleton," *Los Angeles Times*, July 25, 2010, http://articles.latimes.com/2010/jul/25/local/la-me-ajax-20100726. Also see "Theatre of War Project: Overview," Outside the Wire, accessed April 1, 2015, http://www.outsidethewirellc.com/projects/theater-of-war/overview.

16. Elizabeth Blair, "In Ancient Dramas, Vital Words for Today's Warriors," *NPR*, November 25, 2008, http://www.npr.org/templates/story/story.php?storyId=97413320.

Chapter Two

1. Ronald Melzack and Patrick D. Wall, *The Challenge of Pain*, rev. ed. (London: Penguin, 1991), 36.

2. Institute of Medicine of the National Academies, *Relieving Pain in America: A Blueprint for Transforming Prevention, Care, Education, and Research* (Report Brief, June 2011), http://www.iom.edu/~/media/Files/Report%20Files/2011/Relieving-Pain-in-America-A-Blueprint-for-Transforming-Prevention-Care-Education-Research/Pain%20Research%202011%20Report%20Brief.pdf.

3. Maurice Natanson, *Edmund Husserl: Philosopher of Infinite Tasks* (Evanston, IL: Northwestern University Press, 1973), 12–19.

4. Elaine Scarry, *The Body in Pain: The Making and Unmaking of the World* (New York: Oxford University Press, 1985), 162.

5. S. Kay Toombs, *The Meaning of Illness: A Phenomenological Account of the Different Perspectives of Physician and Patient* (Dordrecht: Kluwer Academic, 1992), 36–37.

6. Nikola Grahek, *Feeling Pain and Being in Pain*, 2nd ed. (Cambridge, MA: MIT Press, 2007), 81.

7. Patrick Wall, *Pain: The Science of Suffering* (New York: Columbia University Press, 2000), 146.

8. Melzack and Wall, *Challenge of Pain*, 191.

9. Jerome Groopman, *How Doctors Think* (New York: Houghton Mifflin, 2007), 265–66.

10. Hans-Georg Gadamer, *Truth and Method*, trans. and ed. Garrett Barden and John Cumming (New York: Crossroad, 1984), 235–40.

11. Scarry, *Body in Pain*, 13.

12. Emily Dickinson, *The Complete Poems of Emily Dickinson*, ed. Thomas H. Johnson (Boston: Little, Brown, 1960), 323–24.

13. Martin Heidegger, *Being and Time*, trans. John Macquarrie and Edward Robinson (New York: Harper and Row, 1962), 375–80.

14. John B. Brough, "Temporality and Illness: A Phenomenological Perspective," in *Handbook of Phenomenology and Medicine*, ed. S. Kay Toombs (Dordrecht: Kluwer Academic, 2001), 43.

15. Eric J. Cassell, "The Phenomenon of Suffering and Its Relationship to Pain," in Toombs, *Handbook of Phenomenology and Medicine*, 387.

16. Havi Carel, *Illness: The Cry of the Flesh* (Stocksfield, UK: Acumen Press, 2008), 134.

17. Fredrik Svenaeus, *The Hermeneutics of Medicine and the Phenomenology of Health: Steps Towards a Philosophy of Medical Practice*, 2d rev. ed. (Dordrecht: Kluwer Academic, 2001).

18. Cassell, "Phenomenon of Suffering," 387.

19. Friedrich Nietzsche, *A Nietzsche Reader*, ed. and trans. R. J. Hollingdale (London: Penguin, 1977), 249-62.

20. Alphonse Daudet, *In the Land of Pain*, ed. and trans. Julian Barnes (New York: Alfred A. Knopf, 2002), 19.

21. J. C. Couceiro-Bueno, "The Phenomenology of Pain: An Experience of Life," in *Phenomenology and Existentialism in the Twentieth Century*, ed. Anna-Teresa Tymieniecka (Dordrecht: Springer, 2009), 297.

22. Carl G. Jung, *The Portable Jung*, ed. Joseph Campbell (New York: Penguin, 1976), 17.

23. Arthur Kleinman et al., "Pain as a Human Experience: An Introduction," in *Pain as a Human Experience: An Anthropological Perspective*, ed. Mary-Jo Delvecchio Good, Paul E. Brodwin, Byron J. Good, and Arthur Kleinman (Berkeley: University of California Press, 1992), 10.

24. "IASP Taxonomy," International Association for the Study of Pain, accessed June 17, 2014, http://www.iasp-pain.org/Education/Content.aspx?ItemNumber=1698.

25. Byron J. Good, "A Body in Pain—The Making of a World of Chronic Pain," in Good et al., *Pain as a Human Experience*, 46.

26. Bruce M. Eimer, *Hypnotize Yourself Out of Pain Now!* 2d ed. (Bethel, CT: Crown House, 2008).

27. Jean E. Jackson, "'After a While No One Believes You': Real and Unreal Pain," in Good et al., *Pain as a Human Experience*, 160.

28. Maurice Merleau-Ponty, *Phenomenology of Perception*, trans. Colin Smith (London: Routledge and Kegan Paul, 1962), 146.

29. Drew Leder, *The Absent Body* (Chicago: University of Chicago Press, 1990).

30. Richard M. Zaner, *The Context of Self: A Phenomenological Inquiry Using Medicine as a Clue* (Athens: Ohio University Press, 1981), 54.

31. Scarry, *Body in Pain*, 52.

32. David Bakan, *Disease, Pain, and Sacrifice* (Chicago: University of Chicago Press, 1968), 76-77.

33. Toombs, *Meaning of Illness*, 75.

34. Jenny Slatman, *Our Strange Body: Philosophical Reflections on Identity and Medical Interventions* (Amsterdam: Amsterdam University Press, 2015).

35. Bakan, *Disease, Pain, and Sacrifice*, 78.

36. Frederik J. J. Buytendijk, *Pain*, trans. Eda O'Shiel (Westport, CT: Greenwood Press, 1961), 27.

37. Scarry, *Body in Pain*, 4.

38. Maria-Liisa Honkasalo, "Space and Embodied Experience: Rethinking the Body in Pain," *Body & Society* 4, no. 2 (1998): 35-57.

39. Marcel Proust, *The Guermantes Way*, trans. Mark Treharne (New York: Penguin, 1992), 114.

40. Good, "Body in Pain," 47. Also see Toombs, *Meaning of Illness*, 67.

41. Heidegger, *Being and Time*, 172-79.

42. Good, "Body in Pain," 36.

43. Arthur W. Frank, *At the Will of the Body: Reflections on Illness* (Boston: Houghton Mifflin, 1991), 58.

44. Toombs, *Meaning of Illness*, 94.

45. Ibid., 59.

46. Melzack and Wall, *Challenge of Pain*, 25.

47. Arthur Kleinman, "Pain and Resistance: The Delegitimation and Relegitimation of Local Worlds," in Good et al., *Pain as a Human Experience*, 186.

48. Melzack and Wall, *Challenge of Pain*, 36.

49. Kleinman, "Pain and Resistance," 179.

50. Buytendijk, *Pain*, 20.

51. Scarry, *Body in Pain*, 29.

52. Arthur Frank, *The Wounded Storyteller: Body, Illness, and Ethics* (Chicago: University of Chicago Press, 1995), 54–55.

53. Matt. 27:46 (King James Version).

54. Marcel Proust, *Time Regained: In Search of Lost Time*, ed. D. J. Enright and Joanna Kilmartin, trans. Andreas Mayor and Terence Kilmartin (New York: Random House, 1993), 6:315.

55. Paul Brand and Philip Yancey, *Pain: The Gift Nobody Wants* (Darby, CT: Diane, 1999).

56. Drew Leder and Kirsten Jacobson, "Health and Disease: The Experience of Health and Illness," *Encyclopedia of Bioethics* 3 (2014): 1434–43. Also see Carel, *Illness*, 77–88.

57. Honkasalo, "Space and Embodied Experience," 35–57.

58. Victor Turner, *The Forest of Symbols* (IthacaNY: Cornell University Press, 1967), 97.

Chapter Three

1. Keith Thomas, *Religion and the Decline of Magic: Studies in Popular Beliefs in Sixteenth and Seventeenth Century England* (New York: Oxford University Press, 1997). Also see Roy Porter, "The Rise of Physical Examination," in *Medicine and the Five Senses*, ed. W. F. Bynum and Porter Roy (Cambridge: Cambridge University Press, 1993), 179–97.

2. H. Tristram Engelhardt Jr., *The Foundations of Bioethics* (New York: Oxford University Press, 1986). Also see Michel Foucault, *The Birth of the Clinic*, trans. A. M. Sheridan Smith (New York: Vintage Books, 1973), 124–48.

3. Porter, "Rise of Physical Examination," 179–97.

4. Richard Baron, "An Introduction to Medical Phenomenology: 'I Can't Hear You While I'm Listening,'" *Annals of Internal Medicine* 103, no. 4 (1985): 606–11.

5. Stanley Reiser, *Medicine and the Reign of Technology* (Cambridge: Cambridge University Press, 1978). Also see Merriley Borell, "Training the Senses, Training the Mind," in Bynum and Roy *Medicine and the Five Senses*, 244–61.

6. Edwin A. Burtt, *The Metaphysical Foundations of Modern Science* (Atlantic Highlands, NJ: Humanities Press, 1952).

7. Abraham Verghese, "A Touch of Sense," *Health Affairs* 28, no. 4 (2009): 1178–79.

8. Martin Buber, *I and Thou* (New York: Free Press, 1971).

9. Sally Gadow, "Touch and Technology: Two Paradigms of Patient Care," *Journal of Religion Health* 23, no. 1 (1984): 63–69.

10. Francisco J. Varela, "Intimate Distances: Fragments for a Phenomenology of Organ Transplantation," *Journal of Consciousness Studies* 8, no. 5–7 (2001): 266.

11. Matthew Ratcliffe, "Touch and Situatedness," *International Journal of Philosophical Studies* 16, no. 3 (2008): 299–322.

12. Erwin Straus, *Phenomenological Psychology*, trans. Erling Eng (New York: Basic, 1966).

13. Hans Jonas, *The Phenomenon of Life: Toward a Philosophical Biology* (Chicago: University of Chicago Press, 1966).

14. Constance Classen, ed., *The Book of Touch* (Oxford: Berg, 2005).

15. Jonas, *Phenomenon of Life*.

16. Maurice Merleau-Ponty, *Phenomenology of Perception*, trans. Colin Smith (London: Routledge and Kegan Paul, 1962), 92. Also see his *The Visible and the Invisible*, ed. Claude Lefort, trans. Alphonso Lingis (Evanston, IL: Northwestern University Press, 1968), 147–48.

17. Ratcliffe, "Touch and Situatedness," 317.

18. Fredrik Svenaeus, *The Hermeneutics of Medicine and the Phenomenology of Health: Steps Towards a Philosophy of Medical Practice*, 2d rev. ed. (Dordrecht: Kluwer Academic, 2001). Also see his "What is Phenomenology of Medicine? Embodiment, Illness and Being-in-the-World," in *Health, Illness and Disease*, ed. Havi Carel and Rachel Cooper (Durham, UK: Acumen Press, 2013).

19. Hans-Georg Gadamer, *The Enigma of Health* (Stanford, CA: Stanford University Press, 1996), 125–26.

20. Richard Selzer, *Mortal Lessons: Notes on the Art of Surgery* (New York: Simon and Schuster, 1974), 34.

21. Verghese, "Touch of Sense," 1180.

22. Valera, "Intimate Distances," 269.

23. Drew Leder, *The Absent Body* (Chicago: University of Chicago Press, 1990).

24. Marguerite O'Haire, "Companion Animals and Human Health: Benefits, Challenges, and the Road Ahead," *Journal of Veterinary Behavior* 5 (2010): 226–34.

25. Eva Marie Simms, "Milk and Flesh: A Phenomenological Reflection on Infancy and Coexistence," *Journal of Phenomenological Psychology* 32, no. 1 (2001): 22–40.

26. Ruth Feldman and Arthur Eidelman, "Skin-to-Skin Contact (Kangaroo Care) Accelerates Autonomic and Neurobehavioural Maturation in Preterm Infants," *Developmental Medicine & Child Neurology* 45 (2003): 274–81. Also see Tiffany Field et al., "Massage Therapy by Parents Improves Early Growth and Development," *Infant Behavior and Development* 27, no. 4 (2004): 435–42, and Tiffany Field, "Massage Therapy Facilitates Weight Gain in Preterm Infants," *Current Directions in Psychological Science* 10 (2001): 51–54.

27. Kim Jobst et al., "Diseases of Meaning, Manifestations of Health, and Metaphor," *Journal of Alternative and Complementary Medicine* 5, no. 6 (1999): 495–502.

28. Lance Hosey, *The Shape of Green: Aesthetics, Ecology and Design* (Washington, DC: Island Press, 2013), 65.

Chapter Four

1. Jeremy Greene, *Prescribing by Numbers: Drugs and the Definition of Disease* (Baltimore: Johns Hopkins University Press, 2007).

2. Ibid.

3. "Global Drug Sales to Top $1 Trillion in 2014—IMS," *Reuters*, April 20, 2010, http://www.reuters.com/article/2010/04/20/pharmaceuticals-forecast-idUSN1921921520100420/.

4. Steven Manners, *Super Pills: The Prescription Drugs We Love to Take* (Vancouver: Raincoast, 2006), 2.

5. Greene, *Prescribing by Numbers*; Manners, *Super Pills*, 2. Also see Howard Brody, *Hooked: Ethics, the Medical Profession, and the Pharmaceutical Industry* (Lanham, MD: Rowman and

Littlefield, 2007); Ivan Illich, *Limits to Medicine: Medical Nemesis—The Expropriation of Health* (London: Calder and Boyars, 1975); Jonathan Liebeneau, Gregory Higby, and Elaine Stroud, eds., *Pill Peddlers: Essays on the History of the Pharmaceutical Industry* (Madison, WI: American Institute of the History of Pharmacy, 1990).

6. Maurice Merleau-Ponty, *Phenomenology of Perception*, trans. Colin Smith (London: Routledge and Kegan Paul, 1962). Also see Drew Leder, *The Absent Body* (Chicago: University of Chicago Press, 1990); Erwin Straus, *The Primary World of Senses: A Vindication of Sensory Experience*, trans. Jacob Needleman (New York: Free Press of Glencoe, 1963); S. Kay Toombs, *The Meaning of Illness: A Phenomenological Account of the Different Perspectives of Physician and Patient* (Dordrecht: Kluwer Academic, 1992).

7. "Relief Is Just a Swallow Away," accessed July 10, 2013, http://www.bryanfields.com/samples /alka/mem/speedyad.html.

8. Edwin A. Burtt, *The Metaphysical Foundations of Modern Science* (Atlantic Highlands, NJ: Humanities Press, 1952).

9. Jim Hogshire, *Pills-a-Go-Go: A Fiendish Investigation into Pill Marketing, Art, History and Consumption* (Venice, CA: Feral House, 1999), 50–55.

10. Albert Borgmann, *Technology and the Character of Contemporary Life: A Philosophical Inquiry* (Chicago: University of Chicago Press, 1984), 40–48.

11. Hogshire, *Pills-a-Go-Go*, 51.

12. David Herzberg, *Happy Pills in America: From Miltown to Prozac* (Baltimore: Johns Hopkins University Press, 2009), 1.

13. Peter Kramer, *Listening to Prozac: The Landmark Book About Antidepressants and the Remaking of the Self* (New York: Penguin, 1997).

14. Peter Conrad and Valerie Leiter, "From Lydia Pinkham to Queen Levitra: Direct-to-Consumer Advertising and Medicalization," in *Pharmaceuticals and Society: Critical Discourses and Debates*, ed. Simon Williams, Jonathan Gabe, and Peter Davis (Oxford: Wiley-Blackwell, 2009), 22.

15. Nick Fox and Katie Ward, "Pharma in the Bedroom . . . and the Kitchen . . . the Pharmaceuticalization of Daily Life," in Williams et al., *Pharmaceuticals and Society*, 42.

16. Steven Woloshin and Lisa M. Schwartz, "Sell a Disease to Sell a Drug," *Washington Post*, June 7, 2015, http://www.washingtonpost.com/opinions/the-bulked-up-campaign-around-low -testosterone/2015/06/07/a9abda16-0573-11e5-8bda-c7b4e9a8f7ac_story.html?hpid=z3.

17. Daniel Moerman, *Meaning, Medicine, and "Placebo Effect"* (Cambridge: Cambridge University Press, 2002). Also see Howard Brody and Daralyn Brody, *The Placebo Response: How You Can Release the Body's Inner Pharmacy for Better Health* (New York: HarperCollins, 2000); Dylan Evans, *Placebo: Mind over Matter in Modern Medicine* (New York: Oxford University Press, 2004).

18. Drew Leder and Mitchell Krucoff, "Toward a More Materialistic Medicine: The Value of Authentic Materialism Within Current and Future Medical Practice," *Journal of Alternative and Complementary Medicine* 17 (2011): 859–65.

19. Daniel Moerman, *Meaning, Medicine, and "Placebo Effect"* (Cambridge: Cambridge University Press, 2002), 18–20, 47–48.

20. Stephanie Dutchen, "A Drug by Any Other Name," *Scope*, January 5, 2009, http:// scopeweb.mit.edu/articles/a-drug-by-any-other-name/.

21. Louis Dupre, *Symbols of the Sacred* (Grand Rapids, MI: Eerdmans, 2000).

22. Greene, *Prescribing by Numbers*, 1.

23. Rebecca Waber et al. "Commercial Features of Placebo and Therapeutic Efficacy," *JAMA* 299, no. 9 (2008): 1016–17.

24. Greene, *Prescribing by Numbers*, 237–38.

25. Hogshire, *Pills-a-Go-Go*, 59–62.

26. Brody, *Hooked*.

27. Hogshire, *Pills-a-Go-Go*, 8.

28. Manners, *Super Pills*, 56.

29. Rebecca Tuhus-Dubrow, "The Little Green Pill," *Slate*, January 3, 2011, http://www.slate .com/articles/health_and_science/green_room/2011/01/the_little_green_pill.html.

30. Greene, *Prescribing by Numbers*, 217.

31. David Morris, *Illness and Culture in the Postmodern Age* (Berkeley: University of California Press, 1998), 78–106.

32. Jacques Derrida, *Dissemination*, trans. Barbara Johnson (Chicago: University of Chicago Press, 1981), 61–171.

33. Walter Brogan, "Plato's Pharmakon: Between Two Repetitions," in *Derrida and Deconstruction*, ed. Hugh Silverman (New York: Routledge, 1989), 8.

34. Moerman, *Meaning, Medicine, and "Placebo Effect."*

35. Drew Leder and Kirsten Jacobson, "Health and Disease: The Experience of Health and Illness," in *Encyclopedia of Bioethics*, 4th ed., vol. 3, ed. Bruce Jennings (New York: Macmillan Reference USA, 2014), 1434–43.

36. Moerman, *Meaning, Medicine, and "Placebo Effect"*; Brody and Brody, *Placebo Response*.

37. Wang Yang-ming, *Instructions for Practical Living and Other Neo-Confucian Writings* (New York: Columbia University Press, 1963), 222.

38. Hans-Georg Gadamer, *The Enigma of Health* (Stanford, CA: Stanford University Press, 1996), 125–26.

39. Leder and Krucoff, "Toward a More Materialistic Medicine," 859–65.

Chapter Five

1. Paul Starr, *The Social Transformation of American Medicine* (New York: Basic, 1982).

2. E. Richard Brown, *Rockefeller Medicine Men: Medicine and Capitalism in America* (Berkeley: University of California Press, 1979).

3. Peter Whitehouse and Daniel George, *The Myth of Alzheimer's: What You Aren't Being Told About Today's Most Dreaded Diagnosis* (New York: St. Martin's Press, 2008).

4. Alfred North Whitehead, *Science and the Modern World* (New York: Free Press, 1997), 48–60.

5. Donald Loy, *Money, Sex, War, Karma: Notes for a Buddhist Revolution* (Somerville, MA: Wisdom, 2008).

6. Karl Marx, *Das Kapital: A Critique of Political Economy*, ed. Friedrich Engels (Washington, DC: Regnery Gateway, 1999).

7. Robert Tucker, ed., *The Marx-Engels Reader*, 2nd ed. (New York: W. W. Norton, 1978), 302–29.

8. Ibid., 321.

9. *American Heritage Dictionary*, 4th ed. (New York: Houghton Mifflin Harcourt, 2010).

10. Edwin A. Burtt, *The Metaphysical Foundations of Modern Science* (Atlantic Highlands, NJ: Humanities Press, 1952). Also see Herbert Butterfield, *The Origins of Modern Science* (New York: Free Press, 1997).

11. Rene Descartes, "Discourse on the Method of Rightly Conducting the Reason," in *The Philosophical Works of Descartes*, vol. 1, eds. Elizabeth Haldane and George R. T. Ross (Cambridge: Cambridge University Press, 1911), 119–20.

12. Ibid.

13. Burtt, *Metaphysical Foundations*.

14. Fredrik Svenaeus, *The Hermeneutics of Medicine and the Phenomenology of Health: Steps Towards a Philosophy of Medical Practice*, 2d rev. ed. (Dordrecht: Kluwer Academic, 2001).

15. Edmund Husserl, *Ideas Pertaining to a Pure Phenomenology and to a Phenomenological Philosophy: Second Book. Studies in the Phenomenology of Constitution*, trans. Richard Rojcewicz and André Schuwer (Dordrecht: Kluwer Academic, 1989).

16. Maurice Merleau-Ponty, *Phenomenology of Perception*, trans. Colin Smith (London: Routledge and Kegan Paul, 1962).

17. Shaun Gallagher, *How the Body Shapes the Mind* (Oxford: Clarendon Press, 2005). Also see Alva Noë, *Out of Our Heads: Why You Are Not Your Brain, and Other Lessons from the Biology of Consciousness* (New York: Hill and Wang, 2009).

18. Drew Leder, *The Absent Body* (Chicago: University of Chicago Press, 1990).

19. Whitehead, *Science and the Modern World*, 48–60. Also see Christian de Quincey, *Radical Nature: The Soul of Matter* (Rochester, VT: Park Street Press, 2002); David Ray Griffin, *Unsnarling the World-Knot: Consciousness, Freedom, and the Mind-Body Problem* (Berkeley: University of California Press, 1998).

20. Janet Bristow and Victoria Cole-Galo, *The Prayer Shawl Companion: 38 Knitted Designs to Embrace, Inspire, and Celebrate Life* (Newtown, CT: Taunton Press, 2008). Also see Prayer Shawl Ministry, accessed July 25, 2010, http://www.shawlministry.com/.

21. Katie Zezima, "From Balls of Yarn, Needles and Prayers, a New Ministry," *New York Times*, November 13, 2004, B8.

22. Susan Maddox, "My Mission-Prayer Quilts," accessed July 25, 2010, http://maddox oncology.com/blog/.

23. Zezima, "From Balls of Yarn," B8.

24. Thomas Csordas, ed. *Embodiment and Experience: The Existential Ground of Culture and Self* (Cambridge: Cambridge University Press, 1994). Also see his *Body/Meaning/Healing* (New York: Palgrave Macmillan, 2002); Sudhir Kakar, *Shamans, Mystics and Doctors: A Psychological Inquiry into India and Its Healing Traditions* (Chicago: University of Chicago Press, 1982); Margaret Lock and Judith Farquhar, eds. *Beyond the Body Proper: Reading the Anthropology of Material Life* (Durham, NC: Duke University Press, 2007).

25. James Frazer, *The Golden Bough: A Study in Magic and Religion* (New York: Macmillan, 1922).

26. Larry Dossey, "'Eating Papers' and Other Curious Aspects of Nutrition," *Alternative Therapies in Health and Medicine* 4 (1998): 11–16, 99–104.

27. Daniel Moerman, "Physiology and Symbols: The Anthropological Implications of the Placebo Effect," in *The Anthropology of Medicine: From Culture to Method*, ed. Lola Romanucci-Ross, Daniel Moerman, and Laurence Tancredi (Westport, CT: Bergin and Garvey, 1997).

28. Dossey, "'Eating Papers,'" 11–16, 99–104.

29. Drew Leder, "The Experience of Health and Illness," in *Encyclopedia of Bioethics*, 3rd ed., ed. Stephen Post (New York: Macmillan Reference, 2003), 1081–87.

30. Albert Borgmann, *Technology and the Character of Contemporary Life: A Philosophical Inquiry* (Chicago: University of Chicago Press, 1984), 40–48.

31. Martin Heidegger, "The Thing," in *Poetry, Language, Thought*, trans. Albert Hofstadter (New York: Harper and Row, 1971), 165–82.

32. Jeanne Achterberg et al., *Rituals of Healing: Using Imagery for Health and Wellness* (New York: Bantam, 1994).

33. "World Class Healthcare Totally Free of Charge," Sri Satha Sai Institute of Higher Medical Sciences: Prasanthigram, accessed July 26, 2010, http://psg.sssihms.org.in/.

34. "Sri Satha Sai Central Trust," International Sai Organization, accessed July 26, 2010, http://www.sathyasai.org/ashrams/centraltrust.htm.

35. Martin Heidegger, "The Origin of the Work of Art," in Hofstadter, *Poetry, Language, Thought*, 17–87.

36. William Thomas, *The Eden Alternative: Nature, Hope and Nursing Homes* (Columbia: University of Missouri Press, 1994).

37. Caroline Hsu, "The Greening of Aging," *U.S. News & World Report*, June 19, 2006, 48–52.

38. William Thomas, *What Are Old People For? How Elders Will Save the World* (Acton, MA: VanderWyk and Burnham, 2004).

39. Hsu, "Greening of Aging," 48–52.

40. Melissa Matchett et al., "The Implantable Cardioverter Defibrillator: Its History, Current Psychological Impact and Future," *Expert Review of Medical Devices* 6 (2009): 43–50.

41. Sue Ann Thomas et al., "Quality of Life and Psychosocial Status of Patients with Implantable Cardioverter Defibrillators," *American Journal of Critical Care* 15 (2006): 389–98. Also see J. Michael Bostwick and Christopher Sola, "An Updated Review of Implantable Cardioverter/Defibrillators, Induced Anxiety, and Quality of Life," *Psychiatric Clinics North America* 30, no. 4 (2007): 677–88; Susan Zayac and Nancy Finch, "Recipients' of Implanted Cardioverter-Defibrillators Actual and Perceived Adaptation: A Review of the Literature," *Journal of the American Academy of Nurse Practitioners* 21 (2009): 549–56.

42. Fanny Jacq et al., "A Comparison of Anxiety, Depression and Quality of Life Between Device Shock and Nonshock Groups in Implantable Cardioverter Defibrillator Recipients," *General Hospital Psychiatry* 31 (2009): 266–73.

43. Sandeep Jauhar, "Jolts of Anxiety," *New York Times Magazine*, May 5, 2002, 16–21.

44. Anne Pollock, "The Internal Cardiac Defibrillator," in *The Inner History of Devices*, ed. Sherry Turkle (Cambridge, MA: MIT Press, 2008), 98–111.

45. Zayac and Finch, "Recipients' of Implanted Cardioverter-Defibrillators."

46. Pollock, "Internal Cardiac Defibrillator," 98–111.

47. Jauhar, "Jolts of Anxiety," 16–21.

48. Philip Kapleau, *The Zen of Living and Dying: A Practical and Spiritual Guide* (Boston: Shambhala Press, 1998), 33.

Chapter Six

1. Thomas Kuhn, *The Structure of Scientific Revolutions* (Chicago: University of Chicago Press, 1962). Also see Paul Feyerabend, *Against Method* (London: Verso, 1975); Michael Polanyi, *Personal Knowledge* (Chicago: University of Chicago Press, 1958).

2. Ian R. McWhinney, "Medical Knowledge and the Rise of Technology," *Journal of Medicine and Philosophy* 3 (1978): 293–304.

3. Ronald Munson, "Why Medicine Cannot Be a Science," *Journal of Medicine and Philosophy* 6 (1981): 183–208.

4. Hans-Georg Gadamer, *The Enigma of Health*, trans. Jason Gaiger and Nicholas Walker (Stanford, CA: Stanford University Press, 1996), 34, 39.

5. Stephen Toulmin, "On the Nature of the Physician's Understanding," *Journal of Medicine and Philosophy* 1 (1976): 32–50.

6. Stephen L. Daniel, "The Patient as Text: A Model of Clinical Hermeneutics," *Theoretical Medicine* 7 (1986): 195–210.

7. Eugenie Gatens-Robinson, "Clinical Judgment and the Rationality of the Human Sciences," *Journal of Medicine and Philosophy* 11 (1986): 167–78.

8. Edward Gogel and James Terry, "Medicine as Interpretation: The Uses of Literary Metaphors and Methods," *Journal of Medicine and Philosophy* 12 (1987): 205–17.

9. Byron Good and Mary-Jo Delvecchio Good, "The Meaning of Symptoms: A Cultural Hermeneutic Model for Clinical Practice," in *The Relevance of Social Science for Medicine*, eds. Leon Eisenberg and Arthur Kleinman (Dordrecht: D. Reidel, 1978), 165–96.

10. Fredrik Svenaeus, *The Hermeneutics of Medicine and the Phenomenology of Health: Steps Towards a Philosophy of Medical Practice*, 2nd rev. ed. (Dordrecht: Kluwer Academic, 2001), 134–40.

11. Richard Palmer, *Hermeneutics: Interpretation Theory in Schleiermacher, Dilthey, Heidegger, and Gadamer* (Evanston, IL: Northwestern University Press, 1969).

12. Richard Bernstein, *Beyond Objectivism and Relativism: Science, Hermeneutics, and Praxis* (Philadelphia: University of Pennsylvania Press, 1983).

13. Martin Heidegger, *Being and Time*, trans. John Macquarrie and Edward Robinson (New York: Harper and Row, 1962), 188–95.

14. Daniel, "Patient as Text," 195–210.

15. Svenaeus, *Hermeneutics of Medicine*, 11.

16. Annemarie Mol, *The Body Multiple: Ontology in Medical Practice* (Durham, NC: Duke University Press, 2002), 33.

17. H. Tristram Engelhardt Jr., "Human Well-Being and Medicine: Some Basic Value-Judgments in the Biomedical Sciences," in *Science, Ethics and Medicine*, ed. H. Tristram Engelhardt Jr. and Daniel Callahan (Hastings-on-the-Hudson: The Hastings Center Institute of Society, Ethics and the Life Sciences, 1976), 120–39.

18. David Bakan, *Disease, Pain, and Sacrifice* (Chicago: University of Chicago Press, 1968), 57–58.

19. Good and Good, "Meaning of Symptoms," 165–96.

20. Drew Leder, *The Absent Body* (Chicago: University of Chicago Press, 1990), 36–68.

21. Lewis Thomas, *The Lives of a Cell* (New York: Bantam, 1974), 78.

22. Rita Charon, "Narrative Medicine: A Model for Empathy, Reflection, Profession, and Trust," *Journal of the American Medical Society* 286, no. 15 (2001): 1898.

23. Arthur Frank, *The Wounded Storyteller: Body, Illness, and Ethics* (Chicago: University of Chicago Press, 1995). Also see Drew Leder, "Toward a Phenomenology of Pain," *Review of Existential Psychology and Psychiatry* 19 (1984–1985): 255–66; Elaine Scarry, *The Body in Pain: The Making and Unmaking of the World* (New York: Oxford University Press, 1985), 3–23.

24. Mol, *Body Multiple*, 27.

25. Richard Baron, "An Introduction to Medical Phenomenology: 'I Can't Hear You While I'm Listening,'" *Annals of Internal Medicine* 103, no. 4 (1985): 606–11.

26. Maurice Merleau-Ponty, *Phenomenology of Perception*, trans. Colin Smith (London: Routledge and Kegan Paul, 1962). Also see Herbert Plügge, "Man and His Body," in *The*

Philosophy of the Body, ed. Stuart F. Spicker (Chicago: Quadrangle, 1970), 293–311; Richard Zaner, *The Problem of Embodiment* (The Hague: Martinus Nijhoff, 1964).

27. Drew Leder, "Medicine and Paradigms of Embodiment," *Journal of Medicine and Philosophy* 9 (1984): 29–43.

28. Merleau-Ponty, *Phenomenology of Perception*, 144–46.

29. Gilbert Ryle, *The Concept of Mind* (New York: Barnes and Noble, 1949), 25–61. Also see Michael Polanyi, *Knowing and Being* (Chicago: University of Chicago Press, 1969), 141–42.

30. Don Ihde, *Technics and Praxis* (Dordrecht: D. Reidel, 1979). Also see Patrick Heelan, "The Nature of Clinical Science," *Journal of Medicine and Philosophy* 2 (1977): 20–32.

31. Polanyi, *Knowing and Being*, 138–58.

32. Ibid., 188–89.

33. Stanley Reiser, *Medicine and the Reign of Technology* (Cambridge: Cambridge University Press, 1978), 166–73, 227–31.

34. Ihde, *Technics and Praxis*, 28–39.

35. Mol, *Body Multiple*, 55, 143.

36. Heidegger, *Being and Time*, 191–95.

37. Jerome Groopman, *How Doctors Think* (New York: Houghton Mifflin, 2007), 35.

38. Ibid., 24–40.

39. Ibid., 21.

40. Ibid., 128.

41. Hans-Georg Gadamer, *Truth and Method*, trans. and ed. Garrett Barden and John Cumming (New York: Crossroad, 1984), 325–41.

42. Mol, *Body Multiple*, 53–85.

43. Svenaeus, *Hermeneutics of Medicine*, 146–66.

44. Gadamer, *Enigma of Health*.

45. Frank, *Wounded Storyteller*, 5–6.

46. Ibid., 58.

47. H. Tristram Engelhardt Jr., "Illnesses, Diseases, and Sicknesses," in *The Humanity of the Ill*, ed. Victor Kestenbaum (Knoxville: University of Tennessee Press, 1982), 152.

48. Svenaeus, *Hermeneutics of Medicine*, 147.

49. Anne Fadiman, *The Spirit Catches You and You Fall Down: A Hmong Child, Her American Doctors, and the Collision of Two Cultures* (New York: Farrar, Straus and Giroux, 1997), 262.

50. Gadamer, *Truth and Method*, 274–305.

51. Gadamer, *Enigma of Health*.

52. Heidegger, *Being and Time*, 194–95.

53. Reiser, *Medicine and the Reign of Technology*, 1–6.

54. Hans Jonas, *The Phenomenon of Life: Toward a Philosophical Biology* (Chicago: University of Chicago Press, 1966), 135–56.

55. Michel Foucault, *The Birth of the Clinic*, trans. Alan M. Sheridan Smith (New York: Vintage, 1973).

56. Ibid., 146.

57. H. Tristram Engelhardt Jr., *The Foundations of Bioethics* (New York: Oxford University Press, 1986), 176–84.

58. Reiser, *Medicine and the Reign of Technology*, 30.

59. Ihde, *Technics and Praxis*, 16–27.

60. Groopman, *How Doctors Think*, 156–202.

61. Reiser, *Medicine and the Reign of Technology*, 94.

62. Edwin A. Burtt, *The Metaphysical Foundations of Modern Science* (Atlantic Highlands, NJ: Humanities Press, 1952), 74–90.

63. Svenaeus, *Hermeneutics of Medicine*, 33.

64. Reiser, *Medicine and the Reign of Technology*, 158–95.

65. Delicia Yard, "PSA Testing: Why the U.S. and Europe Differ," *Renal and Urology News*, September 21, 2011, http://www.renalandurologynews.com/prostate-cancer/psa-testing-why-the -us-and-europe-differ/article/212312/.

Chapter Seven

1. Richard E. Palmer, *Hermeneutics: Interpretation Theory in Schleiermacher, Dilthey, Heidegger, and Gadamer* (Evanston, IL: Northwestern University Press, 1969).

2. Wilhelm Dilthey, *Selected Works*, trans. and ed. H. P. Rickman (Cambridge: Cambridge University Press, 1976), 170–245.

3. Martin Heidegger, *Being and Time*, trans. John Macquarrie and Edward Robinson (New York: Harper and Row, 1962), 188–95.

4. Patrick A. Heelan, *Space-Perception and the Philosophy of Science* (Berkeley: University of California Press, 1983).

5. Heidegger, *Being and Time*, 191–92.

6. Hans-Georg Gadamer, *Truth and Method*, trans. and ed. Garrett Barden and John Cumming (New York: Crossroads, 1984), 235–40.

7. Thomas Nagel, *The View from Nowhere* (New York: Oxford University Press, 1986).

8. Heidegger, *Being and Time*, 194–95. Also see Gadamer, *Truth and Method*, 235–38, 258–67, 325–51.

9. Hans-Georg Gadamer, *The Enigma of Health: The Art of Healing in a Scientific Age*, trans. Jason Gaiger and Nicholas Walker (Stanford, CA: Stanford University Press, 1996).

10. Gadamer, *Truth and Method*, 274–305.

11. Immanuel Kant, *Foundations of the Metaphysics of Morals*, trans. Lewis White Beck (Indianapolis: Bobbs Merrill, 1969), 26–72.

12. Leo Tolstoy, *The Death of Ivan Ilych and Other Stories*, trans. Aylmer Maude and J. D. Duff (New York: New American Library, 1960), 121–22.

13. Arthur Frank, *The Wounded Storyteller: Body, Illness, and Ethics* (Chicago: University of Chicago Press, 1995), 10.

14. Harold Alderman, "By Virtue of a Virtue," *Review of Metaphysics* 36 (September 1982): 127–53.

15. Havi Carel, *Illness: The Cry of the Flesh* (Stocksfield, UK: Acumen Press, 2008).

16. Jay Katz, *The Silent World of Doctor and Patient* (New York: Free Press, 1984); Frank, *The Wounded Storyteller*.

17. Angela Woods, "Beyond the Wounded Storyteller: Rethinking Narrativity, Illness and Embodied Self-Experience," in *Health, Illness and Disease: Philosophical Essays*, ed. Havi Carel and Rachel Cooper (Durham, UK: Acumen Press, 2013), 113–28.

18. Arthur Kleinman, *The Illness Narratives* (New York: Basic, 1988). Also see Anne H. Hawkins, *Reconstructing Illness: Studies in Pathography* (West Lafayette, IN: Purdue University Press, 1999).

19. Frank, *Wounded Storyteller*, 53.

20. Hawkins, *Reconstructing Illness*. Also see Howard Brody, *Stories of Sickness* (New Haven, CT: Yale University Press, 1987), 182–92.

21. Susan Sontag, *Illness as Metaphor* (New York: Farrar, Straus and Giroux, 1978).

22. Rita Charon, "Narrative Medicine: A Model for Empathy, Reflection, Profession, and Trust," *Journal of the American Medical Society* 286, no. 15 (2001): 1897.

23. Antonio Casado da Rocha and Arantza Etxeberria, "Towards Autonomy-within-Illness: Applying the Triadic Approach to the Principles of Bioethics," in *Health, Illness and Disease: Philosophical Essays*, ed. Havi Carel and Rachel Cooper (Durham, UK: Acumen Press, 2013), 70.

24. Richard Zaner, *Ethics and the Clinical Encounter* (Englewood Cliffs, NJ: Prentice Hall, 1988), 84–86, 251–55.

25. Erwin Straus, "The Upright Posture," in *Phenomenological Psychology*, trans. Erling Eng (New York: Basic, 1966).

26. Oliver Sacks, *A Leg to Stand On* (New York: HarperCollins, 1994), 129.

27. Iris Marion Young, *On Female Body Experience: Throwing Like a Girl and Other Essays* (Oxford: Oxford University Press, 2005), 27–45.

28. Lisa Diedrich, "Breaking Down: A Phenomenology of Disability," *Literature and Medicine* 20, no. 2 (2001): 209–30.

29. Michel Foucault, *The History of Sexuality*, vol. 1: *An Introduction*, trans. Robert Hurley (New York: Vintage, 1980). Also see his *Discipline and Punish: The Birth of the Prison*, trans. Alan Sheridan (New York: Vintage, 1979); *The Birth of the Clinic*, trans. Alan M. Sheridan Smith (New York: Vintage, 1973); *Madness and Civilization: A History of Insanity in the Age of Reason*, trans. Richard Howard (New York: Vintage, 1973).

30. Jennifer A. Parks and Victoria S. Wike, *Bioethics in a Changing World* (Upper Saddle River, NJ: Prentice Hall, 2010). Also see David Schenck, "The Texture of Embodiment: Foundation for Medical Ethics," *Human Studies* 9, no. 1 (1986): 43–54; Susan Sherwin, "Whither Bioethics? How Feminism Can Help Reorient Bioethics," *International Journal of Feminist Approaches to Bioethics* 1, no. 1 (2008): 7–27.

31. George Agich, *Autonomy and Long-term Care* (New York: Oxford University Press, 1993).

32. Young, *On Female Body Experience*, 155–70.

33. Isabel Dyck et al., "The Home as a Site for Long-term Care: Meanings and Management of Bodies and Spaces," *Health & Place* 11, no. 2 (2005): 173–85.

34. Isabel Dyck, "Hidden Geographies: The Changing Lifeworlds of Women with Multiple Sclerosis," *Social Science and Medicine* 40, no. 3 (1995): 307–20.

35. William May, *The Patient's Ordeal* (Bloomington: Indiana University Press, 1991).

36. Anatole Broyard, *Intoxicated by My Illness and Other Writings on Life and Death* (New York: Fawcett Columbine, 1992). Also see Arthur Frank, *At the Will of the Body: Reflections on Illness* (New York: Houghton Mifflin, 2002).

37. Carel, *Illness*.

38. Sacks, *Leg to Stand On*, 146.

39. Ibid., 148.

40. Frank, *Wounded Storyteller*, 150.

41. Edmund Pellegrino and David Thomasma, *Virtues in Medical Practice* (New York: Oxford University Press, 1993).

42. Schenck, "Texture of Embodiment"; Sherwin, "Whither Bioethics."

43. Casado da Rocha and Etxeberria, "Towards Autonomy-within-illness," 72.

44. Charon, "Narrative Medicine," 1898.

45. Sidney Callahan and Daniel Callahan, "Breaking Through Stereotypes," *Commonweal* 111, no. 017 (1984): 520–23.

46. Paul Ricoeur, *Freud and Philosophy: An Essay on Interpretation*, trans. Denis Savage (New Haven, CT: Yale University Press, 1970), 32–36.

47. Gadamer, *Truth and Method*, 18–43. Also see Georgia Warnke, *Gadamer: Hermeneutics, Tradition and Reason* (Stanford, CA: Stanford University Press, 1987), 107–38.

48. Heidegger, *Being and Time*, 256–73.

49. Dyck et al., "Home as a Site," 173–85.

50. Drew Leder and Kirsten Jacobson, "Health and Disease: The Experience of Health and Illness," in *Bioethics*, 4th ed., vol. 3, ed. Bruce Jennings (Farmington Hills, MI: Macmillan Reference USA, 2014), 1434–43.

51. Patricia Benner et al., *Educating Nurses: A Call for Radical Transformation* (San Francisco: Jossey-Bass, 2010); Sherwin, "Whither Bioethics?" Also see Sandra Thomas and Howard Pollio, *Listening to Patients: A Phenomenological Approach to Nursing Research and Practice* (New York: Springer, 2002); Ian Thompson et al., *Nursing Ethics*, 5th ed. (Edinburgh: Churchill Livingston Elsevier, 2006).

52. Anne Fadiman, *The Spirit Catches You and You Fall Down: A Hmong Child, Her American Doctors, and the Collision of Two Cultures* (New York: Farrar, Straus and Giroux, 1997). Also see Shaun Gallagher and Jesper Sørensen, "Experimenting with Phenomenology," *Consciousness and Cognition* 15, no. 1 (2006): 119–34; Louis Sass et al., "Phenomenological Psychopathology and Schizophrenia: Contemporary Approaches and Misunderstandings," *Philosophy, Psychiatry, & Psychology* 18, no. 1 (2011): 1–23; Esther Sternberg, *Healing Spaces: The Science of Place and Well-Being* (Cambridge, MA: Harvard University Press, 2009); Fredrik Svenaeus, *The Hermeneutics of Medicine and the Phenomenology of Health: Steps Towards a Philosophy of Medical Practice*, 2nd rev. ed. (Dordrecht: Kluwer Academic, 2001).

53. Charon, "Narrative Medicine." Also see her *Narrative Medicine: Honoring the Stories of Illness* (New York: Oxford University Press, 2008).

54. Carel, *Illness*, 43.

55. Sacks, *Leg to Stand On*.

Chapter Eight

1. Fredrik Svenaeus, "The Body as Gift, Resource or Commodity? Heidegger and the Ethics of Organ Transplantation," *Bioethical Inquiry* 7 (2010): 163–72.

2. Renée Fox and Judith Swazey, *Spare Parts: Organ Replacement in American Society* (New York: Oxford University Press, 1992), 8–13.

3. "Statistics About Diabetes," American Association of Diabetes, June 10, 2014, http://www.diabetes.org/diabetes-basics/statistics/?loc=db-slabnav.

4. Giuliano Testa and Mark Siegler, "Increasing the Supply of Kidneys for Transplantation by Making Living Donors the Preferred Source of Donor Kidneys," *Medicine* 93 (2014): 29.

5. Mitra Mahdavi-Mazdeh, "The Iranian Model of Living Renal Transplantation," *Kidney International* 82 (2012): 627–34.

6. Kate Greasley, "A Legal Market in Organs: The Problem of Exploitation," *Journal of Medical Ethics* 40 (2012): 55, doi:10.1136/medethics-2012-100770.

7. Mark Dowie, *We Have a Donor: The Bold New World of Organ Transplanting* (New York: St. Martin's Press, 1988), 131.

8. Rene Descartes, *The Philosophical Writings of Descartes*, vol. 2, trans. John Cottingham, Robert Stoothoff, and Dugald Murdoch (Cambridge: Cambridge University Press, 1984), 54.

9. Richard Zaner, *Ethics and the Clinical Encounter* (Englewood Cliffs, NJ: Prentice Hall, 1988).

10. Carolyn Merchant, *The Death of Nature* (San Francisco: Harper and Row, 1980).

11. Descartes, *Philosophical Writings of Descartes*, 142-43.

12. Ibid., 143.

13. Jack Vrooman, *Rene Descartes: A Biography* (New York: G. P. Putnam's Sons, 1970), 141.

14. Ibid., 142.

15. Allucquère R. Stone, "Will the Real Body Please Stand Up? Boundary Stories About Virtual Cultures," in *Cyberspace: First Steps*, ed. Michael Benedikt (Cambridge, MA: MIT Press, 1991), 90.

16. Jenny Slatman, *Our Strange Body: Philosophical Reflections on Identity and Medical Interventions* (Amsterdam: Amsterdam University Press, 2015), 158.

17. Jean-Luc Nancy, "L'Intrus," trans. Susan Hanson, *New Centennial Review* 2, no. 3 (2002): 6.

18. Merchant, *Death of Nature*, 3-4.

19. Hans Jonas, *The Phenomenon of Life: Toward a Philosophical Biology* (Chicago: University of Chicago Press, 1966), 203-4.

20. Dowie, *We Have a Donor*, 217.

21. Andrew Kimbrell, "Forum: Sacred or For Sale?" *Harper's Magazine*, October 1990, 49.

22. Francisco Varela, "Intimate Distances: Fragments for a Phenomenology of Organ Transplantation," *Journal of Consciousness Studies* 8, no. 5-7 (2001): 264.

23. Nancy, "L'Intrus," 8-9.

24. Fox and Swazey, *Spare Parts*, 68.

25. Kazuo Ishiguro, *Never Let Me Go* (New York: Vintage, 2006).

26. Michel Foucault, *Discipline and Punish: The Birth of the Prison*, trans. Alan Sheridan (New York: Vintage, 1979), 135-41.

27. Barbara Garson, *The Electronic Sweatshop* (New York: Simon and Schuster, 1988), 20.

28. Orlando Figes, *Natasha's Dance: A Cultural History of Russia* (New York: Picador, 2002), 464.

29. H. Tristram Engelhardt Jr., *The Foundations of Bioethics* (New York: Oxford University Press, 1986), 127-30.

30. Karl Marx, *Capital*, vol. 1 (New York: International, 1967), 35.

31. Adam Gollner, "The Immortality Financiers: The Billionaires Who Want to Live Forever," *Daily Beast*, August 20, 2013, http://www.thedailybeast.com/articles/2013/08/20/the-immortality-financiers-the-billionaires-who-want-to-live-forever.html.

32. T. Scott Bentley, "U.S. Organ and Tissue Transplant Cost Estimates and Discussion," *Milliman Research Report*, December 2014, http://www.milliman.com/uploadedFiles/insight/Research/health-rr/1938HDP_20141230.pdf.

33. Henry Hansmann, "The Economics and Ethics of Markets for Human Organs," in *Organ Transplantation Policy: Issues and Prospects*, ed. James Blumstein and Frank Sloan (Durham, NC: Duke University Press, 1989).

34. Mark Cherry, *Kidney for Sale by Owner: Human Organs, Transplantation, and the Market* (Washington DC: Georgetown University Press, 2005), 151-52.

35. H. Tristram Engelhardt Jr., "The Body for Fun, Beneficence, and Profit: A Variation on a Post-modern Theme," in *Persons and Their Bodies: Rights, Responsibilities, Relationships*, ed. Mark Cherry (Dordrecht: Kluwer Academic, 1999), 277–301.

36. Alisdair MacIntyre, *After Virtue* (Notre Dame, IN: University of Notre Dame Press, 1981).

37. Cherry, *Kidney for Sale*, 147–62.

38. Julian Savulescu, "Is the Sale of Body Parts Wrong?" *Journal of Medical Ethics* 29 (2003): 138–39. Also see Sarah McGrath, "Organ Procurement, Altruism, and Autonomy," *Journal of Value Inquiry* 40 (2006): 297–309; Cherry, *Kidney for Sale*.

39. Greasley, "Legal Market in Organs," 51.

40. Simon Rippon, "Imposing Options on People in Poverty: The Harm of a Live Donor Organ Market," *Journal of Medical Ethics* 40 (2014): 145–50.

41. Arthur Caplan, *If I Were a Rich Man Could I Buy a Pancreas? And Other Essays on the Ethics of Health Care* (Bloomington: Indiana University Press, 1992) 158–77.

42. William May, *The Patient's Ordeal* (Bloomington: Indiana University Press, 1991), 180.

43. Greasely, "Legal Market in Organs," 52–53.

44. Ronald Bailey, "Should I Be Allowed to Buy Your Kidney?" *Forbes*, May 28, 1990, 368.

45. Sanjoy Hazarika, "India Debates Ethics of Buying Transplant Kidneys," *New York Times*, August 17, 1992, A20.

46. May, *Patient's Ordeal*, 197.

47. Bailey, "Should I Be Allowed?," 367.

48. Arthur Frank, *The Wounded Storyteller: Body, Illness, and Ethics* (Chicago: University of Chicago Press, 1995), 36.

49. Drew Leder, "A Tale of Two Bodies: The Cartesian Corpse and the Lived Body," in *The Body in Medical Thought and Practice*, ed. Drew Leder (Dordrecht: Kluwer Academic, 1992).

50. Edmund Husserl, *Ideas Pertaining to a Pure Phenomenology and to a Phenomenological Philosophy*, 2nd bk., *Studies in the Phenomenology of Constitution*, trans. Richard Rojcewicz and André Schuwer (Dordrecht: Kluwer Academic, 1989).

51. Maurice Merleau-Ponty, *Phenomenology of Perception*, trans. Colin Smith (London: Routledge and Kegan Paul, 1962).

52. Erwin Straus, *The Primary World of Senses: A Vindication of Sensory Experience*, trans. Jacob Needleman (New York: Free Press of Glencoe, 1963). Also see his *Phenomenological Psychology*, trans. Erling Eng (New York: Basic, 1966).

53. Richard Zaner, *The Context of Self: A Phenomenological Inquiry Using Medicine as a Clue* (Athens: Ohio University Press, 1981). Also see his *Ethics and the Clinical Encounter*.

54. Gilbert Ryle, *The Concept of Mind* (New York: Harper and Row, 1949), 15–16.

55. Drew Leder, *The Absent Body* (Chicago: University of Chicago Press, 1990).

56. Carl Zimmer, "Tending the Body's Microbial Garden," *New York Times*, June 19, 2012, D1.

57. Eula Biss, *On Immunity: An Inoculation* (Minneapolis: Graywolf Press, 2014), 161.

58. Ibid., 76.

59. Carel Havi, *Illness: The Cry of the Flesh* (Stocksfield, UK: Acumen Press, 2008), 56.

60. Mark Dowie, "Transplant Fever," *Mother Jones* 14, no. 3 (1989): 20.

61. Eva Marie Simms, "Milk and Flesh: A Phenomenological Reflection on Infancy and Coexistence," *Journal of Phenomenological Psychology* 32, no. 1 (2001): 25–26.

62. May, *Patient's Ordeal*, 180.

63. Thomas Murray, "Gifts of the Body and the Needs of Strangers," *Hastings Center Report* 17 (1987): 30–38.

64. Marcel Mauss, *The Gift: Forms and Functions of Exchange in Archaic Societies*, trans. Ian Cunnison (Glencoe, IL: Free Press, 1954).

65. Richard Titmuss, *The Gift Relationship: From Human Blood to Social Policy* (London: Allen and Unwin, 1970).

66. May, *Patient's Ordeal*, 187–91.

67. Varela, "Intimate Distances," 267.

68. Kristin Zeiler, "Ethics and Organ Transfer: A Merleau-Pontean Perspective," *Health Care Analysis* 17 (2009): 110–22.

69. May, *Patient's Ordeal*, 182–87.

70. Tu Wei-ming, *Confucian Thought: Selfhood as Creative Transformation* (Albany: State University of New York Press, 1985), 35–50. Also see Wang Yang-ming, "Inquiry on the Great Learning," in *A Sourcebook in Chinese Philosophy*, ed. Wing-tsit Chan (Princeton, NJ: Princeton University Press, 1963).

71. Leder, *Absent Body*, 156–73.

72. David Abram, "The Ecology of Magic," *Orion* 10, no. 3 (1991): 37.

73. Ibid.

74. Martin Heidegger, *Being and Time*, trans. John Macquarrie and Edward Robinson (New York: Harper and Row, 1962).

75. Svenaeus, "Body as Gift," 171.

76. Nancy, "L'Intrus," 8–9.

77. Slatman, *Our Strange Body*, 76.

78. Ibid., 93–105.

79. Murray, "Gifts of the Body," 32.

Chapter Nine

1. Peter Singer, *Animal Liberation* (New York: HarperCollins, 1975; New York: Harper Perennial. 2001). Also see his *In Defense of Animals: The Second Wave* (Malden, MA: Blackwell, 2006).

2. Michael Pollan, *The Omnivore's Dilemma: A Natural History of Four Meals* (New York: Penguin, 2006). Also see David Kirby, *Animal Factory: The Looming Threat of Industrial Pig, Dairy, and Poultry Farms to Humans and the Environment* (New York: St. Martin's Press, 2010).

3. Marc Kaufman, "Guidelines for Treatment of Food Animals Released; Retailers Urge Improved Conditions on Farms," *Washington Post*, June 28, 2002, A3. Also see David Barboza, "Animal Welfare's Unexpected Allies," *New York Times*, June 25, 2003, C1.

4. Karl Marx, "Estranged Labor," in *The Economic and Philosophic Manuscripts of 1844* (New York: International, 1964), 106–19.

5. Ibid., 110.

6. Ibid., 114.

7. Ibid.

8. Barbara Garson, *The Electronic Sweatshop* (New York: Simon and Schuster, 1988), 20.

9. Marx, "Estranged Labor," 108.

10. Jim Mason and Mary Finelli, "Brave New Farm," in *In Defense of Animals: The Second Wave*, ed. Peter Singer (Malden, MA: Blackwell, 2006), 104–22.

11. Temple Grandin and Catherine Johnson, *Animals in Translation: Using the Mysteries of Autism to Decode Animal Behavior* (New York: Harcourt, 2006), 69–81.

12. Ted Benton, "Humanism Equals Speciesism: Marx on Humans and Animals," *Radical Philosophy* 50 (1998): 4–18.

13. Marx, "Estranged Labor," 181.

14. Benton, "Humanism Equals Speciesism," 4–18.

15. Marx, "Estranged Labor," 113.

16. Ibid., 111.

17. Ibid.

18. Jean-Guy Vaillancourt, "Marxism and Ecology: More Benedictine than Franciscan," in *The Greening of Marxism*, ed. Ted Benton (New York: Guilford Press, 1996), 53.

19. Ted Benton, ed., *The Greening of Marxism* (New York: Guilford Press, 1996).

20. James O'Connor, *Natural Causes: Essays in Ecological Marxism* (New York: Guilford Press, 1998).

21. John Barry, "Marxism and Ecology," in *Marxism and Social Science*, ed. Andrew Gamble, David Marsh, and Tony Tant (Urbana: University of Illinois Press, 1999), 259–79.

22. Ibid., 276.

23. Jim Mason, *An Unnatural Order: Uncovering the Roots of Our Domination of Nature and Each Other* (New York: Simon and Schuster, 1993).

24. Richard McKeon, ed., *The Basic Works of Aristotle* (New York: Random House, 1941), 1137.

25. St. Thomas Aquinas, *On the Truth of the Catholic Faith (Summa Contra Gentiles)*, bk. 3: Providence, pt. 2, trans. Vernon J. Bourke (New York: Image, 1956), 115.

26. Aquinas, *Truth of the Catholic Faith*, 119.

27. Immanuel Kant, *Lectures on Ethics*, trans. Louis Infield (London: Methuen, 1963), 239.

28. Richard Austin, *Hope for the Land: Nature in the Bible* (Atlanta: John Knox Press, 1988). Also see Wendell Berry, *The Gift of Good Land: Further Essays Cultural and Agricultural* (Berkeley, CA: Counterpoint, 2009); Stephen Clark, *How to Think About the Earth: Philosophical and Theological Models for Ecology* (New York: Mowbray, 1993); Jeanne Kay, "Concepts of Nature in the Hebrew Bible," *Environmental Ethics* 10 (1988): 309–27; Andrew Linzey, *Animal Theology* (Urbana: University of Illinois Press, 1995); Andrew Linzey, *Christianity and the Rights of Animals* (New York: Crossroad, 1987).

29. Matthew Scully, "Factory Farm Meat Not on Menu for Feast of St. Francis," *Dallas Morning News*, October 4, 2004, http://www.animalliberationfront.com/Philosophy/MathewScully/factoryfarm.htm.

30. Francis, "Encyclical Letter Laudato Si' of the Holy Father Francis on Care for Our Common Home," Section III: 116, accessed on December 17, 2015, http://w2.vatican.va/content/francesco/en/encyclicals/documents/papa-francesco_20150524_enciclica-laudato-si.html.

31. Jonathan Swift, *A Modest Proposal and Other Satirical Works* (Mineola, NY: Dover, 1996), 53.

32. Keith Thomas, *Religion and the Decline of Magic: Studies in Popular Beliefs in Sixteenth and Seventeenth Century England* (New York: Oxford University Press, 1997).

33. Edwin A. Burtt, *The Metaphysical Foundations of Modern Science* (Atlantic Highlands, NJ: Humanities Press, 1952). Also see Herbert Butterfield, *The Origins of Modern Science* (New York: Free Press, 1997).

34. Carolyn Merchant, *The Death of Nature* (San Francisco: Harper and Row, 1980).

35. Rene Descartes, *The Philosophical Works of Descartes*, vol. 1, ed. Elizabeth Haldane and George Ross (Cambridge: Cambridge University Press, 1911), 333.

36. Ibid., 116–18.

37. John Cottingham, "A Brute to the Brutes? Descartes' Treatment of Animals," *Philosophy* 53 (1978): 551–59. Also see Peter Harrison, "Descartes on Animals," *Philosophical Quarterly* 42 (1992): 219–27; Janice Thomas, "Does Descartes Deny Consciousness to Animals?" *Ratio* 19 (2006): 336–63.

38. Gary Steiner, "Descartes on the Moral Status of Animals," *Archiv fur Geschichte der Philosophie* 80 (1988): 268–91.

39. Rene Descartes, *Treatise of Man* (Cambridge, MA: Harvard University Press, 1972), vii–ix.

40. Steiner, "Descartes on the Moral Status of Animals," 288.

41. Sylvia Federici, *Caliban and the Witch: Women, the Body, and Primitive Accumulation* (New York: Autonomedia, 2004), 159.

42. Julien Offray de La Mettrie, *Machine Man and Other Writings*, ed. Ann Thomson (Cambridge: Cambridge University Press, 1996).

43. Michel Foucault, *Discipline and Punish: The Birth of the Prison*, trans. Alan Sheridan (New York: Vintage, 1979), 136.

44. David Abram, *The Spell of the Sensuous: Perception and Language in a More Than Human World* (New York: Pantheon, 1996).

45. Donna Haraway, *Simians, Cyborgs, and Women: The Reinvention of Nature* (New York: Routledge, 1991). Also see Glen Mazis, *Humans, Animals, Machines: Blurring Boundaries* (Albany: State University of New York Press, 2008).

46. Temple Grandin and Catherine Johnson, *Animals Make Us Human: Creating the Best Life for Animals* (Boston: Houghton Mifflin Harcourt, 2009).

Chapter Ten

1. Michelle Alexander, *The New Jim Crow: Mass Incarceration in the Age of Colorblindness* (New York: New Press, 2012).

2. Eric Schlosser, "The Prison-Industrial Complex," *Atlantic Monthly*, December 1998, 51–77.

3. Lauren Glaze and Danielle Kaeble, *Correctional Populations in the United States, 2013* (Washington, DC: U.S. Bureau of Justice Statistics, December 2014), http://www.bjs.gov/content/pub/pdf/cpus13.pdf.

4. *The Punishing Decade: Prison and Jail Estimates at the Millennium* (Washington, DC: Justice Policy Institute, May 2000), http://www.cjcj.org/index.html.

5. Federal Bureau of Investigation, "Uniform Crime Reporting Statistics," accessed June 18, 2015, http://www.bjs.gov/ucrdata/Search/Crime/State/RunCrimeStatebyState.cfm.

6. Glaze and Kaeble, *Correctional Populations*.

7. Michelle Ye Hee Lee, "Does the United States Really Have 5 Percent of the World's Population and One Quarter of the World's Prisoners?" *Washington Post*, April 30, 2015, accessed June 18, 2015, http://www.washingtonpost.com/blogs/fact-checker/wp/2015/04/30/does-the-united-states-really-have-five-percent-of-worlds-population-and-one-quarter-of-the-worlds-prisoners/.

8. Schlosser, "Prison-Industrial Complex," 51–77.

9. Lee, "Does the United States."

10. Rebecca Vallas and Sharon Dietrich, *One Strike and You're Out* (Washington, DC: Center for American Progress, December 2014), https://cdn.americanprogress.org/wp-content/uploads/2014/12/VallasCriminalRecordsReport.pdf.

11. "Fact Sheet: Trends in U.S. Corrections," The Sentencing Project, accessed June 18, 2015, http://sentencingproject.org/doc/publications/inc_Trends_in_Corrections_Fact_sheet.pdf.

12. Vallas and Dietrich, *One Strike*.

13. Jeffrey Toobin, "The Milwaukee Experiment," *New Yorker*, May 11, 2015, 24–32.

14. Drew Leder et al., *The Soul Knows No Bars: Inmates Reflect on Life, Death, and Hope* (Lanham, MD: Rowman and Littlefield, 2000).

15. Michel Foucault, *Discipline and Punish: The Birth of the Prison*, trans. Alan Sheridan (New York: Vintage, 1979), 135–28.

16. Isabel Dyck et al., "The Home as a Site for Long-Term Care: Meanings and Management of Bodies and Spaces," *Health & Place* 11, no. 2 (2005): 173–85.

17. Ibid., 176.

18. Fredrik Svenaeus, "What Is Phenomenology of Medicine? Embodiment, Illness and Being-in-the-World," in *Health, Illness and Disease*, ed. Havi Carel and Rachel Cooper (Durham, UK: Acumen, 2013), 103–4. Also see his *The Hermeneutics of Medicine and the Phenomenology of Health: Steps Towards a Philosophy of Medical Practice*, 2nd rev. ed. (Dordrecht: Kluwer Academic, 2001).

19. Havi Carel, *Illness: The Cry of the Flesh* (Stocksfield, UK: Acumen, 2008), 129.

20. Edmund Husserl, *The Phenomenology of Internal Time-Consciousness*, ed. Martin Heidegger, trans. James S. Churchill (Bloomington: Indiana University Press, 1964).

21. Martin Heidegger, *Being and Time*, trans. John Macquarrie and Edward Robinson (New York: Harper and Row, 1962).

22. Ibid., 378.

23. Eugene Minkowski, *Lived Time: Phenomenological Psychopathological Studies*, trans. N. Metzel (Evanston, IL: Northwestern University Press, 1970), 83.

24. Ibid., 87.

25. Ibid., 89.

26. Ibid., 87.

27. Leder et al., *Soul Knows No Bars*, 86.

28. Heidegger, *Being and Time*, 377.

29. Leder et al., *Soul Knows No Bars*, 86.

30. Heidegger, *Being and Time*, 138–48.

31. Edward S. Casey, *Getting Back into Place; Toward a Renewed Understanding of the Place-World* (Bloomington: Indiana University Press, 1993).

32. O. F. Bollnow, "Lived-Space," *Philosophy Today* 5 (1961): 31–39.

33. Leder et al., *Soul Knows No Bars*, 57–58.

34. Ibid., 56.

35. Ibid., 75–76.

36. Arlando ("Tray") Jones, *Eager Street: A Life on the Corner and Behind Bars* (Baltimore: Apprentice House, 2010).

37. Maurice Merleau-Ponty, *Phenomenology of Perception*, trans. Colin Smith (London: Routledge and Kegan Paul, 1962), 146.

38. Maurice Merleau-Ponty, *The Visible and the Invisible*, ed. Claude Lefort, trans. Alphonso Lingis (Evanston, IL: Northwestern University Press, 1968), 123–24, 130–55.

39. Drew Leder, *The Absent Body* (Chicago: University of Chicago Press, 1990), 70–83.

40. Oliver Sacks, *A Leg to Stand On* (New York: HarperCollins, 1994), 27.

41. Simone de Beauvoir, *The Second Sex*, trans. H. M. Parshley (New York: Vintage, 1974).

42. Marilyn Frye, *Politics of Reality: Essays in Feminist Theory* (Trumansburg, NY: Crossing Press Feminist, 1983), 1–16.

43. Merleau-Ponty, *Phenomenology of Perception*, 137.

44. Iris Marion Young, *On Female Body Experience: Throwing Like a Girl and Other Essays* (Oxford: Oxford University Press, 2005).

45. Kristin Zeiler, "A Phenomenology of Excorporation, Bodily Alienation and Resistance: Rethinking Sexed and Racialized Embodiment," *Hypatia* 28, no. 1 (2013): 69–84.

46. Frantz Fanon, *Black Skin, White Masks*, trans. Richard Philcox (New York: Grove Press, 1967), 111–13. For valuable references, also see Lewis R. Gordon, ed., *Existence in Black: An Anthology of Black Existential Philosophy* (New York: Routledge, 1997).

47. Leder et al., *Soul Knows No Bars*, 56.

48. Merleau-Ponty, *Visible and the Invisible*, 143.

49. Foucault, *Discipline and Punish*, 195–228.

50. Leder et al., *Soul Knows No Bars*, 44–45.

51. Leder, *Absent Body*, 108–25.

52. Lisa Guenther, *Solitary Confinement: Social Death and Its Afterlives* (Minneapolis: University of Minnesota Press, 2013), 3–22.

53. Ibid, 20.

54. Ibid.

55. Christia Mercer, "I Teach Philosophy at Columbia. But Some of My Best Students Are Inmates," *Washington Post*, March 24, 2015, accessed on June 4, 2015, http://www.washington post.com/posteverything/wp/2015/03/24/i-teach-philosophy-at-columbia-but-the-best-students-i-have-are-inmates/.

56. Lois M. Davis et al., *Evaluating the Effectiveness of Correctional Education: A Meta-Analysis of Programs That Provide Education to Incarcerated Adults* (Santa Monica: RAND, 2013), http://www.rand.org/pubs/research_reports/RR266.

Chapter Eleven

1. Drew Leder et al., *The Soul Knows No Bars: Inmates Reflect on Life, Death and Hope* (Lanham, MD: Rowman and Littlefield, 2000).

2. Jessica Benko, "The Radical Humaneness of Norway's Halden Prison," *New York Times*, March 26, 2015.

3. Doran Larson, "Why Scandinavian Prisons Are Superior," *Atlantic*, September 24, 2013, http://www.theatlantic.com/international/archive/2013/09/why-scandinavian-prisons-are-superior /279949/.

4. Dan Rodricks, "Glendening: 'Life Means Life' Absolutism Was Wrong," *Baltimore Sun*, February 20, 2011.

5. Jean-Paul Sartre, *No Exit and Three Other Plays* (New York: Vintage International, 1989), 45.

6. Benko, "Radical Humaneness."

7. Jorge Luis Borges, *Ficciones*, ed. Anthony Kerrigan (New York: Grove Press, 1994), 43.

Chapter Twelve

1. James C. Howell, *Preventing and Reducing Juvenile Delinquency: A Comprehensive Framework*, 2nd ed. (Thousand Oaks, CA: Sage, 2009), 3–16.

2. Jim Mason, *An Unnatural Order: Uncovering the Roots of Our Domination of Nature and Each Other* (New York: Simon and Schuster, 1993), 163.

3. Charles Patterson, *Eternal Treblinka: Our Treatment of Animals and the Holocaust* (New York: Lantern, 2002), 27–50.

4. Michelle Alexander, *The New Jim Crow: Mass Incarceration in the Age of Colorblindness* (New York: New Press, 2010).

5. Helen Taylor Greene and Shaun L. Gabbidon, *Encyclopedia of Race and Crime* (Thousand Oaks, CA: Sage, 2009). Also see Shaun L. Gabbidon, *Criminological Perspectives on Race and Crime* (New York: Routledge, 2007), 109–40.

6. John Sloop, *The Cultural Prison: Discourse, Prisoners, and Punishment* (Tuscaloosa: University of Alabama Press, 1996), 130.

7. Cassandra Shaylor, "'It's Like Living in a Black Hole': Women of Color and Solitary Confinement in the Prison Industrial Complex," *New England Journal on Criminal and Civil Confinement* 24 (Summer 1998): 395–96.

8. Michel Foucault, *Discipline and Punish: Birth of the Prison*, trans. Alan Sheridan (New York: Vintage, 1979), 138.

9. Matthew Cole, "'Animal Machines' to 'Happy Meat'? Foucault's Ideas of Disciplinary and Pastoral Power Applied to 'Animal-Centered' Welfare Discourse," *Animals* 1 (2011): 86.

10. Peter Singer, *Animal Liberation* (New York: HarperCollins, 1975; New York: Harper Perennial, 2001). Also see David Kirby, *Animal Factory: The Looming Threat of Industrial Pig, Dairy, and Poultry Farms to Humans and the Environment* (New York: St. Martin's Press, 2010); Drew Leder, "Old McDonald Had a Farm: The Metaphysics of Factory Farming," *Journal of Animal Ethics* 2, no. 1 (2012): 73–86; Peter Singer, *In Defense of Animals: The Second Wave* (Malden, MA: Blackwell, 2006).

11. *Brown v. Plata*, 131 S. Ct. 1910 (2011).

12. Adam Liptak, "Justices, 5–4, Tell California to Cut Prisoner Population," *New York Times*, May 24, 2011.

13. Jim Mason and Mary Finelli, "Brave New Farm," in *In Defense of Animals: The Second Wave*, ed. Peter Singer (Malden, MA: Blackwell 2006): 104–22.

14. Eric Schlosser, "The Prison Industrial Complex," *Atlantic Monthly*, December 1998, 51–77.

15. George Will, "When Solitude Is Torture," *Washington Post*, February 20, 2013. Also see Lisa Guenther, *Solitary Confinement: Social Death and Its Afterlives* (Minneapolis: University of Minnesota Press, 2013).

16. Peter Singer, *Practical Ethics*, 2nd ed. (Cambridge: Cambridge University Press, 1993), 59–61.

17. Drew Leder et al., *The Soul Knows No Bars: Inmates Reflect on Life, Death, and Hope* (Rowman and Littlefield, 2000), 7.

18. Lisa Guenther, "Beyond Dehumanization: A Post-Humanist Critique of Intensive Confinement," *Journal for Critical Animal Studies* 10, no. 2 (2012): 56.

19. JCI inmate, in our class discussion.

20. Guenther, "Beyond Dehumanization," 56.

21. Alan Mobley, "Killing Time on the Prairie," *Journal for Critical Animal Studies* 10, no. 2 (2012): 115.

22. Gennifer Furst, "Prison-Based Animal Programs: A National Survey," *Prison Journal* 86, no. 4 (2006): 407–30.

23. Janet Lai, "Pet Facilitated Therapy in Correctional Institutions," Office of the Deputy Commissioner for Women, Correctional Service of Canada, April 1998, accessed May 28, 2013,

www.csc-scc.gc.ca/text/prgnn/fsw/pet/pet-eng.shtml. Also see Kirk Johnson, "Raising Frogs for Freedom, Prison Project Opens Doors," *New York Times*, September 28, 2012.

24. Furst, "Prison-Based Animal Programs," 420.

25. Vincent Greco, "Canine Partners for Life Graduation Ceremony," *Jessup Correctional Institution Outback Observer* 2, no. 11 (2012).

26. Furst, "Prison-Based Animal Programs," 422−23.

27. Todd Harkrader et al., "Pound Puppies: The Rehabilitative Uses of Dogs in Correctional Facilities," *Corrections Today* 66, no. 2 (2004): 74−79.

28. Lai, "Pet Facilitated Therapy."

29. Harkrader et al., "Pound Puppies," 74−79.

30. Ibid.

31. David Abram, "Animation, Animals, and Animism," *Parabola* 8, no. 1 (1983): 92−96. Also see David Abram, *The Spell of the Sensuous: Perception and Language in a More Than Human World* (New York: Pantheon, 1996); David Abram, *Becoming Animal: An Earthly Cosmology* (New York: Pantheon, 2010); Ralph R. Acampora, *Corporal Compassion: Animal Ethics and Philosophy of Body* (Pittsburgh: University of Pittsburgh Press, 2006); Drew Leder, "Embodying Otherness: Shape-shifting and the Natural World," *Environmental Philosophy* 9, no. 2 (2012): 123−41.

32. Georg Feuerstein, *The Shambhala Encyclopedia of Yoga* (Boston: Shambhala, 1997), 115−16. Also see Swami Muktananda, *I Am That: The Science of Hamsa from the Vijnana Bhairava* (South Fallsburg, NY: Siddha Yoga, 1992).

33. Anthony J. Nocella II, "Animal Advocates for Prison and Slave Abolition: A Transformative Justice Approach to Movement Politics for an End to Racism," *Journal for Critical Animal Studies* 10, no. 2 (2012): 121.

Chapter Thirteen

1. David Abram, *The Spell of the Sensuous: Perception and Language in a More-Than-Human World* (New York: Pantheon, 1996).

2. Arne Naess, "Notes on the Politics of the Deep Ecology Movement," *Sustaining Gaia: Contributions to Another World View. Papers from the Environment, Ethics, and Ecology II Conference* (Clayton, Australia: Graduate School of Environmental Science, Monash University, 1984), 180.

3. David Abram, "Animation, Animals, and Animism," *Parabola* 8, no. 1 (1983): 92−96.

4. Eva Marie Simms, "Milk and Flesh: A Phenomenological Reflection on Infancy and Coexistence," *Journal of Phenomenological Psychology* 32, no. 1 (2001): 25.

5. Jean-Marie Chauvet et al., *Dawn of Art: The Chauvet Cave* (New York: Harry N. Abrams, 1996).

6. Richard Schechner, *Performance Studies: An Introduction* (New York: Routledge, 2002), 221−25.

7. Jim Mason, *An Unnatural Order: Uncovering the Roots of Our Domination of Nature and Each Other* (New York: Simon and Schuster, 1993), 108−9.

8. Robert Lawlor, *Voices of the First Day: Awakening in the Aboriginal Dreamtime* (Rochester, VT: Inner Traditions, 1991), 302−3.

9. Hans Peter Duerr, *Dreamtime: Concerning the Boundary Between Wilderness and Culture* (Oxford: Basil Blackwell, 1985). Also see Abram, *Spell of the Sensuous*; David Abram, *Becoming Animal: An Earthly Cosmology* (New York: Pantheon, 2010), 244.

10. Abram, *Becoming Animal*, 244–45.

11. Ibid., 238–39.

12. Mark Griffith, "Slaves of Dionysos: Satyrs, Audience, and the Ends of the Oresteia," *Classical Antiquity* 21, no. 2 (2002): 195–258.

13. Georg Feuerstein, *The Shambhala Encyclopedia of Yoga* (Boston: Shambhala, 1997), 114–15, 261. Also see Vanamali, *Shakti: Realm of the Divine Mother* (Rochester, VT: Inner Traditions, 2006), 207–15.

14. Philip Lutgendorf, "My Hanuman Is Bigger Than Yours," *History of Religions* 33, no. 3 (1994): 211–45.

15. Drew Leder, *Sparks of the Divine* (Notre Dame: Sorin, 2004).

16. Swami Nikilananda, *The Upanishads* (New York: Harper Torchbooks, 1963), 114.

17. Feuerstein, *Shambhala Encyclopedia*, 110, 126.

18. Leder, *Sparks of the Divine*, 58–60.

19. Feuerstein, *Shambhala Encyclopedia*, 115–16. Also see Swami Muktananda, *I Am That: The Science of Hamsa from the Vijnana Bhairava* (South Fallsburg, NY: Siddha Yoga, 1992).

20. Roger Jahnke, *The Healing Promise of Qi: Creating Extraordinary Wellness Through Qigong and Tai Chi* (New York: McGraw-Hill, 2002).

21. Douglas Wile, *Lost T'ai-chi Classics from the Late Ch'ing Dynasty* (Albany: State University of New York Press, 1996), 52–53.

22. Narada Mahathera, *The Buddha and His Teachings* (Mumbai: Jaico, 2006), 32–33.

23. Michael Marder, *Plant-thinking: A Philosophy of Vegetal Life* (New York: Columbia University Press, 2013), 12.

24. Ibid., 73–74.

25. Una Chaudhuri, "(De)Facing the Animals: Zooësis and Performance," *Drama Review* 51, no. 1 (2007): 8–20.

26. Schechner, *Performance Studies*, 2.

27. Drew Leder, *The Absent Body* (Chicago: University of Chicago Press, 1990), 36–68.

28. Wang Yang-ming, *Instructions for Practical Living and Other Neo-Confucian Writings* (New York: Columbia University Press, 1963), 222.

29. Edward O. Wilson, "Biophilia and the Conservation Ethic," in *The Biophilia Hypothesis*, ed. Stephen R. Kellert and Edward O. Wilson (Washington, DC: Island Press, 1993), 31–41.

30. Roger Ulrich, "Biophilia, Biophobia, and Natural Landscapes," in *The Biophilia Hypothesis*, ed. Stephen R. Kellert and Edward O. Wilson (Washington, DC: Island Press, 1993), 73–137.

31. Aristotle, "De Anima," in *The Basic Works of Aristotle*, ed. Richard McKeon (New York: Random House, 1941), 535–603.

32. Simms, "Milk and Flesh," 25.

33. Thomas Nagel, "What Is It Like to Be a Bat?" *Philosophical Review* 83, no. 4 (1974): 435–50.

34. Abram, *Becoming Animal*. Also see Ralph R. Acampora, *Corporal Compassion: Animal Ethics and Philosophy of Body* (Pittsburgh: University of Pittsburgh Press, 2006), 86; Jacques Derrida, *The Animal That Therefore I Am*, trans. David Wills, ed. Marie-Louise Mallet (New York: Fordham University Press, 2008), 14; Glen Mazis, *Humans, Animals, Machines: Blurring Boundaries* (Albany: State University of New York Press, 2008).

35. Temple Grandin and Catherine Johnson, *Animals in Translation: Using the Mysteries of Autism to Decode Animal Behavior* (New York: Harcourt, 2006).

36. Ibid., 303–6.

37. Acampora, *Corporal Compassion*, 86.

38. Alexandra Horowitz, *Inside of a Dog: What Dogs See, Smell, and Know* (New York: Scribner, 2010). Also see Clinton Sanders, *Understanding Dogs: Living and Working with Canine Companions* (Philadelphia: Temple University Press, 1999).

39. Erwin Straus, *The Primary World of Senses: A Vindication of Sensory Experience* (New York: Free Press of Glencoe, 1963).

40. Maurice Merleau-Ponty, *Phenomenology of Perception*, trans. Colin Smith (London: Routledge and Kegan Paul, 1962).

41. Ibid., 354.

42. Derrida, *Animal That Therefore I Am*, 14.

43. Maurice Merleau-Ponty, "Husserl at the Limits of Phenomenology," in *Praise of Philosophy and Other Essays*, trans. John Wild and James Edie (Evanston, IL: Northwestern University, 1988), 190.

44. Acampora, *Corporal Compassion*, 86.

45. Abram, *Becoming Animal*, 254.

46. Mason, *Unnatural Order*, 163.

47. Carolyn Merchant, *The Death of Nature* (San Francisco: Harper and Row, 1980). Also see Edwin A. Burtt, *The Metaphysical Foundations of Modern Science* (Atlantic Highlands, NJ: Humanities Press, 1952); Keith Thomas, *Religion and the Decline of Magic: Studies in Popular Beliefs in Sixteenth and Seventeenth Century England* (New York: Oxford University Press, 1997).

48. Abram, *Spell of the Sensuous*, 25.

49. John Berger, *About Looking* (New York: Vintage, 1991), 3-28.

50. Donna Haraway, *Simians, Cyborgs, and Women: The Reinvention of Nature* (New York: Routledge, 1991).

51. Mazis, *Humans, Animals, Machines*, 58-75.

52. Edward O. Wilson, *Biophilia* (Cambridge, MA: Harvard University Press, 1984), 116.

Bibliography

Abram, David. "Animation, Animals, and Animism." *Parabola* 8, no. 1 (1983): 92–96.
———. *Becoming Animal: An Earthly Cosmology.* New York: Pantheon Books, 2010.
———. "The Ecology of Magic." *Orion* 10, no. 3 (1991): 37.
———. *The Spell of the Sensuous: Perception and Language in a More Than Human World.* New York: Pantheon Books, 1996.
Acampora, Ralph. *Corporal Compassion: Animal Ethics and Philosophy of Body.* Pittsburgh: University of Pittsburgh Press, 2006.
Achterberg, Jeanne, Barbara Dossey, and Leslie Kolkmeier. *Rituals of Healing: Using Imagery for Health and Wellness.* New York: Bantam, 1994.
Agich, George. *Autonomy and Long-Term Care.* New York: Oxford University Press, 1993.
Alderman, Harold. "By Virtue of a Virtue." *Review of Metaphysics* 36 (September 1982): 127–53.
Alexander, Michelle. *The New Jim Crow: Mass Incarceration in the Age of Colorblindness.* New York: New Press, 2012.
American Association of Diabetes. "Statistics about Diabetes." *National Diabetes Statistics Report,* June 10, 2014. http://www.diabetes.org/diabetes-basics/statistics/?loc=db-slabnav.
Aquinas, St. Thomas. *On the Truth of the Catholic Faith (Summa Contra Gentiles).* Bk. 3, *Providence,* pt. 2, translated by Vernon J. Bourke, 84–163. New York: Image, 1956.
Aristotle, "De Anima." In *The Basic Works of Aristotle,* edited by Richard McKeon, 535–603. New York: Random House, 1941.
Austin, Richard. *Hope for the Land: Nature in the Bible.* Atlanta: John Knox Press, 1988.
Bailey, Ronald. "Should I Be Allowed to Buy Your Kidney?" *Forbes,* May 28, 1990.
Bakan, David. *Disease, Pain, and Sacrifice.* Chicago: University of Chicago Press, 1968.
Barboza, David. "Animal Welfare's Unexpected Allies." *New York Times,* June 25, 2003.
Baron, Richard. "An Introduction to Medical Phenomenology: 'I Can't Hear You While I'm Listening.'" *Annals of Internal Medicine* 103, no. 4 (1985): 606–11.
Barry, John. "Marxism and Ecology." In *Marxism and Social Science,* edited by Andrew Gamble, David Marsh, and Tony Tant, 259–79. Urbana: University of Illinois Press, 1999.
Benko, Jessica. "The Radical Humaneness of Norway's Halden Prison." *New York Times,* March 26, 2015.
Benner, Patricia, Molly Sutphen, Victoria Leonard, and Lisa Day. *Educating Nurses: A Call for Radical Transformation.* San Francisco: Jossey-Bass, 2010.

Bentley, T. Scott. "U.S. Organ and Tissue Transplant Cost Estimates and Discussion." *Milliman Research Report*, December 2014. http://www.milliman.com/uploadedFiles/insight/Research /health-rr/1938HDP_20141230.pdf.

Benton, Ted, ed. *The Greening of Marxism*. New York: Guilford Press, 1996.

———. "Humanism Equals Speciesism: Marx on Humans and Animals." *Radical Philosophy* 50 (1998): 4–18.

Berger, John. *About Looking*. New York: Vintage, 1991.

Bernstein, Richard. *Beyond Objectivism and Relativism: Science, Hermeneutics, and Praxis*. Philadelphia: University of Pennsylvania Press, 1983.

Berry, Wendell. *The Gift of Good Land: Further Essays Cultural and Agricultural*. Berkeley, CA: Counterpoint, 2009.

Biss, Eula. *On Immunity: An Inoculation*. Minneapolis: Graywolf Press, 2014.

Blair, Elizabeth. "In Ancient Dramas, Vital Words for Today's Warriors." *NPR*, November 25, 2008. http://www.npr.org/templates/story/story.php?storyId=97413320.

Bollnow, O. F. "Lived-Space." *Philosophy Today* 5 (1961): 31–39.

Borell, Merriley. "Training the Senses, Training the Mind." In *Medicine and the Five Senses*, edited by W. F. Bynum and Porter Roy, 244–61. Cambridge: Cambridge University Press, 1993.

Borges, Jorge Luis. *Ficciones*. Edited by Anthony Kerrigan. New York: Grove Press, 1994.

Borgmann, Albert. *Technology and the Character of Contemporary Life: A Philosophical Inquiry*. Chicago: University of Chicago Press, 1984.

Bostwick, J. Michael, and Christopher Sola. "An Updated Review of Implantable Cardioverter/ Defibrillators, Induced Anxiety, and Quality of Life." *Psychiatric Clinics North America* 30, no. 4 (2007): 677–88.

Brand, Paul, and Philip Yancey. *Pain: The Gift Nobody Wants*. Darby, CT: Diane, 1999.

Bristow, Janet, and Victoria Cole-Galo. *The Prayer Shawl Companion: 38 Knitted Designs to Embrace, Inspire, and Celebrate Life*. Newtown, CT: Taunton Press, 2008.

Brody, Howard. *Hooked: Ethics, the Medical Profession, and the Pharmaceutical Industry*. Lanham, MD: Rowman and Littlefield, 2007.

———. *Stories of Sickness*. New Haven, CT: Yale University Press, 1987.

Brody, Howard, and Daralyn Brody. *The Placebo Response: How You Can Release the Body's Inner Pharmacy for Better Health*. New York: HarperCollins, 2000.

Brogan, Walter. "Plato's Pharmakon: Between Two Repetitions." In *Derrida and Deconstruction*, edited by Hugh Silverman, 8. New York: Routledge, 1989.

Brough, John B. "Temporality and Illness: A Phenomenological Perspective." In *Handbook of Phenomenology and Medicine*, edited by S. Kay Toombs, 29–46. Dordrecht: Kluwer Academic, 2001.

Brown, E. Richard. *Rockefeller Medicine Men: Medicine and Capitalism in America*. Berkeley: University of California Press, 1979.

Broyard, Anatole. *Intoxicated by My Illness and Other Writings on Life and Death*. New York: Fawcett Columbine, 1992.

Buber, Martin. *I and Thou*. New York: Free Press, 1971.

Burtt, Edwin A. *The Metaphysical Foundations of Modern Science*. Atlantic Highlands, NJ: Humanities Press, 1952.

Butterfield, Herbert. *The Origins of Modern Science*. New York: Free Press, 1997.

Buytendijk, Frederik J. J. *Pain*. Translated by Eda O'Shiel. Westport, CT: Greenwood Press, 1961.

Callahan, Sidney, and Daniel Callahan. "Breaking Through Stereotypes." *Commonweal* 111, no. 017 (1984): 520–23.

Caplan, Arthur. *If I Were a Rich Man Could I Buy a Pancreas? And Other Essays on the Ethics of Health Care.* Bloomington: Indiana University Press, 1992.

Carel, Havi. *Illness: The Cry of the Flesh.* Stocksfield, UK: Acumen Press, 2008.

Casado da Rocha, Antonio, and Arantza Etxeberria. "Towards Autonomy-within-Illness: Applying the Triadic Approach to the Principles of Bioethics." In *Health, Illness and Disease: Philosophical Essays*, edited by Havi Carel and Rachel Cooper, 70. Durham, UK: Acumen Press, 2013.

Casey, Edward S. *Getting Back Into Place; Toward a Renewed Understanding of the Place-World.* Bloomington: Indiana University Press, 1993.

Cassell, Eric J. *The Healer's Art: A New Approach to the Doctor-Patient Relationship.* Cambridge, MA: MIT Press, 1985.

———. *The Nature of Suffering and the Goals of Medicine.* New York: Oxford University Press, 1991.

———. "The Phenomenon of Suffering and Its Relationship to Pain." In *Handbook of Phenomenology and Medicine*, edited by S. Kay Toombs, 371–90. Dordrecht: Kluwer Academic, 2001.

Charon, Rita. "Narrative Medicine: A Model for Empathy, Reflection, Profession, and Trust." *Journal of the American Medical Society* 286, no. 15 (2001): 1898.

———. *Narrative Medicine: Honoring the Stories of Illness.* New York: Oxford University Press, 2008.

Chaudhuri, Una. "(De)Facing the Animals: Zooësis and Performance." *Drama Review* 51, no. 1 (2007): 8–20.

Chauvet, Jean-Marie, Eliette Dechamps, and Christian Hillaire. *Dawn of Art: The Chauvet Cave.* New York: Harry N. Abrams, 1996.

Cherry, Mark. *Kidney for Sale by Owner: Human Organs, Transplantation, and the Market.* Washington, DC: Georgetown University Press, 2005.

Clark, Stephen. *How to Think About the Earth: Philosophical and Theological Models for Ecology.* New York: Mowbray, 1993.

Classen, Constance, ed. *The Book of Touch.* Oxford: Berg, 2005.

Cole, Matthew. "'Animal Machines' to 'Happy Meat'? Foucault's Ideas of Disciplinary and Pastoral Power Applied to 'Animal-Centered' Welfare Discourse." *Animals* 1 (2011): 86.

Conrad, Peter. "The Social Meaning of AIDS." *Social Policy* 17 (Summer 1986): 51–56.

Conrad, Peter, and Valerie Leiter. "From Lydia Pinkham to Queen Levitra: Direct-to-Consumer Advertising and Medicalization." In *Pharmaceuticals and Society: Critical Discourses and Debates*, edited by Simon Williams, Jonathan Gabe, and Peter Davis, 22. Oxford: Wiley-Blackwell, 2009.

Cottingham, John. "A Brute to the Brutes? Descartes' Treatment of Animals." *Philosophy* 53 (1978): 551–59.

Couceiro-Bueno, J. C. "The Phenomenology of Pain: An Experience of Life." In *Phenomenology and Existentialism in the Twentieth Century*, edited by Anna-Teresa Tymieniecka, 295–307. Dordrecht: Springer, 2009.

Csordas, Thomas, *Body/Meaning/Healing.* New York: Palgrave Macmillan, 2002.

———. ed., *Embodiment and Experience: The Existential Ground of Culture and Self.* Cambridge: Cambridge University Press, 1994.

Daniel, Stephen L. "The Patient as Text: A Model of Clinical Hermeneutics." *Theoretical Medicine* 7 (1986): 195–210.

Daudet, Alphonse. *In the Land of Pain*. Edited and translated by Julian Barnes. New York: Alfred A. Knopf, 2002.

Davis, Lois M., Robert Bozick, Jennifer L. Steele, Jessica Saunders, and Jeremy N. V. Miles. *Evaluating the Effectiveness of Correctional Education: A Meta-Analysis of Programs That Provide Education to Incarcerated Adults*. Santa Monica: RAND, 2013. http://www.rand.org/pubs /research_reports/RR266.

de Beauvoir, Simone. *The Second Sex*. Translated by H. M. Parshley. New York: Vintage, 1974.

de La Mettrie, Julien Offray. *Machine Man and Other Writings*. Edited by Ann Thomson. Cambridge: Cambridge University Press, 1996.

de Quincey, Christian, *Radical Nature: The Soul of Matter*. Rochester, VT: Park Street Press, 2002.

Derrida, Jacques. *The Animal That Therefore I Am*. Translated by David Wills. Edited by Marie-Louise Mallet. New York: Fordham University Press, 2008.

———. *Dissemination*. Translated by Barbara Johnson. Chicago: University of Chicago Press, 1981.

Descartes, Rene. "Discourse on the Method of Rightly Conducting the Reason." In *The Philosophical Works of Descartes*, vol. 1, edited by Elizabeth Haldane and George R. T. Ross, 119–333. Cambridge: Cambridge University Press, 1911.

———. *The Philosophical Writings of Descartes*, vol. 2. Translated by John Cottingham, Robert Stoothoff, and Dugald Murdoch. Cambridge: Cambridge University Press, 1984.

———. *Treatise of Man*. Edited and translated by Thomas Steele Hall. Cambridge, MA: Harvard University Press, 1972.

Dickinson, Emily. *The Complete Poems of Emily Dickinson*. Edited by Thomas H. Johnson. Boston: Little, Brown, 1960.

Diedrich, Lisa. "Breaking Down: A Phenomenology of Disability." *Literature and Medicine* 20, no. 2 (2001): 209–30.

Dilthey, Wilhelm. *Selected Works*. Translated and edited by H. P. Rickman. Cambridge: Cambridge University Press, 1976.

Dossey, Larry. " 'Eating Papers' and Other Curious Aspects of Nutrition." *Alternative Therapies in Health and Medicine* 4, no. 6 (1998): 11–16, 99–104.

Dowie, Mark. "Transplant Fever." *Mother Jones* 14, no. 3 (1989): 19–20.

———. *We Have a Donor: The Bold New World of Organ Transplanting*. New York: St. Martin's Press, 1988.

Duerr, Hans Peter. *Dreamtime: Concerning the Boundary Between Wilderness and Culture*. Oxford: Basil Blackwell, 1985.

Dupre, Louis. *Symbols of the Sacred*. Grand Rapids, MI: William B. Eerdmans, 2000.

Dutchen, Stephanie. "A Drug by Any Other Name." *Scope*, January 5, 2009. http://scopeweb.mit .edu/articles/a-drug-by-any-other-name/.

Dyck, Isabel. "Hidden Geographies: The Changing Lifeworlds of Women with Multiple Sclerosis." *Social Science and Medicine* 40, no. 3 (1995): 307–20.

Dyck, Isabel, Pia Kontos, Jan Angus, and Patricia McKeever. "The Home as a Site for Long-term Care: Meanings and Management of Bodies and Spaces," *Health & Place* 11, no. 2 (2005): 173–85.

Eimer, Bruce, M. *Hypnotize Yourself Out of Pain Now!* 2nd ed. Bethel, CT: Crown House, 2008.

Engelhardt, H. Tristram, Jr. "The Body for Fun, Beneficence, and Profit: A Variation on a Post-modern Theme." In *Persons and Their Bodies: Rights, Responsibilities, Relationships*, edited by Mark Cherry, 277–301. Dordrecht: Kluwer Academic, 1999.

———. *The Foundations of Bioethics*. New York: Oxford University Press, 1986.

———. "Human Well-being and Medicine: Some Basic Value-Judgments in the Biomedical Sciences." In *Science, Ethics and Medicine*, edited by H. Tristram Engelhardt Jr. and Daniel Callahan, 120–39. Hastings-on-the-Hudson: The Hastings Center Institute of Society, Ethics and the Life Sciences, 1976.

———. "Illnesses, Diseases, and Sicknesses." In *The Humanity of the Ill: Phenomenological Perspectives*, edited by Victor Kestenbaum, 142–56. Knoxville: University of Tennessee Press, 1982.

Epictetus. *Handbook of Epictetus*. Translated by Nicholas White. Indianapolis: Hackett, 1983.

Evans, Dylan. *Placebo: Mind over Matter in Modern Medicine*. New York: Oxford University Press, 2004.

Fadiman, Anne. *The Spirit Catches You and You Fall Down: A Hmong Child, Her American Doctors, and the Collision of Two Cultures*. New York: Farrar, Straus and Giroux, 1997.

Fanon, Frantz. *Black Skin, White Masks*. Translated by Richard Philcox. New York: Grove Press, 1967.

Federal Bureau of Investigation. "Uniform Crime Reporting Statistics." Accessed June 18, 2015. http://www.bjs.gov/ucrdata/Search/Crime/State/RunCrimeStatebyState.cfm.

Federici, Sylvia. *Caliban and the Witch: Women, the Body, and Primitive Accumulation*. New York: Autonomedia, 2004.

Feldman, Ruth, and Arthur Eidelman. "Skin-to-Skin Contact (Kangaroo Care) Accelerates Autonomic and Neurobehavioural Maturation in Preterm Infants." *Developmental Medicine & Child Neurology* 45 (2003): 274–81.

Feuerstein, Georg. *The Shambhala Encyclopedia of Yoga*. Boston: Shambhala, 1997.

Feyerabend, Paul. *Against Method*. London: Verso, 1975.

Field, Tiffany. "Massage Therapy Facilitates Weight Gain in Preterm Infants." *Current Directions in Psychological Science* 10 (2001): 51–54.

Field, Tiffany, Maria Hernandez-Reif, and Miguel Diego. "Massage Therapy by Parents Improves Early Growth and Development." *Infant Behavior and Development* 27, no. 4 (2004): 435–42.

Figes, Orlando. *Natasha's Dance: A Cultural History of Russia*. New York: Picador, 2002.

Foucault, Michel. *The Birth of the Clinic*. Translated by Alan M. Sheridan Smith. New York: Vintage. 1973.

———. *Discipline and Punish: The Birth of the Prison*. Translated by Alan Sheridan. New York: Vintage, 1979.

———. *The History of Sexuality*. Vol. 1, *An Introduction*. Translated by Robert Hurley. New York: Vintage, 1980.

———. *Madness and Civilization: A History of Insanity in the Age of Reason*. Translation by Richard Howard. New York: Vintage, 1973.

Fox, Nick, and Katie Ward. "Pharma in the Bedroom . . . and the Kitchen . . . the Pharmaceuticalization of Daily Life." In *Pharmaceuticals and Society: Critical Discourses and Debates*, edited by Simon Williams, Jonathan Gabe, and Peter Davis, 42. Oxford: Wiley-Blackwell, 2009.

Fox, Renée, and Judith Swazey. *Spare Parts: Organ Replacement in American Society*. New York: Oxford University Press, 1992.

Francis. "Encyclical Letter Laudato Si' of the Holy Father Francis on Care for Our Common Home," sec. 3, 116. Accessed December 17, 2015. http://w2.vatican.va/content/francesco/en /encyclicals/documents/papa-francesco_20150524_enciclica-laudato-si.html.

Frank, Arthur, W. *At the Will of the Body: Reflections on Illness*. Boston: Houghton Mifflin, 1991.

———. *The Wounded Storyteller: Body, Illness, and Ethics*. Chicago: University of Chicago Press, 1995.

Frazer, James. *The Golden Bough: A Study in Magic and Religion*. New York: Macmillan, 1922.

Frye, Marilyn. *Politics of Reality: Essays in Feminist Theory*. Trumansburg, NY: Crossing Press Feminist, 1983.

Furst, Gennifer. "Prison-Based Animal Programs: A National Survey." *Prison Journal* 86, no. 4 (2006): 407–30.

Gabbidon, Shaun L. *Criminological Perspectives on Race and Crime*. New York: Routledge, 2007.

Gadamer, Hans-Georg. *The Enigma of Health: The Art of Healing in a Scientific Age*. Translated by Jason Gaiger and Nicholas Walker. Stanford, CA: Stanford University Press, 1996.

———. *Truth and Method*. Translated and edited by Garrett Barden and John Cumming, 18–43. New York: Crossroad, 1984.

Gadow, Sally. "Touch and Technology: Two Paradigms of Patient Care." *Journal of Religion Health* 23, no. 1 (1984): 63–69.

Gallagher, Shaun. *How the Body Shapes the Mind*. Oxford: Clarendon Press, 2005.

Gallagher, Shaun, and Jesper Sørensen. "Experimenting with Phenomenology." *Consciousness and Cognition* 15, no. 1 (2006): 119–34.

Garson, Barbara. *The Electronic Sweatshop*. New York: Simon and Schuster, 1988.

Gatens-Robinson, Eugenie. "Clinical Judgment and the Rationality of the Human Sciences." *Journal of Medicine and Philosophy* 11 (1986): 167–78.

Glaze, Lauren, and Danielle Kaeble. *Correctional Populations in the United States, 2013*. Washington, DC: U.S. Bureau of Justice Statistics, December 2014. http://www.bjs.gov/content /pub/pdf/cpus13.pdf.

"Global Drug Sales to Top $1 Trillion in 2014—IMS," *Reuters*, April 20, 2010. http://www.reuters .com/article/2010/04/20/pharmaceuticals- forecast-idUSN1921921520100420/.

Gogel, Edward, and James Terry. "Medicine as Interpretation: The Uses of Literary Metaphors and Methods." *Journal of Medicine and Philosophy* 12 (1987): 205–17.

Gollner, Adam. "The Immortality Financiers: The Billionaires Who Want to Live Forever." *Daily Beast*, August 20, 2013. http://www.thedailybeast.com/articles/2013/08/20/the-immortality -financiers-the-billionaires-who-want-to-live-forever.html.

Good, Byron, J. "A Body in Pain—The Making of a World of Chronic Pain." In *Pain as a Human Experience: An Anthropological Perspective*, edited by Mary-Jo Delvecchio Good, Paul E. Brodwin, Byron J. Good, and Arthur Kleinman, 29–48. Berkeley: University of California Press, 1992.

Good, Byron, and Mary-Jo Delvecchio Good. "The Meaning of Symptoms: A Cultural Hermeneutic Model for Clinical Practice." In *The Relevance of Social Science for Medicine*, edited by Leon Eisenberg and Arthur Kleinman, 165–96. Dordrecht: D. Reidel, 1978.

Gordon, Lewis R., ed. *Existence in Black: An Anthology of Black Existential Philosophy*. New York: Routledge, 1997.

Grahek, Nikola. *Feeling Pain and Being in Pain.* 2nd ed. Cambridge. MA: MIT Press, 2007.

Grandin, Temple, and Catherine Johnson. *Animals in Translation: Using the Mysteries of Autism to Decode Animal Behavior.* New York: Harcourt, 2006.

———. *Animals Make Us Human: Creating the Best Life for Animals.* Boston: Houghton Mifflin Harcourt, 2009.

Greasley, Kate. "A Legal Market in Organs: The Problem of Exploitation." *Journal of Medical Ethics* 40 (2012): 51–56. doi:10.1136/medethics-2012-100770.

Greco, Vincent. "Canine Partners for Life Graduation Ceremony." *Jessup Correctional Institution Outback Observer* 2, no. 11 (2012).

Greene, Helen Taylor, and Shaun L. Gabbidon. *Encyclopedia of Race and Crime.* Thousand Oaks, CA: Sage, 2009.

Greene, Jeremy. *Prescribing by Numbers: Drugs and the Definition of Disease.* Baltimore: Johns Hopkins University Press, 2007.

Griffin, David Ray. *Unsnarling the World-Knot: Consciousness, Freedom, and the Mind-Body Problem.* Berkeley: University of California Press, 1998.

Griffith, Mark. "Slaves of Dionysos: Satyrs, Audience, and the Ends of the Oresteia." *Classical Antiquity* 21, no. 2 (2002): 195–258.

Groopman, Jerome. *How Doctors Think.* New York: Houghton Mifflin, 2007.

Guenther, Lisa. "Beyond Dehumanization: A Post-Humanist Critique of Intensive Confinement." *Journal for Critical Animal Studies* 10, no. 2 (2012): 69–100.

———. *Solitary Confinement: Social Death and Its Afterlives.* Minneapolis: University of Minnesota Press, 2013.

Hansmann, Henry. "The Economics and Ethics of Markets for Human Organs." In *Organ Transplantation Policy: Issues and Prospects,* edited by James Blumstein and Frank Sloan. Durham, NC: Duke University Press, 1989.

Haraway, Donna. *Simians, Cyborgs, and Women: The Reinvention of Nature.* New York: Routledge, 1991.

Harkrader, Todd, Tod W. Burke, and Stephen S. Owen. "Pound Puppies: The Rehabilitative Uses of Dogs in Correctional Facilities." *Corrections Today* 66, no. 2 (2004): 74–79.

Harrison, Peter. "Descartes on Animals." *Philosophical Quarterly* 42 (1992): 219–27.

Hawkins, Anne H. *Reconstructing Illness: Studies in Pathography.* West Lafayette, IN: Purdue University Press, 1999.

Hazarika, Sanjoy. "India Debates Ethics of Buying Transplant Kidneys." *New York Times,* August 17, 1992.

Heelan, Patrick A. "The Nature of Clinical Science." *Journal of Medicine and Philosophy* 2 (1977): 20–32.

———. *Space-Perception and the Philosophy of Science.* Berkeley: University of California Press, 1983.

Heidegger, Martin. *Being and Time.* Translated by John Macquarrie and Edward Robinson. New York: Harper and Row, 1962.

———. "The Origin of the Work of Art." In *Poetry, Language, Thought,* translated by Albert Hofstadter. New York: Harper and Row, 1971.

———. "The Thing." In *Poetry, Language, Thought,* translated by Albert Hofstadter. New York: Harper and Row, 1971.

Herzberg, David. *Happy Pills in America: From Miltown to Prozac.* Baltimore: Johns Hopkins University Press, 2009.

Hogshire, Jim. *Pills-a-Go-Go: A Fiendish Investigation into Pill Marketing, Art, History and Consumption.* Venice, CA: Feral House, 1999.

Honkasalo, Maria-Liisa. "Space and Embodied Experience: Rethinking the Body in Pain." *Body & Society* 4, no. 2 (1998): 35–57.

Horowitz, Alexandra. *Inside of a Dog: What Dogs See, Smell, and Know.* New York: Scribner, 2010.

Hosey, Lance. *The Shape of Green: Aesthetics, Ecology and Design.* Washington, DC: Island Press, 2013.

Howell, James C. *Preventing and Reducing Juvenile Delinquency: A Comprehensive Framework.* 2nd ed. Thousand Oaks, CA: Sage, 2009.

Hsu, Caroline. "The Greening of Aging." *U.S. News & World Report,* June 19, 2006.

Husserl, Edmund. *Ideas Pertaining to a Pure Phenomenology and to a Phenomenological Philosophy.* Bk. 2, *Studies in the Phenomenology of Constitution.* Translated by Richard Rojcewicz and André Schuwer. Dordrecht: Kluwer Academic, 1989.

———. *The Phenomenology of Internal Time-Consciousness.* Edited by Martin Heidegger. Translated by James S. Churchill. Bloomington: Indiana University Press, 1964.

IASP Taxonomy. International Association for the Study of Pain. Last updated May 22, 2012. http://www.iasp-pain.org/Education/Content.aspx?ItemNumber=1698.

Ihde, Don. *Technics and Praxis.* Dordrecht: D. Reidel, 1979.

Illich, Ivan. *Limits to Medicine: Medical Nemesis—The Expropriation of Health.* London: Calder and Boyars, 1975.

Institute of Medicine of the National Academies. *Relieving Pain in America: A Blueprint for Transforming Prevention, Care, Education, and Research.* Washington, DC: Institute of Medicine, June 2011; revised March 2012. http://www.iom.edu/~/media/Files/Report%20Files/2011 /Relieving-Pain-in-America-A-Blueprint-for-Transforming-Prevention-Care-Education -Research/Pain%20Research%202011%20Report%20Brief.pdf.

International Sai Organization. Sri Satha Sai Central Trust. Accessed July 26, 2010. http://www .sathyasai.org/ashrams/centraltrust.htm.

Ishiguro, Kazuo. *Never Let Me Go.* New York: Vintage, 2006.

Jackson, Jean, E. "'After a While No One Believes You': Real and Unreal Pain." In *Pain as a Human Experience: An Anthropological Perspective,* edited by Mary-Jo Delvecchio Good, Paul E. Brodwin, Byron J. Good, and Arthur Kleinman, 138–68. Berkeley: University of California Press, 1992.

Jacq, Fanny, Gael Foulldrin, Arnaud Savouré, Frédéric Anselme, Audrey Baguelin-Pinaud, Alain Cribier, and Florence Thibaut. "A Comparison of Anxiety, Depression and Quality of Life Between Device Shock and Nonshock Groups in Implantable Cardioverter Defibrillator Recipients." *General Hospital Psychiatry* 31 (2009): 266–73.

Jahnke, Roger. *The Healing Promise of Qi: Creating Extraordinary Wellness Through Qigong and Tai Chi.* New York: McGraw-Hill, 2002.

Jauhar, Sandeep. "Jolts of Anxiety." *New York Times,* May 5, 2002.

Jobst, Kim, Daniel Shostak, and Peter Whitehouse. "Diseases of Meaning, Manifestations of Health, and Metaphor." *Journal of Alternative and Complementary Medicine* 5, no. 6 (1999): 495–502.

Johnson, Kirk. "Raising Frogs for Freedom, Prison Project Opens Doors." *New York Times.* September 28, 2012.

Jonas, Hans. *The Phenomenon of Life: Toward a Philosophical Biology*. Chicago: University of Chicago Press, 1966.

Jones, Arlando ("Tray"). *Eager Street: A Life on the Corner and Behind Bars*. Baltimore: Apprentice House, 2010.

Jung, Carl, G. *The Portable Jung*. Edited by Joseph Campbell. New York: Penguin, 1976.

Justice Policy Institute. *The Punishing Decade: Prison and Jail Estimates at the Millennium*. Washington, DC: Justice Policy Institute, May 2000. http://www.justicepolicy.org/images/upload /00-05_rep_punishingdecade_ac.pdf.

Kakar, Sudhir. *Shamans, Mystics and Doctors: A Psychological Inquiry into India and Its Healing Traditions*. Chicago: University of Chicago Press, 1982.

Kant, Immanuel. *Foundations of the Metaphysics of Morals*. Translated by Lewis White Beck. Indianapolis: Bobbs Merrill, 1969.

———. *Lectures on Ethics*. Translated by Louis Infield. London: Methuen, 1963.

Kapleau, Philip. *The Zen of Living and Dying: A Practical and Spiritual Guide*. Boston: Shambhala, 1998.

Katz, Jay. *The Silent World of Doctor and Patient*. New York: Free Press, 1984.

Kaufman, Marc. "Guidelines for Treatment of Food Animals Released; Retailers Urge Improved Conditions on Farms." *Washington Post*, June 28, 2002.

Kay, Jeanne. "Concepts of Nature in the Hebrew Bible." *Environmental Ethics* 10 (1988): 309–27.

Keith, Thomas. *Religion and the Decline of Magic: Studies in Popular Beliefs in Sixteenth and Seventeenth Century England*. New York: Oxford University Press, 1997.

Kimbrell, Andrew. "Forum: Sacred or For Sale?" *Harper's Magazine*, October 1990.

Kirby, David. *Animal Factory: The Looming Threat of Industrial Pig, Dairy, and Poultry Farms to Humans and the Environment*. New York: St. Martin's Press, 2010.

Kleinman, Arthur. *The Illness Narratives*. New York: Basic, 1988.

———. "Pain and Resistance: The Delegitimation and Relegitimation of Local Worlds." In *Pain as a Human Experience: An Anthropological Perspective*, edited by Mary-Jo Delvecchio Good, Paul E. Brodwin, Byron J. Good, and Arthur Kleinman, 138–68. Berkeley: University of California Press, 1992.

Kleinman, Arthur, Paul E. Brodwin, Byron J. Good, Mary-Jo Delvecchio Good. "Pain as a Human Experience: An Introduction." In *Pain as a Human Experience: An Anthropological Perspective*, edited by Mary-Jo Delvecchio Good, Paul E. Brodwin, Byron J. Good, and Arthur Kleinman, 1–28. Berkeley: University of California Press, 1992.

Kopelman, Loretta. "The Punishment Concept of Disease." In *AIDS: Ethics and Public Policy*, edited by Christine Pierce and Donald VanDeVeer, 49–55. Belmont, CA: Wadsworth, 1988.

Kramer, Peter. *Listening to Prozac: The Landmark Book About Antidepressants and the Remaking of the Self*. New York: Penguin, 1997.

Kuhn, Thomas. *The Structure of Scientific Revolutions*. Chicago: University of Chicago Press, 1962.

Lai, Janet. *Pet Facilitated Therapy in Correctional Institutions*. Ottawa: Office of the Deputy Commissioner for Women, Correctional Service of Canada, April 1998. http://www.csc-scc.gc.ca /text/prgnn/fsw/pet/pet-eng.shtml.

Larson, Doran. "Why Scandinavian Prisons Are Superior." *Atlantic*, September, 24, 2013. http:// www.theatlantic.com/international/archive/2013/09/why-scandinavian-prisons-are-superior /279949/.

Lawlor, Robert. *Voices of the First Day: Awakening in the Aboriginal Dreamtime.* Rochester, VT: Inner Traditions, 1991.

Leder, Drew. *The Absent Body.* Chicago: University of Chicago Press, 1990.

———. "Embodying Otherness: Shape-shifting and the Natural World." *Environmental Philosophy* 9, no. 2 (2012): 123–41.

———. "The Experience of Health and Illness." In *Encyclopedia of Bioethics,* 3rd ed., edited by Stephen Post, 1081–87. New York: Macmillan Reference, 2003.

———. "Medicine and Paradigms of Embodiment." *Journal of Medicine and Philosophy* 9 (1984): 29–43.

———. "Old McDonald Had a Farm: The Metaphysics of Factory Farming." *Journal of Animal Ethics* 2, no. 1 (2012): 73–86.

———. *Sparks of the Divine.* Notre Dame: Sorin Books, 2004.

———. "A Tale of Two Bodies: The Cartesian Corpse and the Lived Body." In *The Body in Medical Thought and Practice,* edited by Drew Leder. Dordrecht: Kluwer Academic, 1992.

———. "Toward a Phenomenology of Pain." *The Review of Existential Psychology and Psychiatry* 19 (1984–1985): 255–66.

Leder, Drew, Charles Baxter, Wayne Brown, Tony Chatman-Bey, Jack Cowan, Michael Green, Gary Huffman, H. B. Johnson Jr., O'Donald Johnson, Arlando Jones III, Mark Medley, "Q", Donald Thompson, Selvyn Tillett, and John Woodland. *The Soul Knows No Bars: Inmates Reflect on Life, Death, and Hope.* Lanham, MD: Rowman and Littlefield, 2000.

Leder, Drew, and Kirsten Jacobson. "Health and Disease: The Experience of Health and Illness." In *Bioethics,* 4th ed., vol. 3, edited by Bruce Jennings, 1434–43. Farmington Hills, MI: Macmillan Reference USA, 2014.

Leder, Drew, and Mitchell Krucoff. "Toward a More Materialistic Medicine: The Value of Authentic Materialism Within Current and Future Medical Practice." *Journal of Alternative and Complementary Medicine* 17 (2011): 859–65.

Lee, Michelle Ye Hee. "Does the United States Really Have 5 Percent of the World's Population and One Quarter of the World's Prisoners?" *Washington Post,* April 30, 2015. https://www .washingtonpost.com/blogs/fact-checker/wp/2015/04/30/does-the-united-states-really -have-five-percent-of-worlds-population-and-one-quarter-of-the-worlds-prisoners/.

Liebeneau, Jonathan, Gregory Higby, and Elaine Stroud, eds. *Pill Peddlers: Essays on the History of the Pharmaceutical Industry.* Madison, WI: American Institute of the History of Pharmacy, 1990.

Linzey, Andrew. *Animal Theology.* Urbana: University of Illinois Press, 1995.

———. *Christianity and the Rights of Animals.* New York: Crossroad, 1987.

Liptak, Adam. "Justices, 5–4, Tell California to Cut Prisoner Population." *New York Times,* May 24, 2011.

Lock, Margaret, and Judith Farquhar, eds. *Beyond the Body Proper: Reading the Anthropology of Material Life.* Durham, NC: Duke University Press, 2007.

Loy, Donald. *Money, Sex, War, Karma: Notes for a Buddhist Revolution.* Somerville, MA: Wisdom, 2008.

Lutgendorf, Philip. "My Hanuman Is Bigger Than Yours." *History of Religions* 33, no. 3 (1994): 211–45.

MacIntyre, Alisdair. *After Virtue.* Notre Dame, IN: University of Notre Dame Press, 1981.

Maddox, Susan. "My Mission-Prayer Quilts." Accessed July 25, 2010. http://maddoxoncology.com /blog/.

Mahathera, Narada. *The Buddha and His Teachings.* Mumbai: Jaico, 2006.

Mahdavi-Mazdeh, Mitra. "The Iranian Model of Living Renal Transplantation." *Kidney International* 82 (2012): 627–34.

Manners, Steven. *Super Pills: The Prescription Drugs We Love to Take.* Vancouver: Raincoast, 2006.

Marder, Michael. *Plant-thinking: A Philosophy of Vegetal Life.* New York: Columbia University Press, 2013.

Marx, Karl. *Capital.* Vol. 1. New York: International, 1967.

———. *Das Kapital: A Critique of Political Economy.* Edited by Friedrich Engels. Washington, DC: Regnery Gateway, 1999.

———. "Estranged Labor." In *The Economic and Philosophic Manuscripts of 1844.* New York: International, 1964.

Mason, Jim. *An Unnatural Order: Uncovering the Roots of Our Domination of Nature and Each Other.* New York: Simon and Schuster, 1993.

Mason, Jim, and Mary Finelli. "Brave New Farm." In *In Defense of Animals: The Second Wave,* edited by Peter Singer, 104–22. Malden, MA: Blackwell, 2006.

Matchett, Melissa, Samuel Sears, Garrett Hazelton, Kari Kirian, Elynor Wilson, and Rajasekhar Nekkanti. "The Implantable Cardioverter Defibrillator: Its History, Current Psychological Impact and Future." *Expert Review of Medical Devices* 6 (2009): 43–50.

Mauss, Marcel. *The Gift: Forms and Functions of Exchange in Archaic Societies.* Translated by Ian Cunnison. Glencoe, IL: Free Press, 1954.

May, William. *The Patient's Ordeal.* Bloomington: Indiana University Press, 1991.

Mazis, Glen. *Humans, Animals, Machines: Blurring Boundaries.* Albany: State University of New York Press, 2008.

McGrath, Sarah. "Organ Procurement, Altruism, and Autonomy." *Journal of Value Inquiry* 40 (2006): 297–309.

McKeon, Richard, ed. *The Basic Works of Aristotle.* New York: Random House, 1941.

McWhinney, Ian R. "Medical Knowledge and the Rise of Technology." *Journal of Medicine and Philosophy* 3 (1978): 293–304.

Melzack, Ronald, and Patrick D. Wall. *The Challenge of Pain.* Rev. ed. London: Penguin, 1991.

Mercer, Christia. "I Teach Philosophy at Columbia. But Some of My Best Students are Inmates," *Washington Post,* March 24, 2015. https://www.washingtonpost.com/posteverything/wp /2015/03/24/i-teach-philosophy-at-columbia-but-the-best-students-i-have-are-inmates/.

Merchant, Carolyn. *The Death of Nature.* San Francisco: Harper and Row, 1980.

Merleau-Ponty, Maurice. "Husserl at the Limits of Phenomenology." In *Praise of Philosophy and Other Essays,* translated by John Wild and James Edie. Evanston, IL: Northwestern University Press, 1988.

———. *Phenomenology of Perception.* Translated by Colin Smith. London: Routledge and Kegan Paul, 1962.

———. *The Visible and the Invisible.* Edited by Claude Lefort. Translated by Alphonso Lingis. Evanston, IL: Northwestern University Press, 1968.

Minkowski, Eugene. *Lived Time: Phenomenological Psychopathological Studies.* Translated by N. Metzel. Evanston, IL: Northwestern University Press, 1970.

Mobley, Alan. "Killing Time on the Prairie." *Journal for Critical Animal Studies* 10, no. 2 (2012): 114–18.

Moerman, Daniel. *Meaning, Medicine, and "Placebo Effect."* Cambridge: Cambridge University Press, 2002.

――――. "Physiology and Symbols: The Anthropological Implications of the Placebo Effect." In *The Anthropology of Medicine: From Culture to Method*, edited by Lola Romanucci-Ross, Daniel Moerman, and Laurence Tancredi, 156–68. Westport, CT: Bergin and Garvey, 1997.

Mol, Annemarie. *The Body Multiple: Ontology in Medical Practice*. Durham, NC: Duke University Press, 2002.

Morris, David. *Illness and Culture in the Postmodern Age*. Berkeley: University of California Press, 1998.

Muktananda, Swami. *I Am That: The Science of Hamsa from the Vijnana Bhairava*. South Fallsburg, NY: Siddha Yoga, 1992.

Munson, Ronald. "Why Medicine Cannot Be a Science." *Journal of Medicine and Philosophy* 6 (1981): 183–208.

Murray, Thomas. "Gifts of the Body and the Needs of Strangers." *Hastings Center Report* 17 (1987): 30–38.

Naess, Arne. "Notes on the Politics of the Deep Ecology Movement." In *Sustaining Gaia: Contributions to Another World View*. Papers from the Environment, Ethics, and Ecology II Conference. Clayton, Australia: Graduate School of Environmental Science, Monash University, 1984.

Nagel, Thomas. *The View from Nowhere*. New York: Oxford University Press, 1986.

――――. "What Is It Like to Be a Bat?" *Philosophical Review* 83, no. 4 (1974): 435–50.

Nancy, Jean-Luc. "L'Intrus," translated by Susan Hanson. *New Centennial Review* 2, no. 3 (2002): 1–14.

Natanson, Maurice. *Edmund Husserl: Philosopher of Infinite Tasks*. Evanston, IL: Northwestern University Press, 1973.

Nietzsche, Friedrich. *A Nietzsche Reader*. Edited and translated by R. J. Hollingdale. London: Penguin, 1977.

Nikilananda, Swami. *The Upanishads*. New York: Harper Torchbooks, 1963.

Nocella, Anthony J., II. "Animal Advocates for Prison and Slave Abolition: A Transformative Justice Approach to Movement Politics for an End to Racism." *Journal for Critical Animal Studies* 10, no. 2 (2012): 119–26.

Noë, Alva. *Out of Our Heads: Why You Are not Your Brain, and Other Lessons from the Biology of Consciousness*. New York: Hill and Wang, 2009.

O'Connor, James. *Natural Causes: Essays in Ecological Marxism*. New York: Guilford Press, 1998.

O'Haire, Marguerite. "Companion Animals and Human Health: Benefits, Challenges, and the Road Ahead." *Journal of Veterinary Behavior* 5 (2010): 226–34.

Palmer, Richard. *Hermeneutics: Interpretation Theory in Schleiermacher, Dilthey, Heidegger, and Gadamer*. Evanston, IL: Northwestern University Press, 1969.

Parks, Jennifer A., and Victoria S. Wike. *Bioethics in a Changing World*. Upper Saddle River, NJ: Prentice Hall, 2010.

Patterson, Charles. *Eternal Treblinka: Our Treatment of Animals and the Holocaust*. New York: Lantern, 2002.

Pellegrino, Edmund, and David Thomasma. *Virtues in Medical Practice*. New York: Oxford University Press, 1993.

Perry, Tony. "Greek Classic Resonates at Camp Pendleton." *Los Angeles Times*, July 25, 2010. http://articles.latimes.com/2010/jul/25/local/la-me-ajax-20100726.

Plügge, Herbert. "Man and His Body." In *The Philosophy of the Body*, edited by Stuart F. Spicker, 293–311. Chicago: Quadrangle, 1970.

Polanyi, Michael. *Knowing and Being.* Chicago: University of Chicago Press, 1969.

———. *Personal Knowledge.* Chicago: University of Chicago Press, 1958.

Pollan, Michael. *The Omnivore's Dilemma: A Natural History of Four Meals.* New York: Penguin, 2006.

Pollock, Anne. "The Internal Cardiac Defibrillator." In *The Inner History of Devices,* edited by Sherry Turkle, 98–111. Cambridge, MA: MIT Press, 2008.

Prayer Shawl Ministry. Accessed July 25, 2010. http://www.shawlministry.com/.

Proust, Marcel. *The Guermantes Way.* Translated by Mark Treharne. New York: Penguin, 1992.

———. *Time Regained: In Search of Lost Time.* Vol. VI, edited by D. J. Enright and Joanna Kilmartin. Translated by Andreas Mayor and Terence Kilmartin. New York: Random House, 1993.

Ratcliffe, Matthew. "Touch and Situatedness." *International Journal of Philosophical Studies* 16, no. 3 (2008): 299–322.

Reiser, Stanley. *Medicine and the Reign of Technology.* Cambridge: Cambridge University Press, 1978.

"Relief is Just a Swallow Away." Accessed July 10, 2013. http://www.bryanfields.com/samples /alka/mem/speedyad.html.

Ricoeur, Paul. *Freud and Philosophy: An Essay on Interpretation.* Translated by Denis Savage. New Haven, CT: Yale University Press, 1970.

Rippon, Simon. "Imposing Options on People in Poverty: The Harm of a Live Donor Organ Market." *Journal of Medical Ethics* 40 (2014): 145–50.

Rodricks, Dan. "Glendening: 'Life Means Life' Absolutism was Wrong." *Baltimore Sun,* February 20, 2011.

Roy, Porter. "The Rise of Physical Examination." In *Medicine and the Five Senses,* edited by W. F. Bynum and Porter Roy, 179–197. Cambridge: Cambridge University Press, 1993.

Ryle, Gilbert. *The Concept of Mind.* New York: Barnes and Noble, 1949.

Sacks, Oliver. *A Leg to Stand On.* New York: HarperCollins, 1994.

Sanders, Clinton. *Understanding Dogs: Living and Working with Canine Companions.* Philadelphia: Temple University Press, 1999.

Sartre, Jean-Paul. *No Exit and Three Other Plays.* New York: Vintage International, 1989.

Sass, Louis, Josef Parnas, and Dan Zahavi. "Phenomenological Psychopathology and Schizophrenia: Contemporary Approaches and Misunderstandings." *Philosophy, Psychiatry, & Psychology* 18, no. 1 (2011): 1–23.

Savulescu, Julian. "Is the Sale of Body Parts Wrong?" *Journal of Medical Ethics* 29 (2003): 138–39.

Scarry, Elaine. *The Body in Pain: The Making and Unmaking of the World.* New York: Oxford University Press, 1985.

Schechner, Richard. *Performance Studies: An Introduction.* New York: Routledge, 2002.

Schenck, David. "The Texture of Embodiment: Foundation for Medical Ethics." *Human Studies* 9, no. 1 (1986): 43–54.

Schlosser, Eric. "The Prison-Industrial Complex." *Atlantic Monthly,* December 1998, 51–77.

Scully, Matthew. "Factory Farm Meat Not on Menu for Feast of St. Francis." *Dallas Morning News,* October 4, 2004. http://www.animalliberationfront.com/Philosophy/MathewScully/factory farm.htm.

Seligmann, Jean, and Nikki Finke Greenberg. "Only Months to Live and No Place to Die." *Newsweek,* August 12, 1985.

Selzer, Richard. *Mortal Lessons: Notes on the Art of Surgery.* New York: Simon and Schuster, 1974.

Shaylor, Cassandra. "'It's Like Living in a Black Hole': Women of Color and Solitary Confinement in the Prison Industrial Complex." *New England Journal on Criminal and Civil Confinement* 24 (Summer 1998): 395–96.

Sherwin, Susan. "Whither Bioethics? How Feminism Can Help Reorient Bioethics." *International Journal of Feminist Approaches to Bioethics* 1, no. 1 (2008): 7–27.

Simms, Eva Marie. "Milk and Flesh: A Phenomenological Reflection on Infancy and Coexistence." *Journal of Phenomenological Psychology* 32, no. 1 (2001): 22–40.

Singer, Peter. *Animal Liberation*. New York: HarperCollins, 1975; New York: Harper Perennial, 2001.

———. ed. *In Defense of Animals: The Second Wave*. Malden, MA: Blackwell, 2006.

———. *Practical Ethics*. 2nd ed. Cambridge: Cambridge University Press, 1993.

Slatman, Jenny. *Our Strange Body: Philosophical Reflections on Identity and Medical Interventions*. Amsterdam: Amsterdam University Press, 2015.

Sloop, John. *The Cultural Prison: Discourse, Prisoners, and Punishment*. Tuscaloosa: University of Alabama Press, 1996.

Sontag, Susan. *Illness as Metaphor*. New York: Farrar, Straus and Giroux, 1978.

Sophocles. *Philoctetes*. In *The Complete Greek Tragedies*, edited by David Grene and Richmond Lattimore, 2:401–60. Chicago: University of Chicago Press, 1959–1960.

Sri Satha Sai Institute of Higher Medical Sciences: Prasanthigram. "World Class Healthcare Totally Free of Charge." Accessed July 26, 2010. http://psg.sssihms.org.in/.

Starr, Paul. *The Social Transformation of American Medicine*. New York: Basic, 1982.

Steiner, Gary. "Descartes on the Moral Status of Animals." *Archiv fur Geschichte der Philosophie* 80 (1988): 268–91.

Sternberg, Esther. *Healing Spaces: The Science of Place and Well-Being*. Cambridge, MA: Harvard University Press, 2009.

Stone, Allucquère R. "Will the Real Body Please Stand Up? Boundary Stories About Virtual Cultures." In *Cyberspace: First Steps*, edited by Michael Benedikt, 90. Cambridge, MA: MIT Press, 1991.

Straus, Erwin. *Phenomenological Psychology*. Translated by Erling Eng. New York: Basic, 1966.

———. *The Primary World of Senses: A Vindication of Sensory Experience*. Translated by Jacob Needleman. New York: Free Press of Glencoe, 1963.

———. "The Upright Posture." In *Phenomenological Psychology*, translated by Erling Eng. New York: Basic, 1966.

Svenaeus, Fredrik. "The Body as Gift, Resource or Commodity? Heidegger and the Ethics of Organ Transplantation." *Bioethical Inquiry* 7 (2010): 163–72.

———. *The Hermeneutics of Medicine and the Phenomenology of Health: Steps Towards a Philosophy of Medical Practice*. 2nd rev. ed. Dordrecht: Kluwer Academic, 2001.

———. "What is Phenomenology of Medicine? Embodiment, Illness and Being-in-the-World." In *Health, Illness and Disease*, edited by Havi Carel and Rachel Cooper. Durham, UK: Acumen Press, 2013.

Swift, Jonathan. *A Modest Proposal and Other Satirical Works*. Mineola, NY: Dover, 1996.

Testa, Giuliano, and Mark Siegler. "Increasing the Supply of Kidneys for Transplantation by Making Living Donors the Preferred Source of Donor Kidneys." *Medicine* 93, no. 29 (2014): e318.

"Theatre of War Project: Overview." Outside the Wire. Accessed April 1, 2015. http://www.outsidethewirellc.com/projects/theater-of-war/overview.

Thomas, Janice. "Does Descartes Deny Consciousness to Animals?" *Ratio* 19 (2006): 336–63.

Thomas, Keith. *Religion and the Decline of Magic: Studies in Popular Beliefs in Sixteenth and Seventeenth Century England*. New York: Oxford University Press, 1997.

Thomas, Lewis. *The Lives of a Cell*. New York: Bantam, 1974.

Thomas, Sandra, and Howard Pollio. *Listening to Patients: A Phenomenological Approach to Nursing Research and Practice*. New York: Springer, 2002.

Thomas, Sue Ann, Erika Friedmann, Chi-Wen Kao, Pia Inguito, Matthew Metcalf, Frances J. Kelley, and Steven S. Gottlieb. "Quality of Life and Psychosocial Status of Patients with Implantable Cardioverter Defibrillators." *American Journal of Critical Care* 15 (2006): 389–98.

Thomas, William. *The Eden Alternative: Nature, Hope and Nursing Homes*. Columbia: University of Missouri, 1994.

———. *What Are Old People For? How Elders Will Save the World*. Acton, MA: VanderWyk and Burnham, 2004.

Thompson, Ian, Kath Melia, Kenneth Boyd, and Dorothy Horsburgh. *Nursing Ethics*. 5th ed. Edinburgh: Churchill Livingston Elsevier, 2006.

Titmuss, Richard. *The Gift Relationship: From Human Blood to Social Policy*. London: Allen and Unwin, 1970.

Tolstoy, Leo. *The Death of Ivan Ilych and Other Stories*. Translated by Aylmer Maude and J. D. Duff. New York: New American Library, 1960.

Toobin, Jeffrey. "The Milwaukee Experiment." *New Yorker*, May 11, 2015.

Toombs, S. Kay. *The Meaning of Illness: A Phenomenological Account of the Different Perspectives of Physician and Patient*. Dordrecht: Kluwer Academic, 1992.

Toulmin, Stephen. "On the Nature of the Physician's Understanding." *Journal of Medicine and Philosophy* 1 (1976): 32–50.

Trends in U.S. Corrections: Fact Sheet. The Sentencing Project. Accessed June 18, 2015. http://sentencingproject.org/doc/publications/inc_Trends_in_Corrections_Fact_sheet.pdf.

Tucker, Robert, ed. *The Marx-Engels Reader*. 2nd ed. New York: W. W. Norton, 1978.

Tuhus-Dubrow, Rebecca. "The Little Green Pill." *Slate*, January 3, 2011. http://www.slate.com/articles/health_and_science/green_room/2011/01/the_little_green_pill.html.

Turner, Victor. *The Forest of Symbols*. Ithaca, NY: Cornell University Press, 1967.

Ulrich, Roger. "Biophilia, Biophobia, and Natural Landscapes." In *The Biophilia Hypothesis*, edited by Stephen R. Kellert and Edward O. Wilson, 73–137. Washington, DC: Island Press, 1993.

Vaillancourt, Jean-Guy. "Marxism and Ecology: More Benedictine than Franciscan." In *The Greening of Marxism*, edited by Ted Benton, 53. New York: Guilford Press, 1996.

Vallas, Rebecca, and Sharon Dietrich. *One Strike and You're Out*. Washington, DC: Center for American Progress, December 2014. https://cdn.americanprogress.org/wp-content/uploads/2014/12/VallasCriminalRecordsReport.pdf.

Vanamali. *Shakti: Realm of the Divine Mother*. Rochester, VT: Inner Traditions, 2006.

van den Berg, J. H. *The Psychology of the Sickbed*. Pittsburgh: Duquesne University Press, 1966.

Varela, Francisco J. "Intimate Distances: Fragments for a Phenomenology of Organ Transplantation." *Journal of Consciousness Studies* 8, no. 5–7 (2001): 259–71.

Verghese, Abraham. "A Touch of Sense." *Health Affairs* 28, no. 4 (2009): 1178–79.

Vrooman, Jack. *Rene Descartes: A Biography*. New York: G. P. Putnam's Sons, 1970.

Waber, Rebecca, Baba Shiv, Ziv Carmon, and Dan Ariely. "Commercial Features of Placebo and Therapeutic Efficacy." *JAMA* 299, no. 9 (2008): 1016–17.

Wall, Patrick. *Pain: The Science of Suffering*. New York: Columbia University Press, 2000.

Wang, Yang-ming. "Inquiry on the Great Learning." In *A Sourcebook in Chinese Philosophy*, edited by Wing-tsit Chan, 659–67. Princeton, NJ: Princeton University Press, 1963.

———. *Instructions for Practical Living and Other Neo-Confucian Writings*. New York: Columbia University, 1963.

Warnke, Georgia. *Gadamer: Hermeneutics, Tradition and Reason*. Stanford, CA: Stanford University Press, 1987.

Wei-ming, Tu. *Confucian Thought: Selfhood as Creative Transformation*. Albany: State University of New York Press, 1985.

Whitehead, Alfred North. *Science and the Modern World*. New York: Free Press, 1997.

Whitehouse, Peter, and Daniel George. *The Myth of Alzheimer's: What You Aren't Being Told About Today's Most Dreaded Diagnosis*. New York: St. Martin's Press, 2008.

Wile, Douglas. *Lost T'ai-chi Classics from the Late Ch'ing Dynasty*. Albany: State University of New York Press, 1996.

Will, George. "When Solitude is Torture." *Washington Post*, February 20, 2013.

Wilson, Edward O. *Biophilia*. Cambridge, MA: Harvard University Press, 1984.

———. "Biophilia and the Conservation Ethic." In *The Biophilia Hypothesis*, edited by Stephen R. Kellert and Edward O. Wilson, 31–41. Washington, DC: Island Press, 1993.

Woloshin, Steven, and Lisa M. Schwartz, "Sell a Disease to Sell a Drug," *Washington Post*, June 7, 2015. https://www.washingtonpost.com/opinions/the-bulked-up-campaign-around -low-testosterone/2015/06/07/a9abda16-0573-11e5-8bda-c7b4e9a8f7ac_story.html?hpid=z3.

Woods, Angela. "Beyond the Wounded Storyteller: Rethinking Narrativity, Illness and Embodied Self-Experience." In *Health, Illness and Disease: Philosophical Essays*, edited by Havi Carel and Rachel Cooper, 113–28. Durham, UK: Acumen Press, 2013.

Yard, Delicia. "PSA Testing: Why the U.S. and Europe Differ." *Renal and Urology News*, September 21, 2011. http://www.renalandurologynews.com/prostate-cancer/psa-testing-why-the-us -and-europe-differ/article/212312/.

Young, Iris Marion. *On Female Body Experience: Throwing Like a Girl and Other Essays*. Oxford: Oxford University Press, 2005.

Zaner, Richard M. *The Context of Self: A Phenomenological Inquiry Using Medicine as a Clue*. Athens: Ohio University Press, 1981.

———. *Ethics and the Clinical Encounter*. Englewood Cliffs, NJ: Prentice Hall, 1988.

———. *The Problem of Embodiment*. The Hague: Martinus Nijhoff, 1964.

Zayac, Susan, and Nancy Finch. "Recipients' of Implanted Cardioverter-defibrillators Actual and Perceived Adaptation: A Review of the Literature." *Journal of the American Academy of Nurse Practitioners* 21 (2009): 549–56.

Zeiler, Kristin. "Ethics and Organ Transfer: A Merleau-Pontean Perspective." *Health Care Analysis* 17 (2009): 110–22.

———. "A Phenomenology of Excorporation, Bodily Alienation and Resistance: Rethinking Sexed and Racialized Embodiment." *Hypatia* 28, no. 1 (2013): 69–84.

Zezima, Katie. "From Balls of Yarn, Needles and Prayers, a New Ministry." *New York Times*, November 13, 2004.

Zimmer, Carl. "Tending the Body's Microbial Garden." *New York Times*, June 19, 2012.

Index

Lightning Source UK Ltd.
Milton Keynes UK
UKOW06f0826031117

312077UK00006B/330/P

9 780226 396101